Procedures in Gastrointestinal Radiology

J. Dobranowski D.A. Stringer
S. Somers G.W. Stevenson

Procedures in Gastrointestinal Radiology

With a Contribution by Lynne McLean
With a Foreword by William M. Thompson

With 175 Illustrations in 335 Parts

Springer-Verlag New York Berlin Heidelberg
London Paris Tokyo Hong Kong

Julian Dobranowski, MD
Staff Radiologist, St. Joseph's Hospital; Assistant Clinical Professor, McMaster University, Hamilton, Ontario L8N 4A6, Canada

David A. Stringer, MD
Head, Ultrasound and Gastrointestinal Radiology, The Hospital for Sick Children, Toronto, Ontario M5G 1X8, Canada; Associate Professor, University of Toronto

Sat Somers, MD
Head, Gastrointestinal Radiology, Chedoke-McMaster Hospitals, Associate Professor, Department of Radiology, McMaster University, Hamilton, Ontario L8N 3Z5, Canada

Giles W. Stevenson, MD
Professor and Chairman, Department of Radiology, Chedoke-McMaster Hospitals and McMaster University, Hamilton, Ontario L8N 3Z5, Canada

Contributor of Chapter 7:
Lynne McLean, RT
Chief Technologist, Department of Radiology, Chedoke-McMaster Hospitals, McMaster Division, Hamilton, Ontario L8N 3Z5, Canada

On the front cover: Fig. 3.14 B *see p.* 55; Fig. 6.11 *see p.* 175.

Library of Congress Cataloging-in-Publication Data
Procedures in gastrointestinal radiology/J. Dobranowski . . . [et al.]
; with a contribution by Lynne McLean ; with a foreword by William M. Thompson.
p. cm.
Includes bibliographical references.

ISBN-13: 978-1-4612-7961-7 e-ISBN-13: 978-1-4612-3308-4
DOI: 10.1007/978-1-4612-3308-4

1. Gastrointestinal system—Diseases—Diagnosis.
2. Gastrointestinal system—Radiography. 3. Gastroscopy.
I. Dobranowski, J. (Julian)
[DNLM: 1. Gastrointestinal System—radiography. 2. Technology, Radiologic. WI 141 P9631]
RC804.R6P76 1990
616.3'307'57—dc20
DNLM/DLC
for Library of Congress 89-21752

Softcover reprint of the hardcover 1st edition 1990

Typeset by TCSystems, Inc., Shippensburg, Pennsylvania.

9 8 7 6 5 4 3 2 1

J. DOBRANOWSKI	To Jolanta, Magdalena, Alexander, and to my parents
D.A. STRINGER	To my wife and children, Judy, Charles, Rosemary, and Henry, and to my parents
S. SOMERS	To my wife Susan and children, Kris and Vijay
G.W. STEVENSON	To GI technologists, radiology residents and GI radiology fellows who over the years have stimulated my interest in this subject

Foreword

Dr. Dobranowski and his associates are to be highly commended for this excellent manual. I am not aware of a similar text covering the subject. Although all of us perform gastrointestinal studies in a different manner, this text provides an excellent overview. The reader will discover that the text is especially well written and focuses on the important issues relating to GI contrast studies. Because Dr. Stevenson's group performs endoscopic procedures, they are included in the manual.

These authors are recognized scholars and leaders in gastrointestinal radiology. Thus, it is easy to understand why the manual is so well done. I am particularly impressed with the emphasis placed on the patient–radiologist relationship before, during, and after completion of a study.

All of us who teach gastrointestinal radiology are concerned about the decline in the number of gastrointestinal contrast studies. We are not sure how we can continue to teach our residents the proper techniques and maintain high-quality teaching programs in gastrointestinal radiology. A manual of this type is thus timely and appropriate. The manual will be a valuable addition to the library of all radiologists. It will be particularly useful for residents who are learning how to perform GI contrast studies.

William M. Thompson, MD
Professor and Chairman
Department of Radiology
University of Minnesota
Minneapolis, MN 55455

Preface

Modern medicine, with its emphasis on early disease detection and treatment, has set new goals for modern gastrointestinal radiology. To be able to make early and accurate diagnoses, radiologists must be acquainted with the various imaging techniques and be able to select the most appropriate study for the presenting clinical problem. The introduction of fiberoptic endoscopy has revealed many shortcomings in gastrointestinal imaging, but this knowledge has subsequently led to improvements in the accuracy of barium studies.

Endoscopy has become the primary method of imaging in some situations, but quality barium radiology remains the initial investigation of choice for routine colon examination, for esophageal symptoms, and for most small bowel disease. For gastric and duodenal disease, barium radiology can be almost as accurate as endoscopy in cooperative patients and is often much cheaper. There remains a clinical need for high-quality barium radiology.

The purpose of this book is to provide a detailed step-by-step description of the various examinations in GI radiology, with emphasis on the barium studies that have primary indications and have been proven to provide the most useful and accurate clinical information. Endoscopic procedures have also been described in the hope that a knowledge of endoscopy will allow the radiologist a more thorough understanding of barium examinations and also allow for a closer interaction between radiology and endoscopy.

We hope that the step-by-step approach of the book will help clarify practical aspects of the various techniques, making it useful to radiology residents and technologists as well as a valuable reference for practicing radiologists.

Acknowledgments. We would like to thank Monika Ferrier for her advice and unending help in the preparation of the manuscript. We thank Richard F. Zazulak for his excellent illustrations, and E-Z-Em Canada, Winthrop Canada, Cook Canada, and Lafayette Canada for their generous financial support. Special thanks to the production and editorial staff of Springer-Verlag for all their work and excellent advice.

J. Dobranowski
D.A. Stringer
S. Somers
G.W. Stevenson

Contents

CHAPTER 1

Introduction

Radiologists should ensure that patients coming for gastrointestinal (GI) radiology procedures receive an adequate description of the procedure that they are about to undergo. This should have been done initially by the referring physician, but when the patient arrives for the examination the technician will usually describe the major points such as drinking of liquids, tilting of the table, and the possibility of an injection that may cause temporary blurring of vision. For courtesy's sake, the radiologist should repeat briefly the highlights of the examination and ask whether the patient has any questions. It is wise, in addition, to confirm the salient points of the history and elicit any other important information. For example, if the requisition states that the patient has difficulty swallowing, it is helpful to establish whether it is a transport or transfer problem; that is, can the patient initiate a swallow satisfactorily although the food then gets stuck in the throat, or is the patient aware that he is not able to transfer the food from the mouth to the gullet. The technician should introduce the radiologist by name, because many patients leave a radiology department not knowing the name of the doctor who has examined them.

Many patients are apprehensive about x-ray examinations, and will be appreciative if both the technologist and radiologist encourage them and keep them at ease during the fluoroscopic procedure. Instructions on how to turn, when to drink, and how much to drink should be given very clearly with an economy of words so that there is the least possible chance of misunderstanding.

Individuals may be divided psychologically into two groups, blunters and monitors [1]. Seventy to 80% of the population are monitors, which means they cope best with difficult situations when given information as to what is going to happen and an explanation of what is being done while the procedure is being performed. A minority of patients cope better with a minimal explanation—"don't tell me about it, doctor, just get on and do it." Radiologists, therefore, need to be sensitive to a patient's needs and attempt to gauge the amount of information each patient desires.

At the end of a procedure, all patients wonder whether the radiologist has found anything wrong, although few ask directly. It is a kindness to give the patient some information at this stage. Most radiologists, however, are not in a position to discuss the full diagnosis and implications with the patient. A compromise, therefore, must be achieved. For many patients it will suffice to say that the examination does not show anything serious, and that you will get in touch with the referring doctor following closer review of the x-rays. If the study revealed an obvious carcinoma, the patient may be told by the radiologist that the trouble has been found, and that it looks like an ulcer, but the radiologist will get in touch with the referring doctor and discuss the ulcer. In other words, the radiologist should always give the patient some information to take away but should usually avoid giving a specific diagnosis, particularly with more serious disease. This is partly because this information should come from the referring physician, and partly because the initial impression from fluoroscopy is not always correct. Review of the films may result in a different diagnosis in the written report. Serious findings, such as malignancy or acute disease, are best communicated by telephone to the referring doctor, particularly if the examination has been performed toward the end of the work week when there may be delay over the weekend before the written report is received.

Patients of the pediatric age group also require special consideration, as is discussed separately in Chapter 5.

References

1. Shipley RH, Butt JH, Horwitz B, Farbry JE (1978). Preparation for a stressful medical procedure: effect of amount of stimulus preexposure and coping style. J Consult Clin Psychol 46:499–507.

CHAPTER 2

Upper Gastrointestinal Tract

Routine Barium Meal

Indications

Esophagus
- Dysphagia
- Odynophagia
- Heartburn
- Hematemesis
- Globus Hystericus

Stomach
- Pain
- Weight Loss
- Abdominal Mass
- Hematemesis
- Melena
- Vomiting

Duodenum
- Pain
- Weight Loss
- Hematemesis
- Melena
- Vomiting

There is continuing controversy over whether endoscopy or barium meal should be performed for examination of the upper gastrointestinal (GI) tract [1]. For gastroesophageal reflux disease, the barium swallow study is the preferred initial examination and often the only investigation required [2,3]. Barium swallow better detects motor abnormalities [2], but encoscopy is needed for barium-negative dysphagia and for biopsy of strictures [4]. In acute odynophagia or food impaction, endoscopy should be the initial examination (when possible) because barium destroys the endoscopic view and endoscopy often is required in these patients for foreign body removal. Endoscopy can, however, miss tumors of the gastroesophageal junction. If endoscopy is used as the initial esophageal investigation in a patient with dysphagia and this study is negative, a follow-up barium swallow should be performed.

For gastric and duodenal disease, in patients who are bleeding, who have had surgery, or who are immobile, endoscopy is a superior examination [1]. For mobile patients, barium meal can be almost as accurate [5,6] as endoscopy. Where there is no difference in cost, endoscopy is the procedure of choice for gastroduodenal pathology. Where endoscopy costs more, barium meal should be performed as the initial investigation for mobile adults who are not bleeding and who have not had previous gastroduodenal surgery [7].

Contraindications and Precautions

1. Suspected perforation: use water-soluble contrast (p. 30).
2. Swallowing disorder that may lead to aspiration. If a patient is suspected of having a swallowing disorder, the examination is started by asking the patient to swallow small sips of barium, using fluoroscopy to observe the pharynx. If aspiration occurs, a decision must be made whether to terminate the examination or to proceed cautiously to define the nature of the abnormality. The severity of obstruction and degree of aspiration and ability of the patient to clear the aspiration will help in the decision.
3. Bowel obstruction, especially partial large bowel obstruction that may convert into complete obstruction.
4. Allergy to barium preparations, although rare, has been described [8,9].
5. Clinical settings in which this test has a low diagnostic yield and other tests are much better, such as hematemesis or severe immobility

Materials

1. A suitable high-density barium
2. Distilled water
3. Effervescent granules, enough to produce adequate gastric distention. Adequate gastric distension varies from patient to patient because of differences in gastric volume. Adequate distention is obtained when gastric folds are separated from each other but not obliterated (approximately 400–800 ml)
4. Antifoam (simethicone), used to prevent bubble formation when the effervescent granules dissolve [10]
5. Intravenous glucagon, 0.3 mg
6. Intravenous Buscopan, 20 mg
7. Ovol (antiflatulent)

We are presently using E-Z HD 98% barium sulfate, 340 g, and Baros effervescent granules. A variety of other materials can give good results (Xopaque, bubbly barium mixture, Baritop granules, EZ gas, see Appendix 1, page 221).

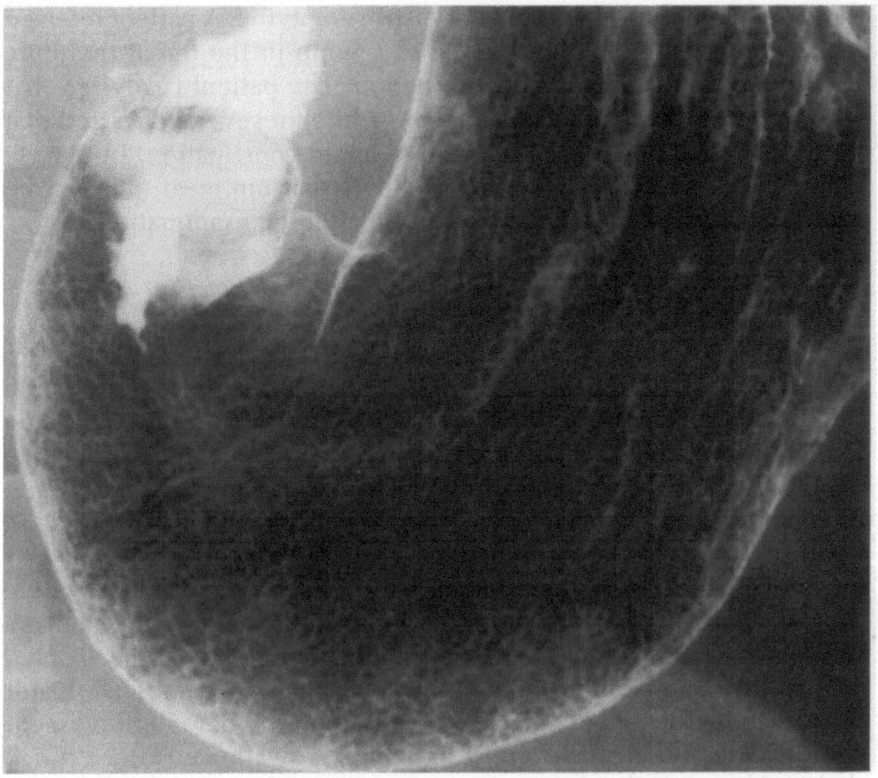

Fig. 2.1. Good coating of gastric mucosa shows surface detail of areae gastricae, small areas of epithelium separated by crevices that fill with thin meniscus of barium. Thick layer of gastric mucus will prevent visualization of the areae gastricae; these are enlarged in patients with gastritis or duodenal ulceration.

Preparation

1. The high-density barium is mixed with 67 ml of distilled water* [11]. Three drops of ovol may be added.
2. Five milliliters of antifoam is mixed with 5–10 ml of distilled water.

Patient Preparation

Nothing by mouth (NPO) after 10:00 P.M. the evening before examination. A barium swallow can be performed without previous fasting; however, this type of study without preparation should be performed only in patients with already diagnosed esophageal disease or having a limited follow-up examination for a specific purpose. A new patient with esophageal symptoms should also have the stomach and duodenum examined, because symptoms in the throat can be caused

* Not all combinations of these products work together, and you may have to experiment to find a suitable combination; we believe it is difficult to obtain uniform results by using tap water because its mineral content varies from city to city, and thus recommend using distilled water. Adequate coating of the stomach is obtained if the areae gastricae are clearly visualized (Fig. 2.1).

by gastroesophageal reflux, which in turn may be exacerbated by duodenal pathology that prevents gastric emptying. A patient referred for barium swallow with a feeling of a lump in the throat therefore should have a full upper GI examination. The patient is advised that after the examination the stool may be white for several days and that fluids and laxatives should be used to avoid constipation. In elderly patients, severe constipation may follow a barium meal; this can be avoided by giving 50 g of oral Lactulose after the examination.

Esophagus

Step 1. Film size, 14 × 14 in. (3 split). The examination is started with the patient in erect position (see discussion on page 21), right side forward (RAO), holding prepared barium in the left hand. The degree of obliquity should be enough to project the esophagus off the spine. A quick fluoroscopic assessment of neck, chest, and abdomen is made to identify any possible abnormalities such as soft-tissue masses, air–fluid levels, or free intraperitoneal air (Fig. 2.2). Under fluoroscopic control, a single small swallow of barium is followed into the stomach to ensure there is no major esophageal obstruction [12]. If no esophageal obstruction is found, the patient takes cup with antifoam/water mixture into the right hand. Two containers of Baros effervescent granules are added to the antifoam, which is swallowed after a quick shake. Alternatively the patient may empty the granules into the

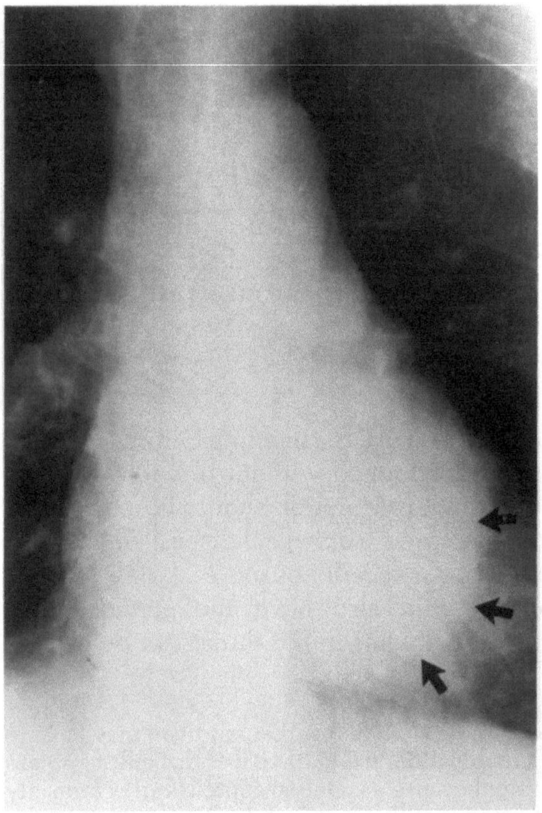

Fig. 2.2. Large retrosternal mass (*arrows*), identified by fluoroscopic examination before barium study in a patient with symptoms of esophageal dysphagia was subsequently found to be a large bronchogenic carcinoma.

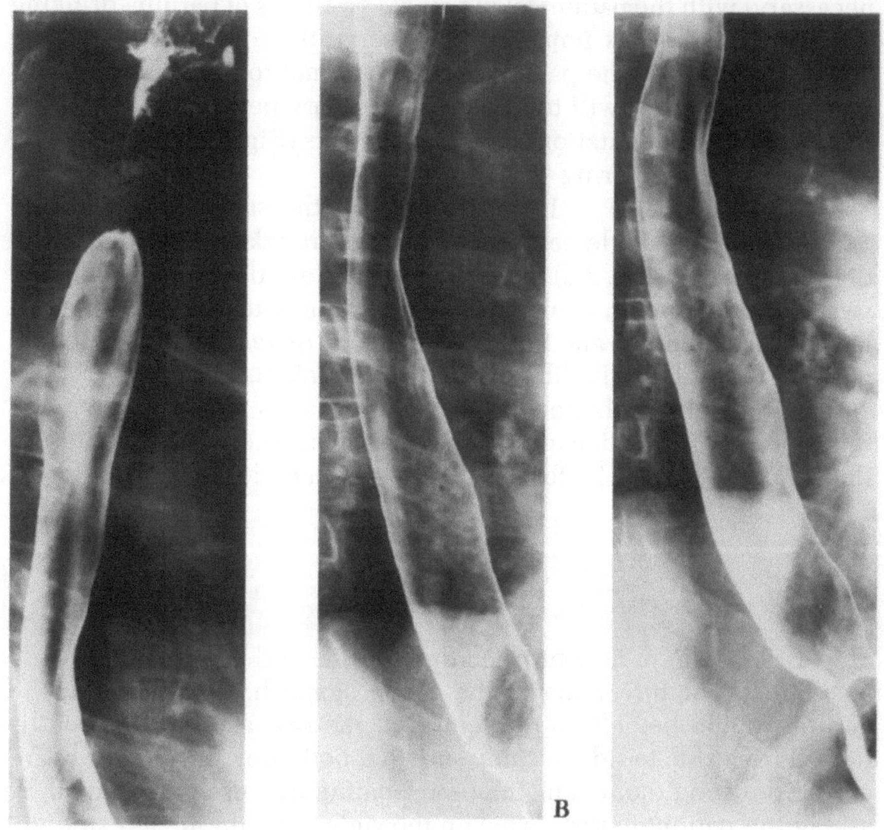

A B C

Fig. 2.3. Double-contrast esophagus. Immediately after swallowing of effervescent granules and barium, and under fluoroscopic control, exposures are obtained that include hypopharynx and upper esophagus (**A**), midesophagus (**B**), and lower esophagus, gastroesophageal junction (**C**).

mouth dry and use the antifoam to wash the granules down. With the patient now swallowing continuously from the cup with barium, three exposures of the distended esophagus are obtained (Fig. 2.3). If Baros tablets are used, the patient puts all the tablets into the back of the mouth, washing the tablets down with the antifoam/water mixture. Usually air swallowed along with the barium and gas refluxing from the stomach gives adequate distention of the esophagus for a double-contrast examination. To prevent belching, the patient is asked to continue dry swallowing when the sensation of imminent belching is developing.

Correct timing of exposure is essential. If the exposure is taken too early, a column of barium will be present in the lower esophagus and will obscure mucosal detail. If the exposure is taken too late, the esophagus can lose both the barium and air, resulting in inadequate distention.

Step 2. The patient is now quickly lowered into the supine position, still with the right side forward. Speed is important; if the patient is allowed to stand too long, gastric emptying of barium will prevent adequate visualization of the stomach and duodenum. Esophageal motility is examined under fluoroscopic control (use video-recording if necessary) with the patient taking *single* swallows of barium, drinking through a straw. It is important to observe the entire swallow from mouth to stomach. The patient is instructed not to double swallow as the second swallow will terminate the primary peristaltic wave. Normal anatomical indentations on the esophagus (Fig. 2.4) should not be confused with stricturing.

Step 3. Film size, 14 × 14 in. (3 split). In the same position, three exposures of the single-contrast esophagus are taken with the patient drinking barium (Fig. 2.5). It can be useful to ask the patient to double swallow at this point, using the second swallow to terminate the primary peristaltic wave and thus allowing good distention of the esophagus long enough for the film exposure to be taken.

One exposure is obtained with the esophagus collapsed (mucosal relief) (Fig. 2.5c), which allows assessment of the esophageal folds for thickening. See page 22 for discussion of prone view.

Stomach

Step 4. The patient now turns on the left side and then into the prone position to obtain coating of the entire stomach. (At this point the barium should be only in the fundus of the stomach.) The patient is rocked from side to side, making sure that both hips and shoulders are elevated during the rocking motion. Coating can also be obtained by asking the patient to turn twice on the right side, prone, left side up, and then supine. If the patient is elderly or debilitated this movement may be difficult, however, and any delay in moving from the right-side-down position to prone may result in filling of small bowel loops with barium, which will interfere with obtaining adequate unobscured films of the antrum. The patient must be turned prone to coat the anterior wall of the stomach.

Step 5. Film size, 10 × 12 in. (single split). The patient is now turned back on the left side and then supine oblique, right side forward. This will bring the barium into the fundus of the stomach (Fig. 2.6A,B). A film is taken now of the antrum and body of the stomach (Fig. 2.6C). If filling of small bowel loops has occurred, angling of the tube cephalad may separate the antrum from the small bowel.

Step 6. Film size, 10 × 12 in. (single split). The patient lies completely supine. This position again allows proper exposure of the antrum and body of the stomach (Fig. 2.7). In some patients, especially if there is a delay between exposures, it may be necessary to recoat the mucosa to obtain adequate mucosal detail.

Fig. 2.5. Single-contrast esophagus with patient supine. Two exposures of esophagus are obtained with esophagus distended with barium (**A, B**) and one exposure with esophagus collapsed (mucosal relief) (**C**).

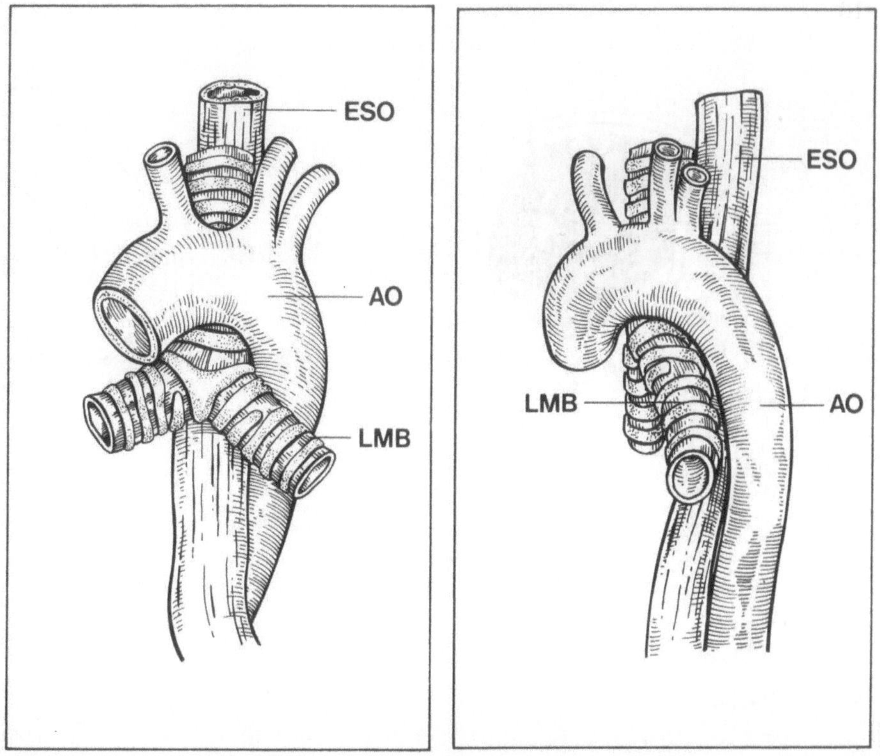

A B

Fig. 2.4. Relationship between esophagus, aorta, and airways is illustrated in anteroposterior (**A**) and lateral (**B**) positions. Normal impressions on esophagus (ESO) are caused by aorta (AO), left mainstem bronchus (LMB), and left atrium.

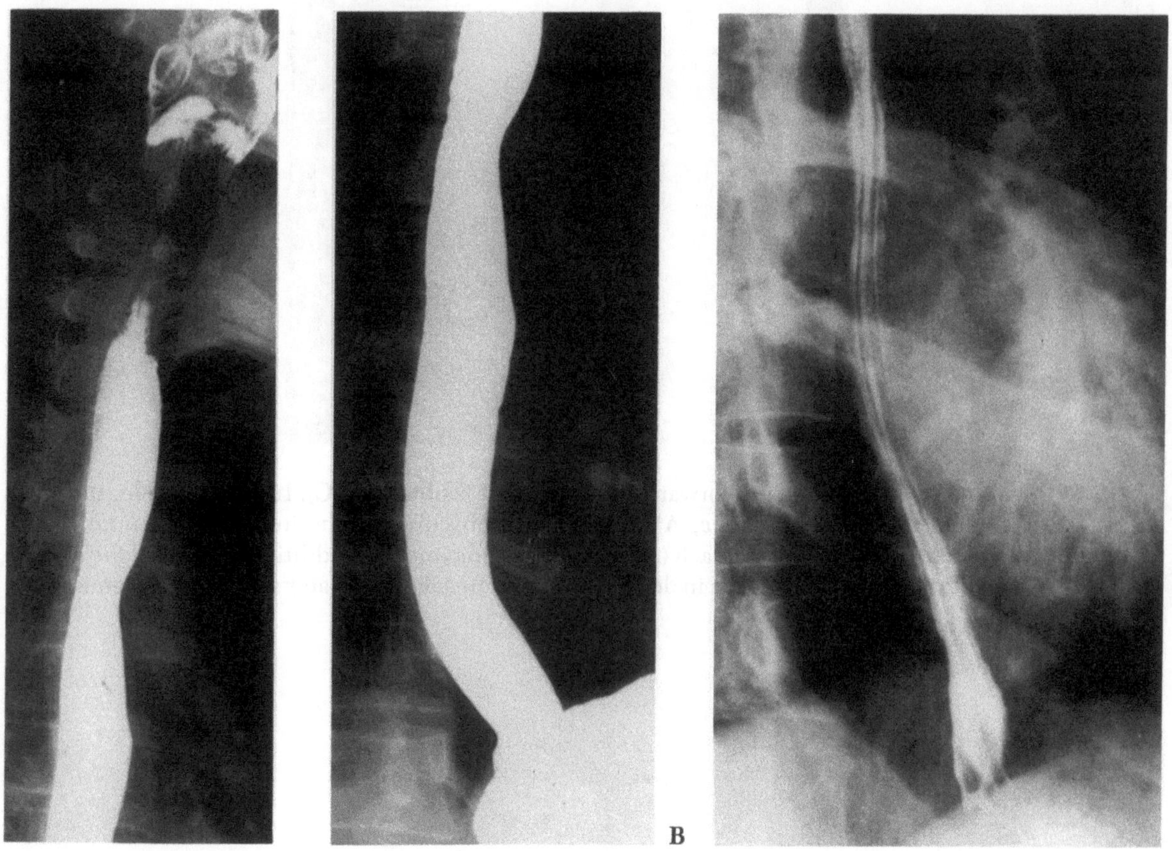

A B C

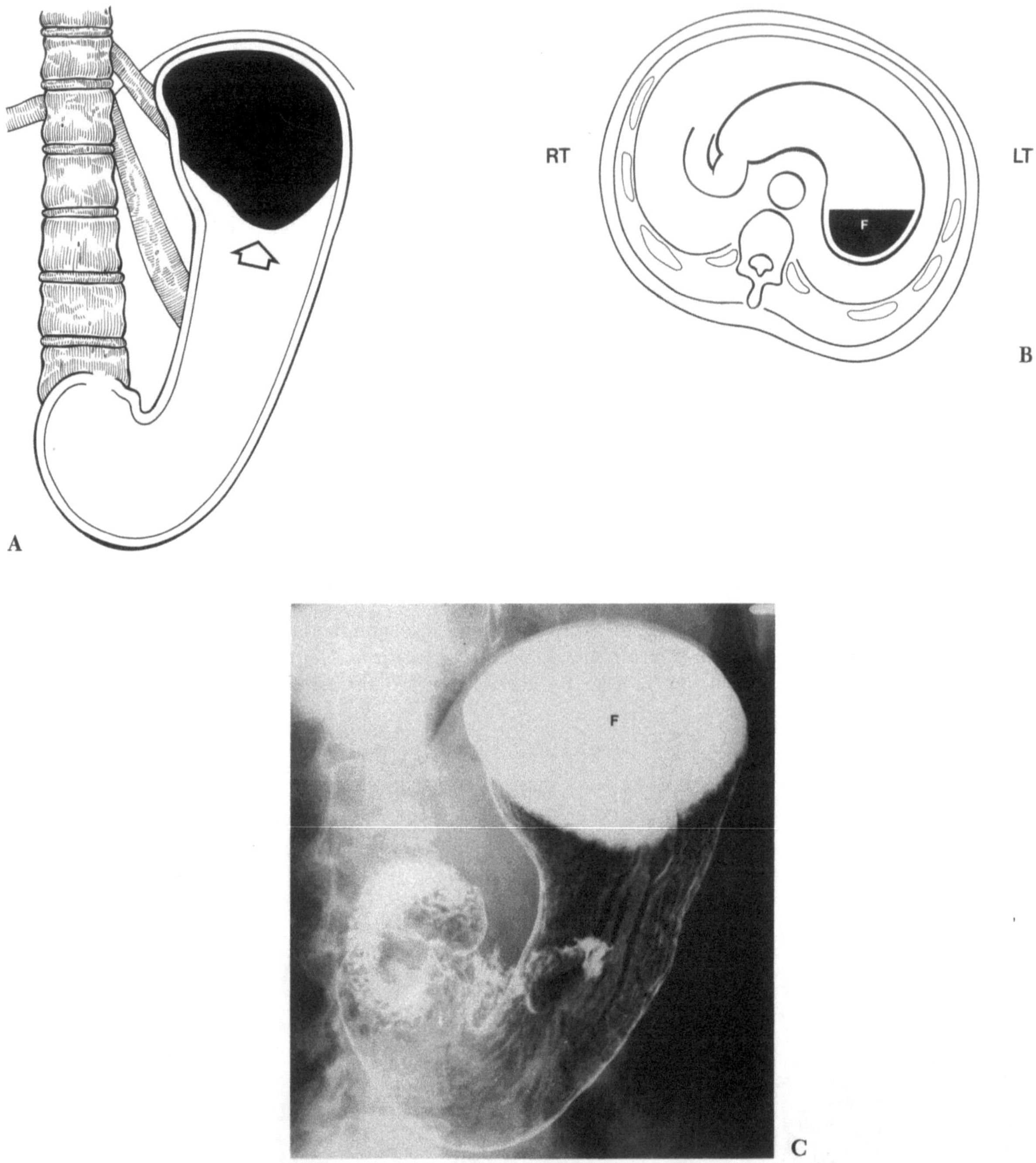

Fig. 2.6. In supine oblique right-side-forward position, barium (shown in *black*) (*arrow*, **A**) will drop with gravity into fundus (**F**) of stomach (**A, B**). Exposure of antrum and body of stomach in double contrast is obtained (**C**). In this example, antrum is partly obscured by barium in duodenum. When this is unavoidable, additional views of the antrum should be taken at a later stage of the examination.

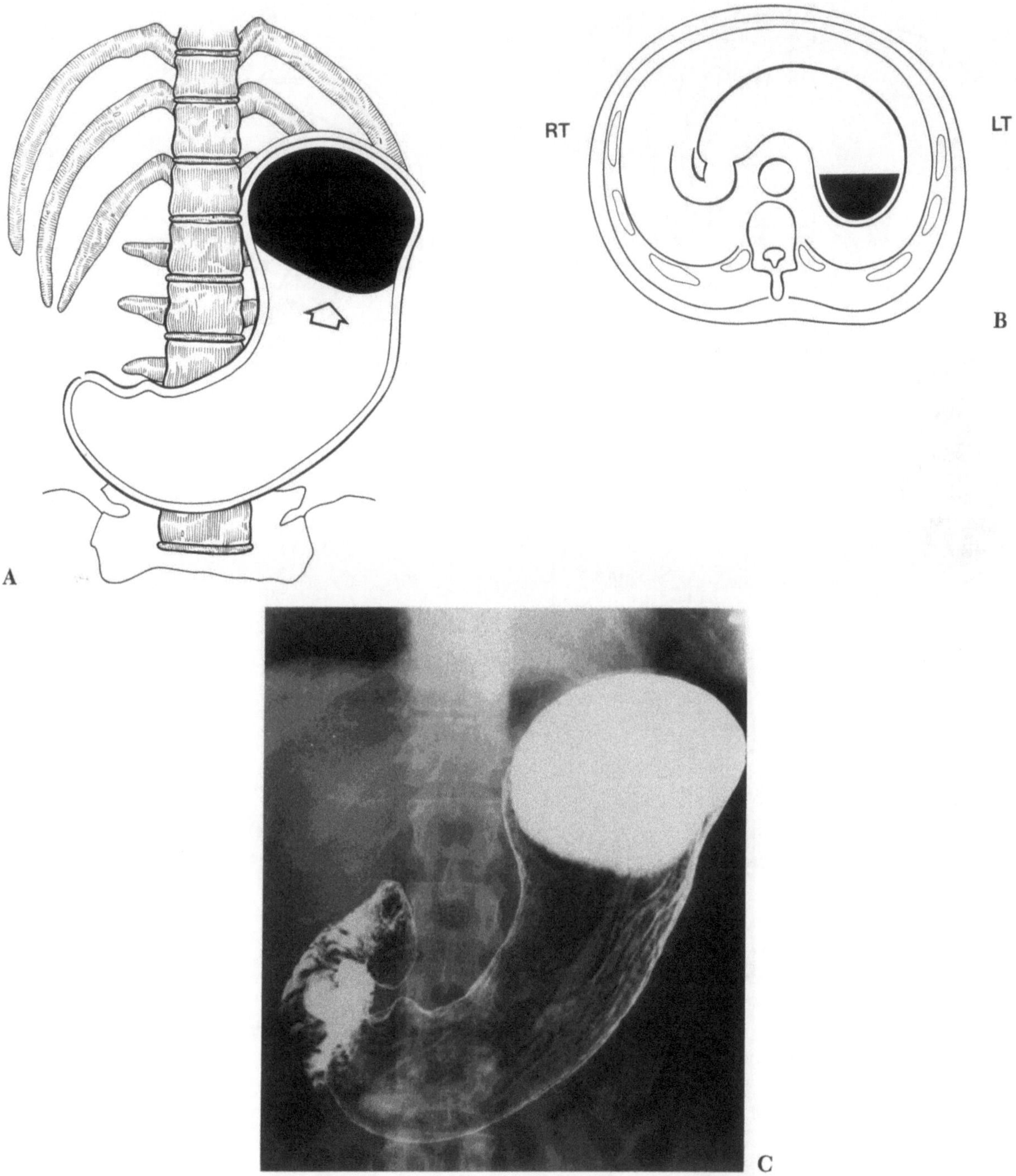

Fig. 2.7. With patient supine, barium (*arrow*, **A**) will remain in fundus (**A, B**) allowing clear visualization of mid and distal stomach (**C**). This film should be taken immediately after preceding one and before coating deteriorates. If delay has occured, rotate patient left and prone again, then return to supine position, to recoat mucosa before film is exposed.

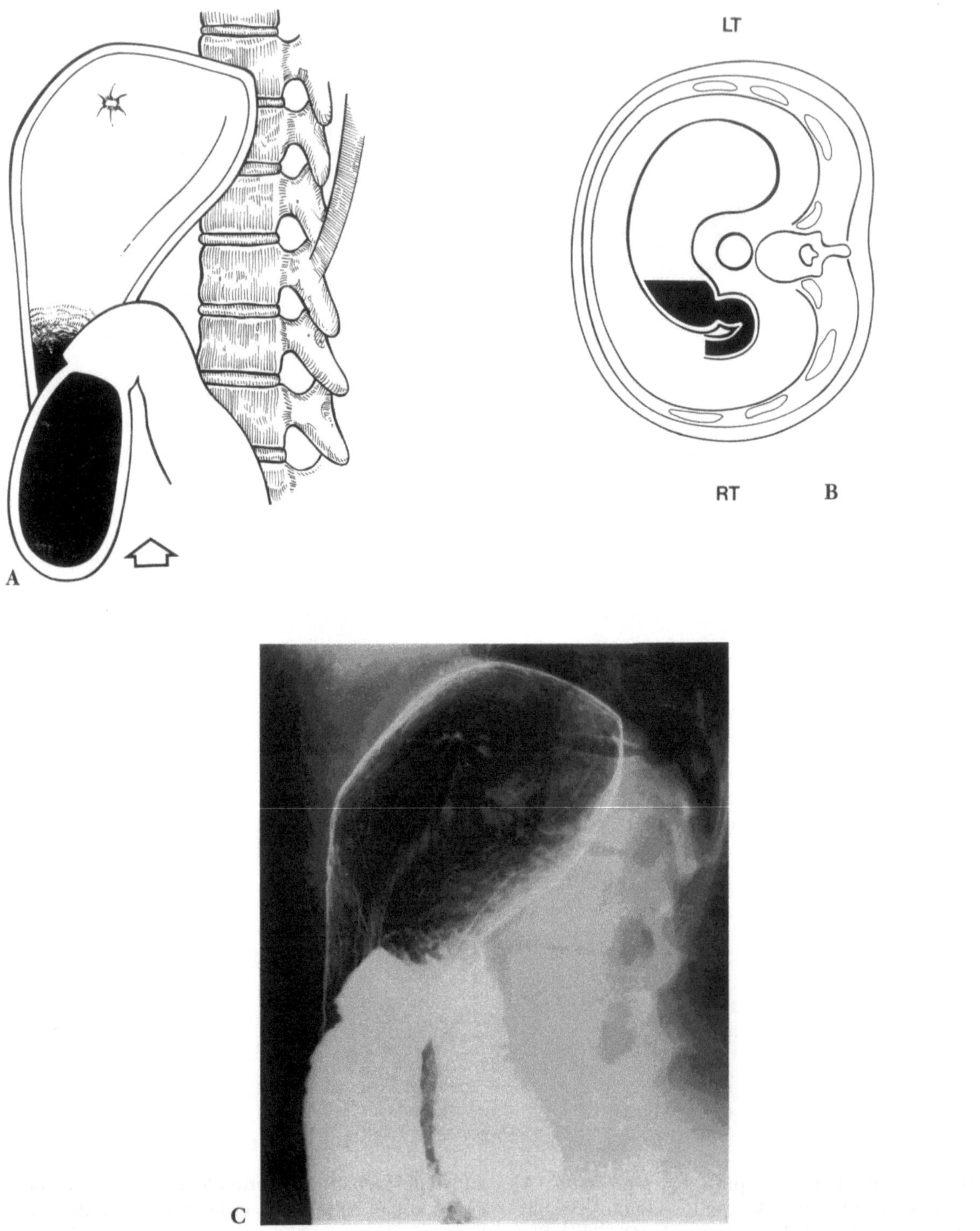

Fig. 2.8. Barium (*black*) will drain into antrum (*arrow*, **A**) by turning patient in to right lateral position (**A, B**). Cardia (**C**) of stomach is visualized. Obliquity of patient is changed so that cardia is seen between anterior and posterior walls of fundus.

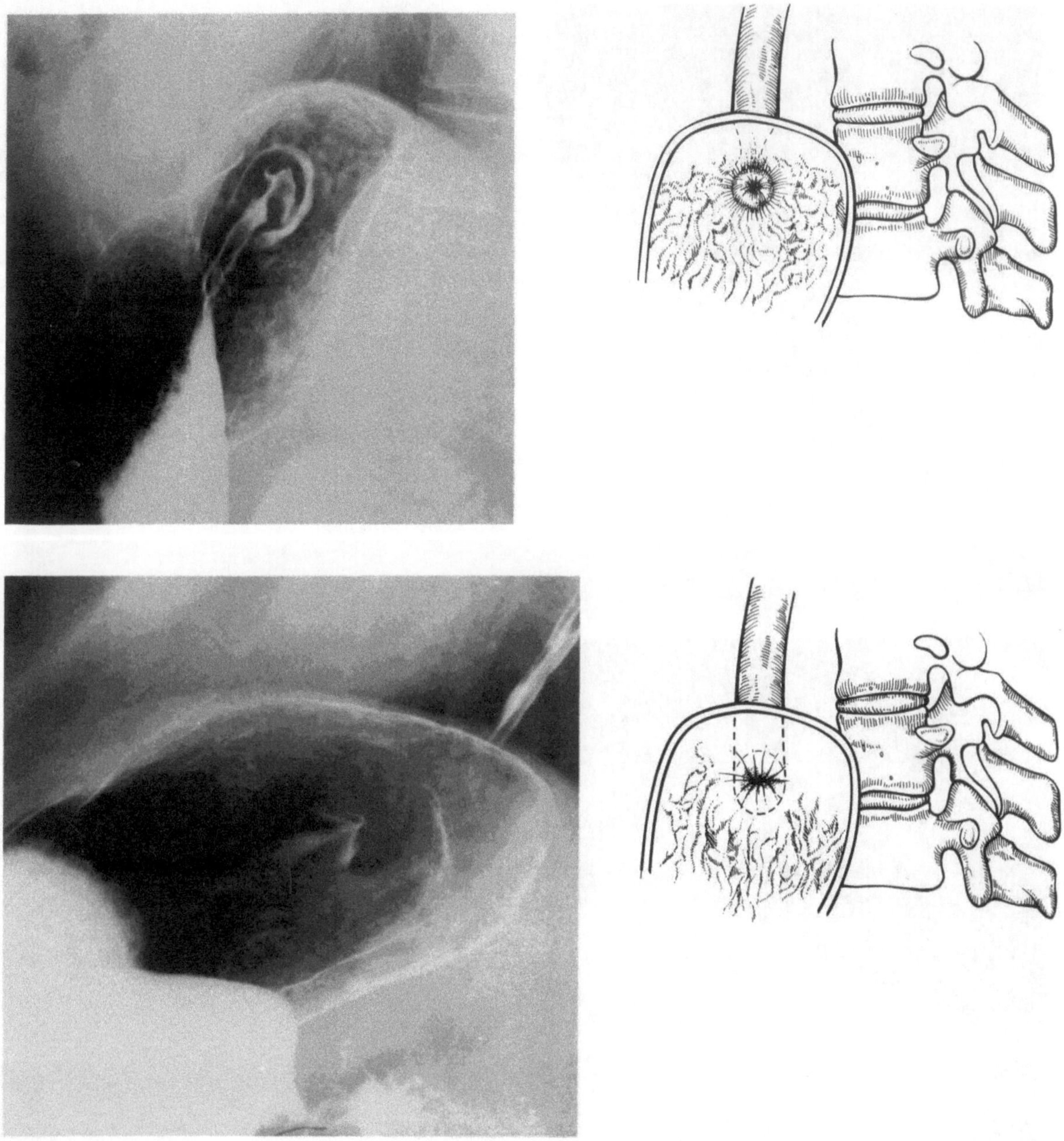

Fig. 2.9. Types of cardia. When lower esophageal sphincter is tightly closed, a mass effect is produced at cardia with mucosal junction at center of mass (type 1) (**A, B**). With relaxation, either from drugs or naturally low pressure, radiating folds are present but no mass (type 2) (**C, D**). (*Continued.*)

Step 7. Film size, 10 × 12 in. (single split). The patient turns into the lateral position on the right side. Because the spine causes an impression on the stomach posteriorly, it is usually necessary to have the patient turn completely lateral on the right side to drain the fundus and to visualize the cardia (Fig. 2.8). In this position barium will also be seen flowing into the duodenum. The head of the table may also be elevated, usually about 45°. Four basic patterns of the cardia have been described [13] (Fig. 2.9).

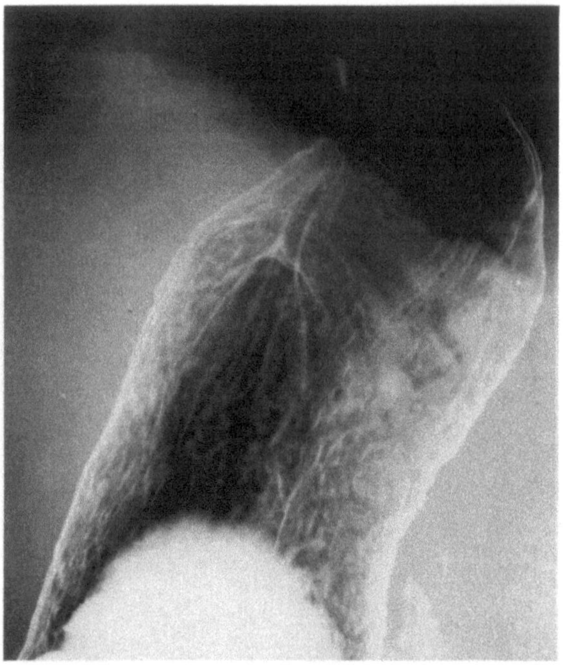
E

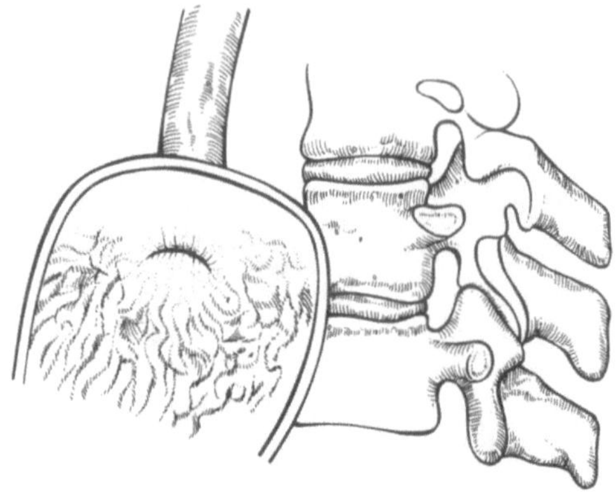
F

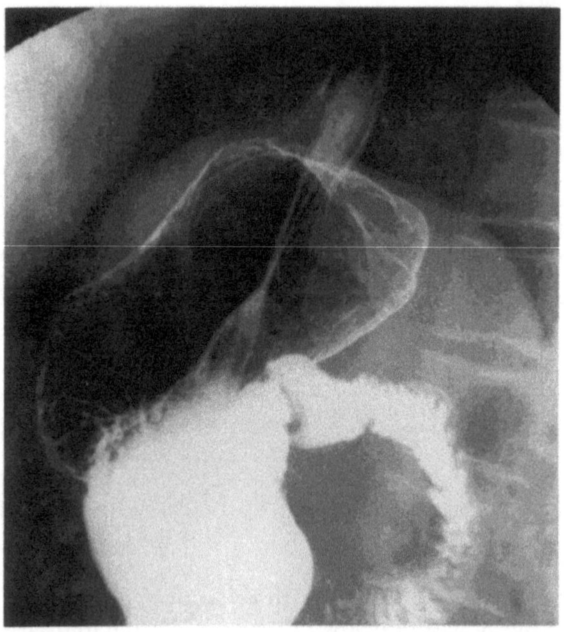
G

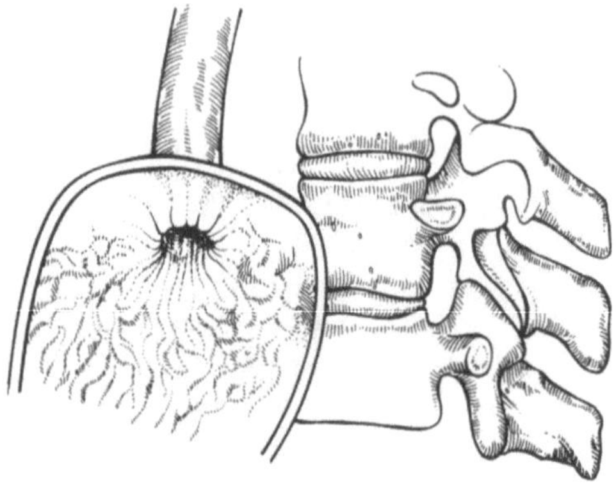
H

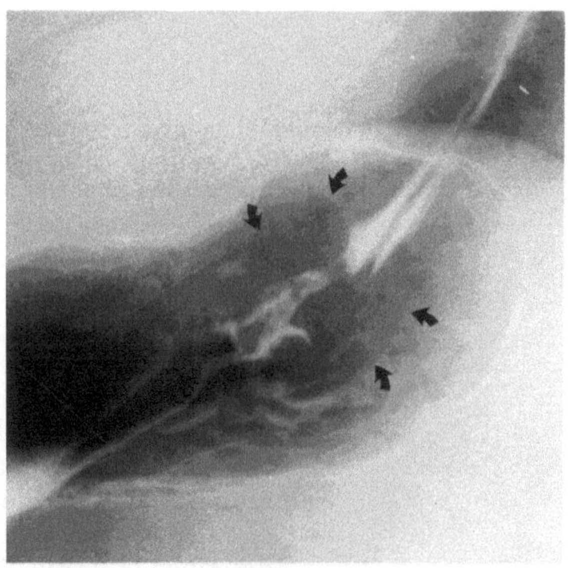
I

Fig. 2.9. With lax sphincter, crescent shadow is seen from partly open sphincter (type 3) (**E, F**). With further relaxation, the junction is wide open and rugal folds may be seen running up through the hiatus (type 4) (**G, H**). Carcinoma of cardia (**I**) can mimic type 1, but folds are distorted and disrupted, and mass (*arrows*) is usually eccentric.

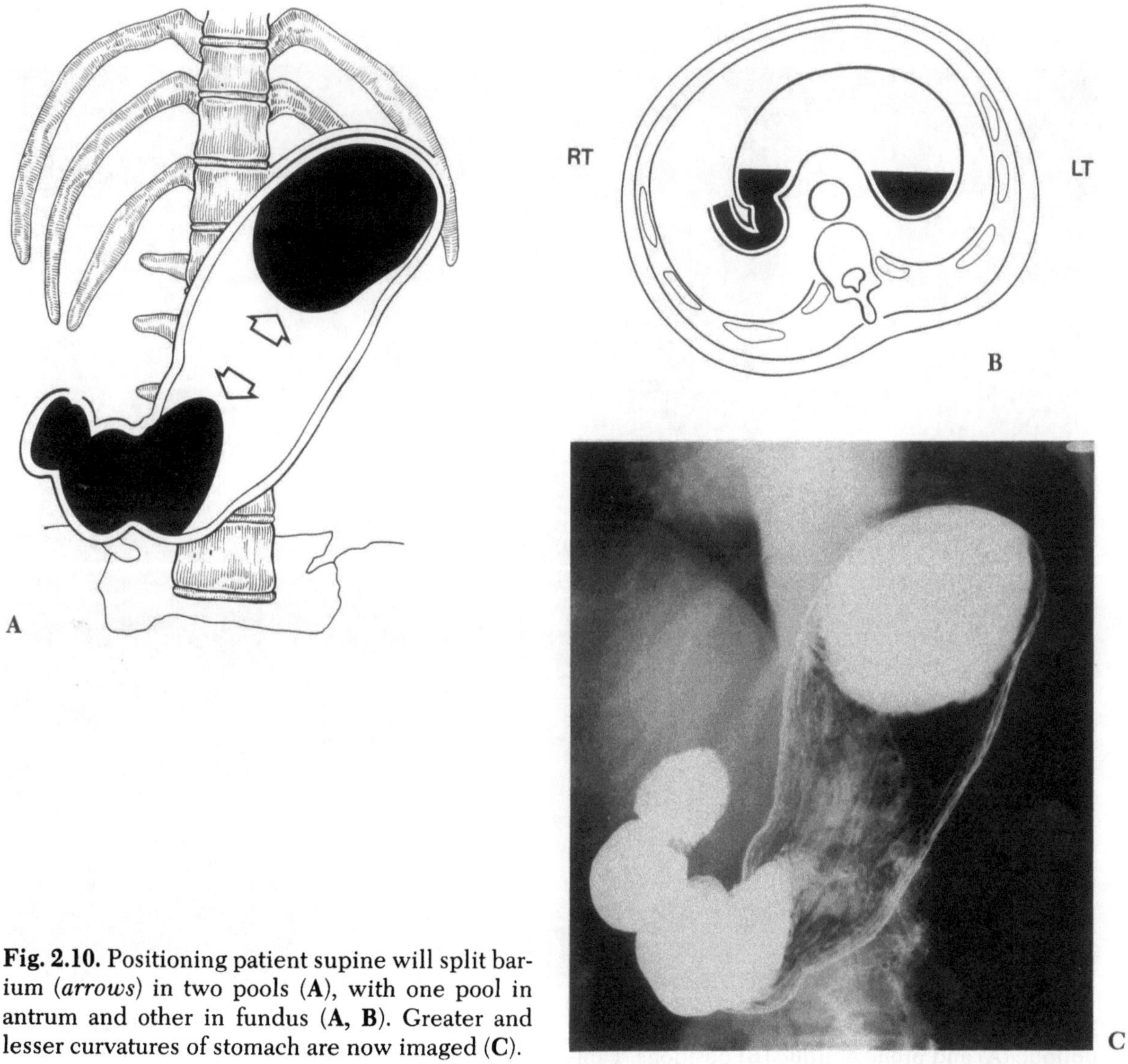

Fig. 2.10. Positioning patient supine will split barium (*arrows*) in two pools (**A**), with one pool in antrum and other in fundus (**A, B**). Greater and lesser curvatures of stomach are now imaged (**C**).

Step 8. Film size, 10 × 12 in. (single split). With the patient still on the right side, the table is brought down into horizontal position. The patient now is put into oblique left-side-forward position. This maneuver will split the barium into two pools, one pool flowing into the fundus and the second staying within the antrum, giving good visualization of the lesser and greater curvatures (Fig. 2.10).

A "flow technique" has been described that allows slightly elevated or depressed lesions, previously unrecognized, to be identified as a thin layer of barium flows over them. Thus, additional spot films of the posterior wall of the body and antrum can be obtained as a thin layer of barium flows "uphill" over the posterior wall. The lesser curvature and posterior wall of the antrum can be observed as a thin layer of barium flows "downhill" by turning the patient subsequently oblique right side down [14]. If the patient has a high transverse stomach, the lesser curvature may be better visualized by an additional cephalic angled view [15].

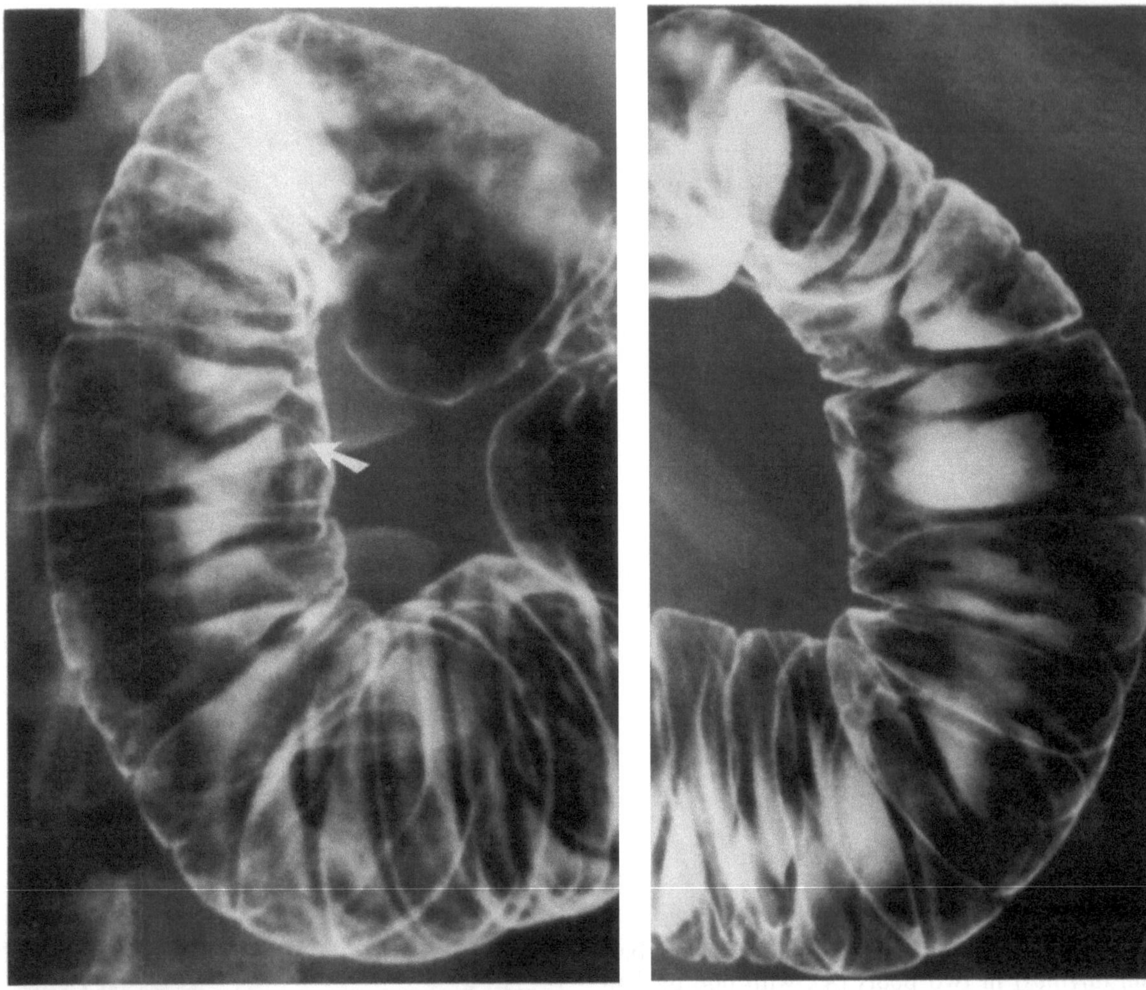

Fig. 2.11. Duodenal loop is imaged in supine oblique (**A**) and prone oblique (**B**) positions. Papilla of Vater (*arrow,* **A**) is seen on medial wall in prone films, and just adjacent to medial wall in supine oblique spots. Minor papilla is visible radiographically in only 20% of patients, but major papilla can be identified in 70% if relaxants are used.

Duodenum (Hypotonic Duodenography) [16]

Step 9. If there are no contraindications, the patient is given an intravenous injection of glucagon (0.3 mg) or Buscopan [17] (see Chapter 8). The dose of Buscopan varies with the speed of the radiologist, and the more experienced radiologist may need only 5–10 mg while the junior radiology resident uses 20 mg. The injection should be given only when an adequate amount of barium has drained into the duodenum; otherwise, the use of an antispasmodic may prevent barium from entering into the duodenum for the duration of its smooth muscle effect.

Step 10. The patient is turned on the left side and then into prone position. To obtain good coating of the duodenum, turn or rock the patient as described in Step 4.

Step 11. Film size, 8 × 10 in. (2 split). The patient is now turned on the left side and slightly supine oblique exposing the duodenal loop (Fig. 2.11A). First exposure is taken.

Fig. 2.12. Pad is positioned under patient's upper abdomen such that barium (*black*) in antrum is displaced toward fundus and air is driven into duodenum.

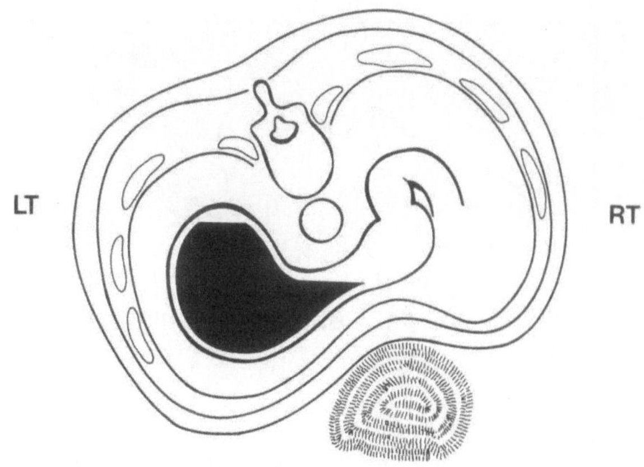

Step 12. The patient is turned back into the left lateral position and then prone. A pad is positioned under the patient's epigastric region. The full duodenal loop is again seen and the second exposure is taken. The incidence of pathology in the third and fourth parts of the duodenum is low. However, if present these abnormalities are quite obvious on double-contrast barium examination. The purpose of the pad is twofold; it drives air into the duodenum and also displaces barium from the antrum allowing visualization of the prone duodenal loop. The pad therefore must be positioned accurately at the level of the antrum, usually in or slightly to the right of the patient's midline (Fig. 2.12). Such a pad can be made simply by rolling up a towel tightly and securing it with tape. Figure 2.13 presents several variations in appearance of the normal ampulla of Vater [18].

Step 13. Film size, 8 × 10 in. (4 split). Four exposures of the duodenal cap are obtained, one in prone position (Fig. 2.14A) (patient still prone from Step 11) and three exposures in various supine oblique (Fig. 2.14B, C, D) right-side-forward position. If the duodenum has a steep anterioposterior course, it may be difficult to visualize the cap without a superimposed second portion. In this situation it may be helpful to film the duodenum in the window between the stomach and loops of jejunum. Angling of the tube, if available, may also be invaluable. If a pool of barium remains in the cap after coating the duodenum, this pool can be cleared by turning the patient supine, elevating the head of the table 45°, and then turning patient on the left side. The normal mucosal pattern of the duodenal cap is shown in Fig. 2.15.

Step 14. Film size, 10 × 12 in. (single split). The patient is now elevated into the erect position. An erect stomach film is obtained in a slightly obliqued position to show the angulus. The entire stomach should be visualized (Fig. 2.16).

Step 15. Film size, 8 × 10 in. (4 split). In the erect position, right side forward, the antrum and duodenum are compressed. Exposures taken as needed. In obese patients compression may not be possible in the erect position but may be successful with the table down 45°, weight off the patient's feet. If compression is still not possible, the prone position with a paddle may be tried. Although double-contrast assessment of the duodenum is frequently good, compression is still important, and some lesions may be identified only in this manner (Fig. 2.17).

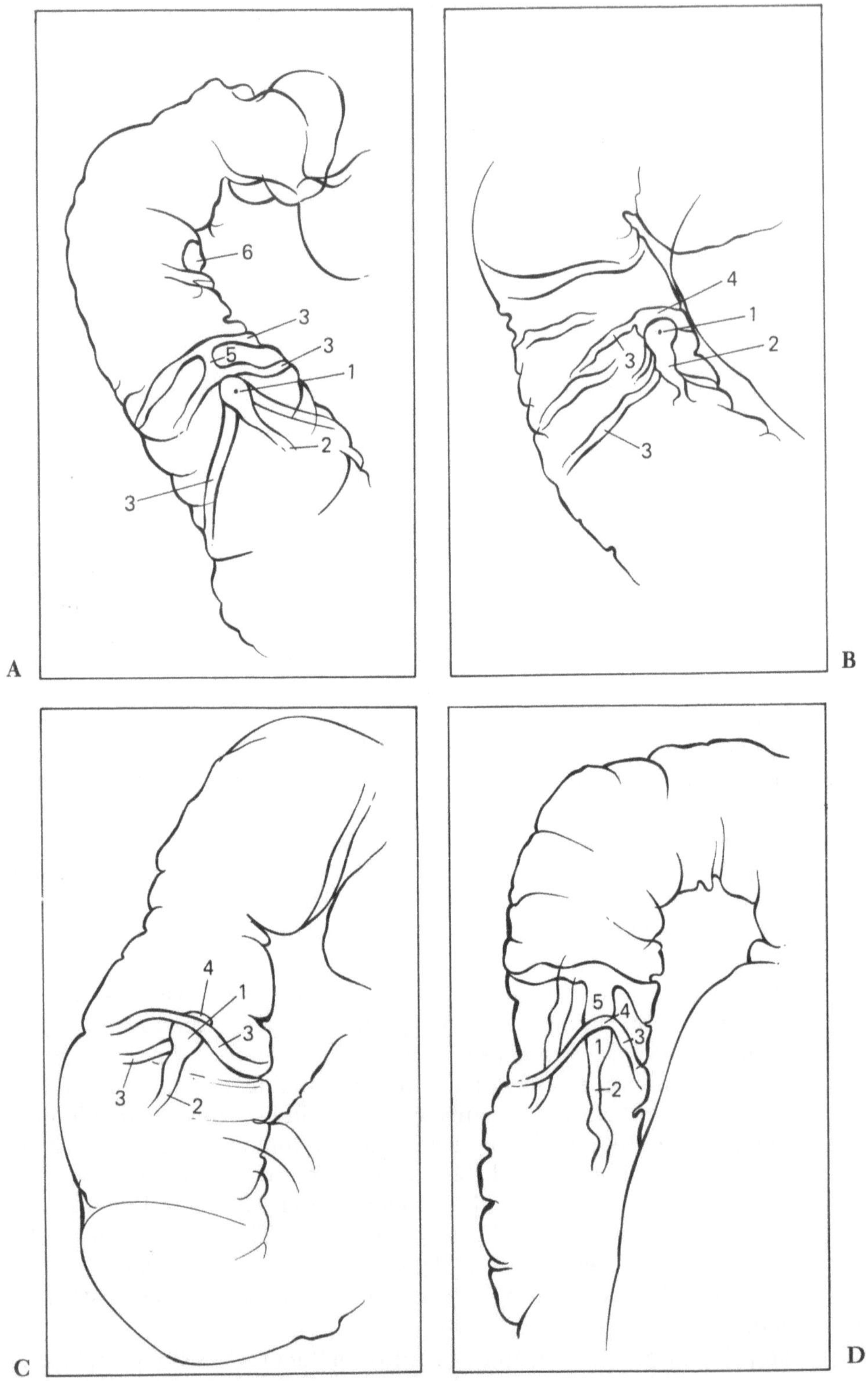

Fig. 2.13.A–D. Normal variations in ampulla of Vater. Ampulla of Vater (*1*), distal longitudinal fold (*2*), oblique fold (*3*), hooded fold (*4*), short proximal longitudinal fold (*5*), and accessory papilla (*6*).

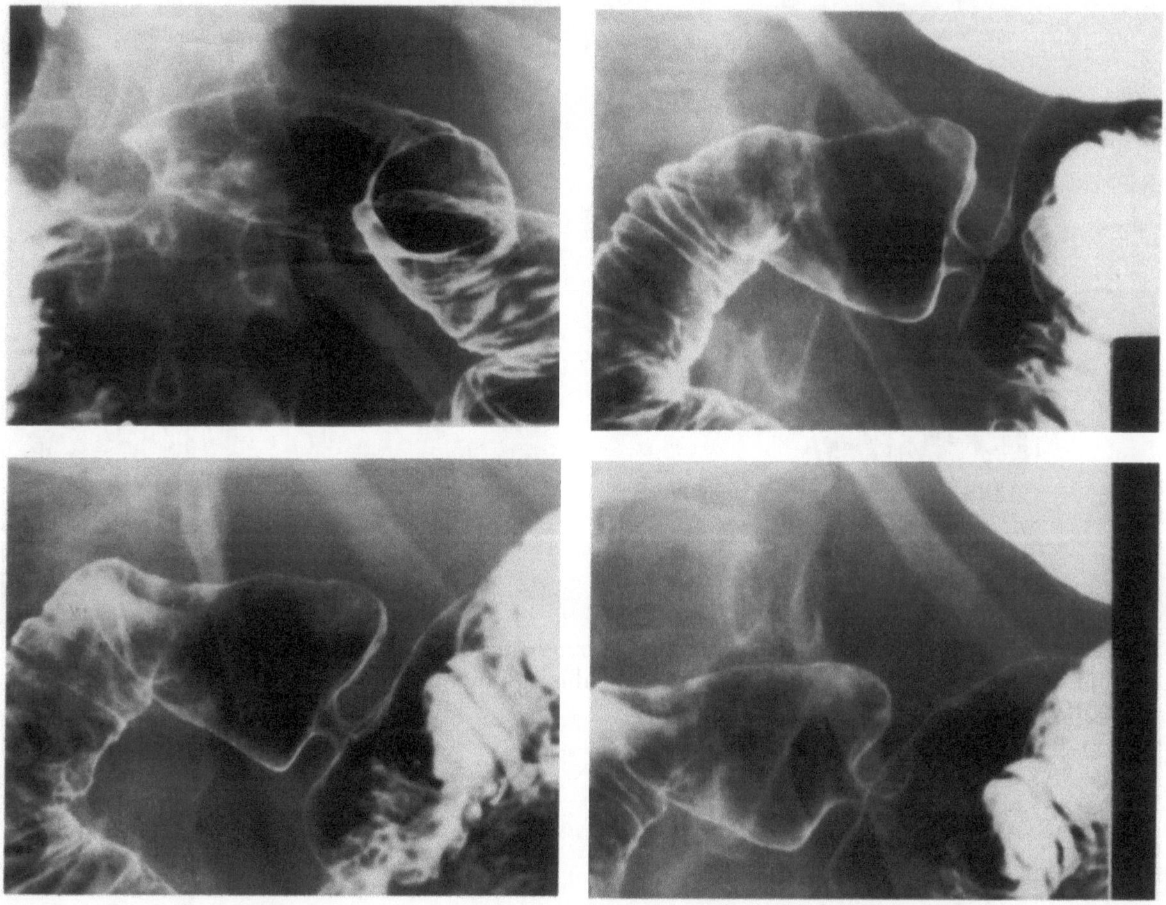

A B C D

Fig. 2.14. Double-contrast examination of duodenal cap in prone (**A**) and various supine right-side-forward obliquities (**B, C, D**).

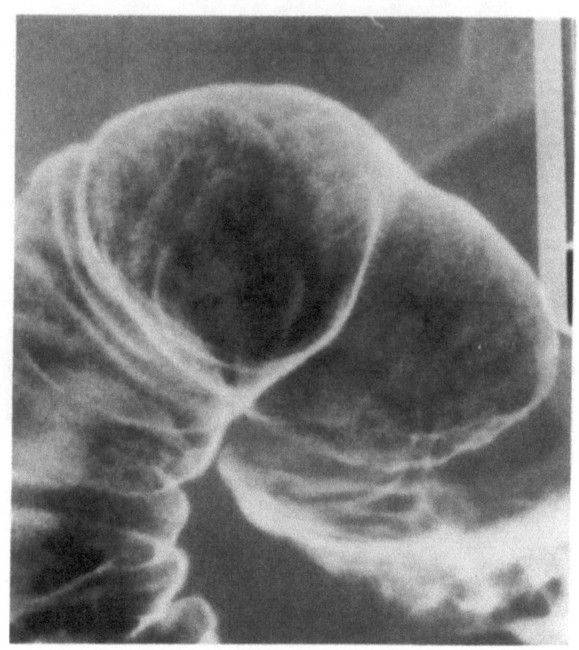

Fig. 2.15. Normal villous pattern of mucosa in duodenal cap.

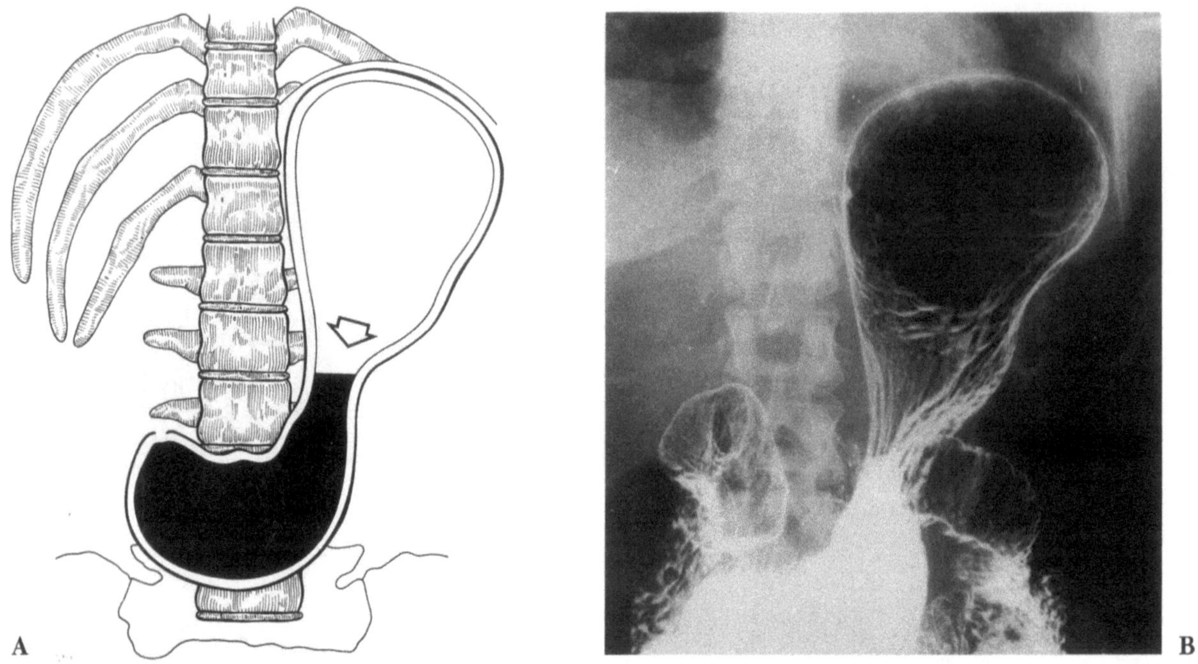

Fig. 2.16. In patient erect position, barium (*black; arrow* in **A**) flows down into antrum and air rises to fundus and cardia (**A**); angulus and fundus are visualized (**B**).

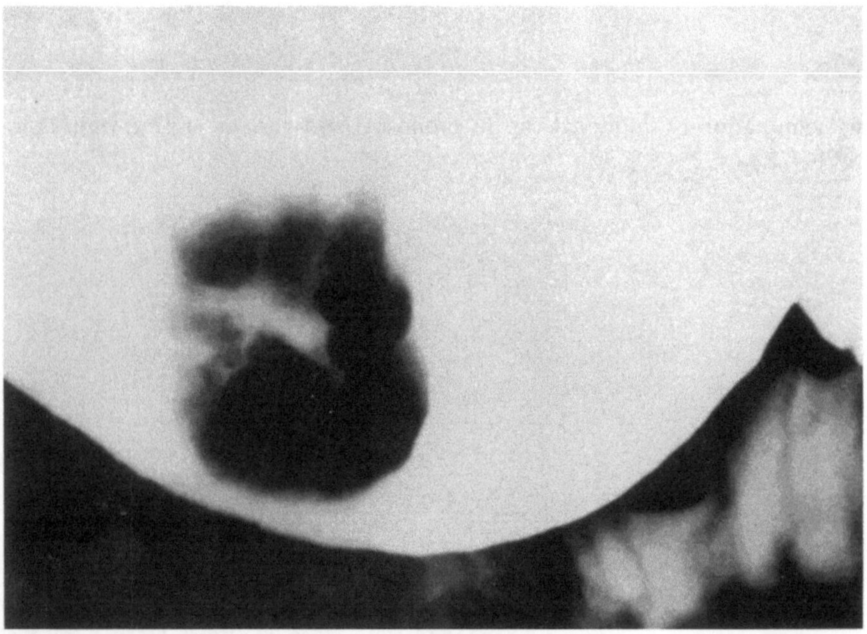

Fig. 2.17. Compression film demonstrates target lesion (metastatic deposit) in antrum.

Table 2.1. Routine upper GI series

Area to examine	Patient position	Film size	Purpose
1. Esophagus	Erect right side forward	14" × 14" (3 split)	Double contrast esophagus
2. Esophagus	Supine right side forward	14" × 14" (3 split)	Single contrast esophagus and mucosal relief
3. Stomach	Supine right side forward	10" × 12" (1 split)	Antrum-body
4. Stomach	Supine	10" × 12" (1 split)	Antrum-body
5. Stomach	Lateral lying on right side	10" × 12" (1 split)	Cardia-fundus
6. Stomach	Supine right side forward	10" × 12" (1 split)	Curvatures
Injection of Buscopan			
7. Duodenum	a) Supine left side forward b) Prone with pad	10" × 12" (1 split)	Hypotonic duodenography
8. Duodenum	a) Prone with pad b) Supine left forward	10" × 12" (4 split)	Duodenal cap
9. Duodenum antrum	Erect	Compression	To visualize anterior duodenal or antral ulcers
10. Stomach	Erect	10" × 12" (1 split)	Fundus

The stomach can usually be examined without Buscopan or glucagon; however, in many patients, a proper examination of the duodenum is impossible without smooth muscle relaxants. When the esophagus is examined without drugs, extra distention for better double contrast may be obtained by using chilled barium [19]. The cold temperature, however, will inhibit primary peristaltic activity. Cold barium should therefore not be used to assess esophageal motility.

The foregoing sequence of films represents a satisfactory routine examination (Table 2.1). The sequence can be varied and there are alternative methods of examining the upper GI tract. For example, the double-contrast films of the esophagus may be taken at the end of the examination, with the patient erect, rather than at the beginning. For this purpose, additional barium and gas granules have to be swallowed with the patient erect after all other films have been obtained. Nevertheless, some radiologists find they obtain better coating of the esophagus by doing the double-contrast examination at the end rather than the beginning. In addition, by starting the examination with the table horizontal, and with the patient resting on the left elbow while drinking, it is easier to prevent barium entering the duodenum until gastric films have been completed.

Patients who are unable to hold the barium cup in the left hand (previous stroke) can have the esophagus examined while standing and holding the cup in the right hand and reversing the obliquity so now the left side is forward.

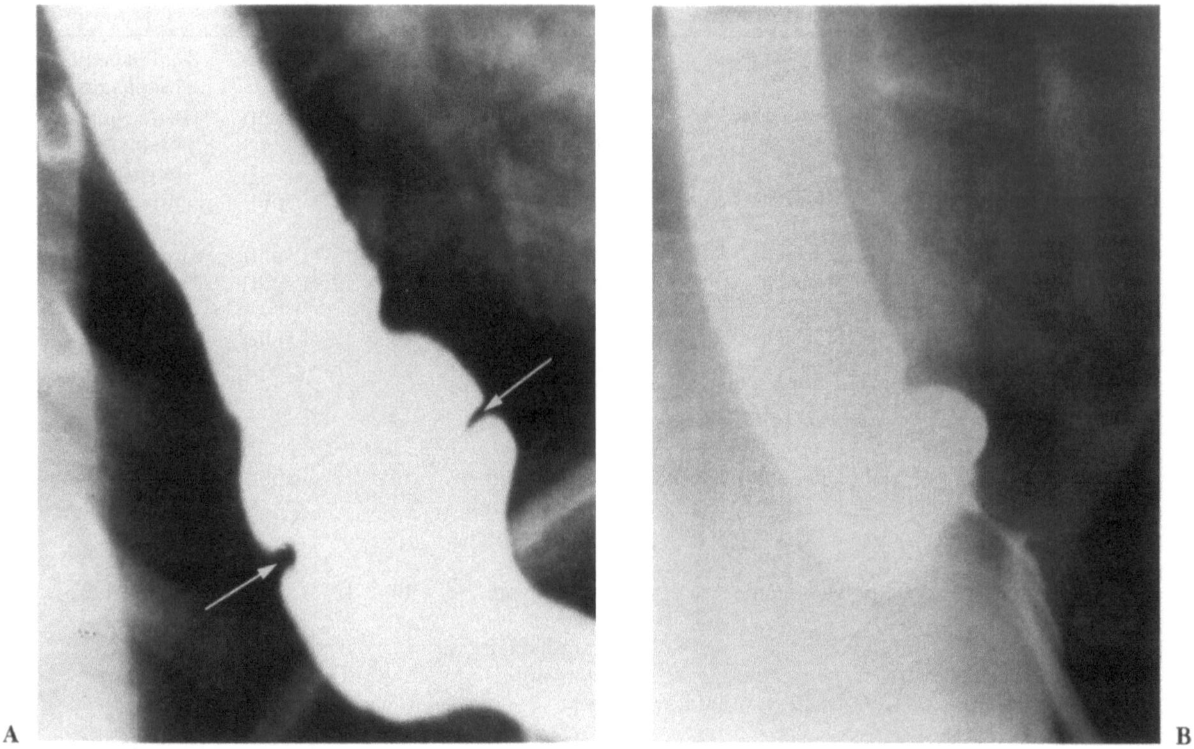

Fig. 2.18. Prone esophageal study. Schatzki ring (*arrows*) is identified easily in prone position (**A**) because of distention associated with increased pressures, but is less clear with patient supine (**B**).

A double-contrast examination of the esophagus can also be achieved if the patient swallows the effervescent granules, water, and high-density barium, and is then placed in the prone position. In the prone right anterior oblique (RAO) position, with the gas in the proximal stomach, the patient takes further sequential swallows of barium. These swallows relax the lower esophageal sphincter, may permit reflux of gas into the esophagus, and shows the lower esophagus clear of overlying structures. The prone esophageal study is sometimes essential for the assessment of the lower esophagus [20] (Fig. 2.18). Strictures and rings at the gastroesophageal junction are shown more clearly prone than supine. The normal anatomy of the gastroesophageal junction is reviewed in Fig. 2.19.

Water has been advocated for the purpose of producing a double-contrast esophagram [21]. This is done by having the patient swallow a mouthful of barium followed rapidly by a mouthful of water. The water washes down the barium, leaving the esophagus coated and producing a double-contrast effect. Although coating of the esophagus by this method may be adequate, swallowing the extra water would prevent adequate study of the remaining upper GI tract. We have not found this technique useful, but it may play an adjunctive role following a routine examination.

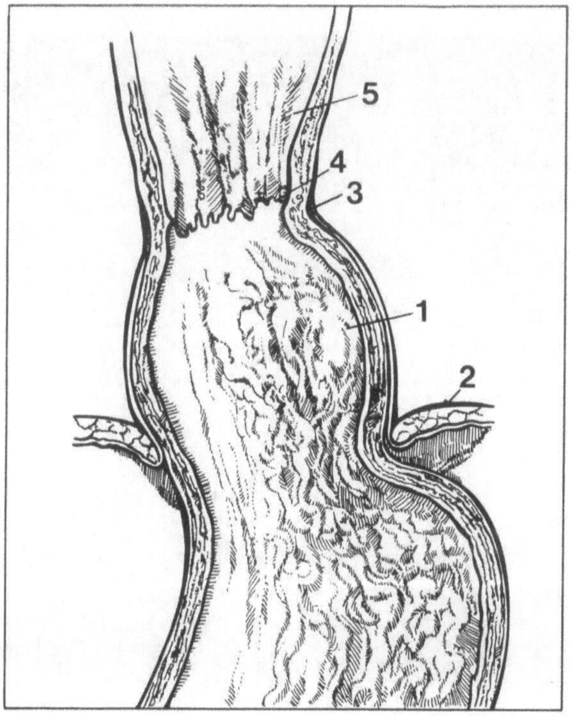

Fig. 2.19. Anatomy of gastroesophageal junction in patient with hiatus hernia (1) above diaphragm (2). Gastroesophageal junction (3), site of B or Schatzki ring, is at same level as mucosal Z line (4), which represents change from columnar to squamous epithelium. In illustration, lower esophageal sphincter (vestibule) is wide open (5).

A double-contrast esophagram can also be obtained with methylcellulose swallowed after barium paste [22]. In this technique, the patient chews and swallows enough barium paste (E-Z paste) to coat the esophagus; esophageal distention is then obtained by drinking 200 ml of chilled hydroxypropyl methylcellulose [1.0% weight per volume (w/v)].

A single-contrast examination of the stomach, although possible, is seldom required unless the patient is too sick to have a double-contrast study or endoscopy. The study is performed with dilute barium (as for a small bowel follow-through), initially with a very low volume. This provides a mucosal relief assessment that is good for evaluation of rugal folds and emptying. Subsequently, enough barium is swallowed to distend the stomach and allow for compression. If the patient is unable to swallow the barium, the study can be performed with the help of a nasogastric tube passed into the stomach. A brief single-contrast examination can be performed at the beginning of a small bowel meal (see page 44).

Many problems can be encountered during an upper GI examination. An inadequate esophageal study can occur: (1) if barium pools in the distal esophagus, preventing a complete double-contrast examination; (2) if foam forms from the effervescent granules; (3) if the patient cannot take large enough swallows to allow air and barium to properly distend the esophagus; or (4) if the patient belches so that no more air is available for controlled reflux into the esophagus from the stomach. The examination of the stomach may also be flawed if the patient belches and loses the gaseous distention. If the patient was slow in swallowing barium in the erect position, barium may have drained into the small bowel, obscuring detail of the antrum and greater curvature.

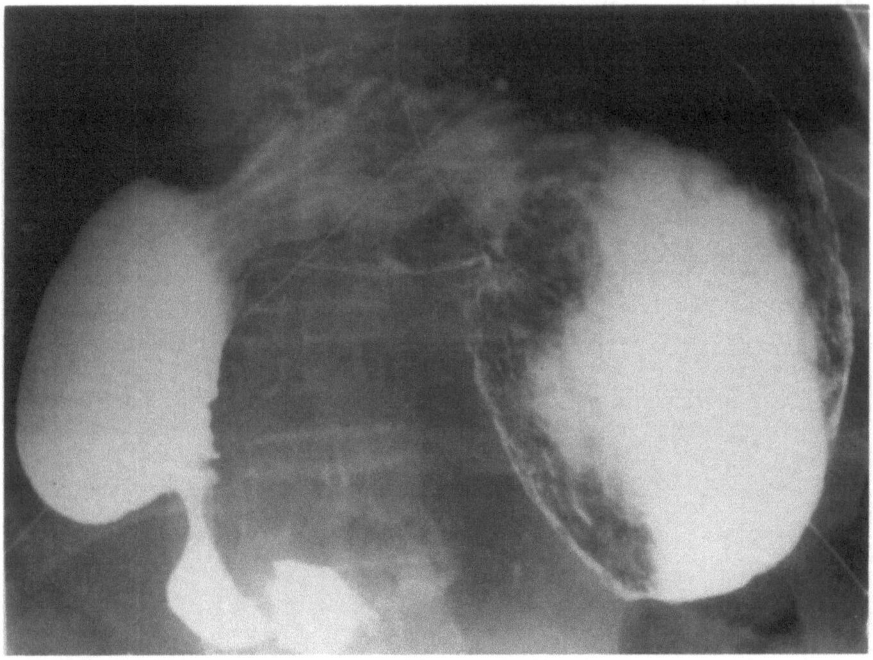

Fig. 2.20. Double-contrast examination in patient with intrathoracic gastric volvulus illustrates difficulties that may arise during routine examination because of changes in anatomy.

The duodenum may not be adequately examined if Buscopan is given before an adequate amount of barium has drained into the duodenum. If inappropriate amounts of water are given with the effervescent granules, adequate coating of the stomach and duodenum will not be achieved. Blurring of films will occur if exposure times are not fast enough, not only because of patient respiration but also because of cardiac motion, especially when examining the cardia. In patients with a large sliding or paraesophageal hiatus hernia, the study must be modified using gravity and patient positioning to achieve adequate barium coating of all parts of the stomach (Fig. 2.20).

Inappropriate barium suspensions used during the study can result in poor mucosal coating, barium precipitation, flaking, and stalactite formation mimicking disease [23].

Esophageal Examination for Specific Problems

Suspected Gastroesophageal Reflux (Water Siphon Test)

A routine examination is carried out until the esophageal and gastric examination has been completed (Step 8, page 15). The duodenum is examined without a hypotonic agent, as this would interfere with esophageal function [24]. Because only 50% of patients with reflux disease will reflux spontaneously during a barium meal, if spontaneous

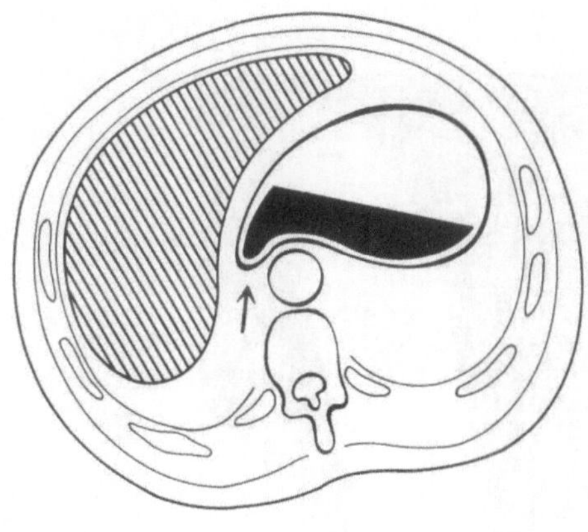

Fig. 2.21. Patient is positioned supine oblique, left side forward, so that barium (*black*) in fundus flows to cover region of cardia.

reflux is not observed it may be provoked to study volume clearance. Reflux occurs more readily with a full stomach, so there should be plenty of barium remaining in the stomach for assessment of reflux. The patient should be positioned so that reflux can occur rather than belching, that is, the cardia must be below the level of the barium–carbon dioxide interface (Fig. 2.21). This means putting the patient on the left side to fill the fundus, then supine and slightly to the right in the position where the cardia is submerged but the barium stays in the fundus and does not run down to the antrum. In this position reflux may occur spontaneously.

The head-down Trendelenburg position is unnecessary unless the configuration of the stomach is such that barium cannot be made to cover the cardia with the table horizontal. If spontaneous reflux is not seen, it may occur if the patient takes a few dry swallows, as the act of swallowing induces lower esophageal sphincter relaxation. Finally, the patient can be given water to drink, while still lying in the same position (water siphon test) [25]. Normal individuals will reflux one or two small puffs of barium into the lower esophagus under these circumstances, with the barium being rapidly cleared by the next peristaltic wave [26]. Reflux patients tend to flood the entire esophagus under this provocation (Fig. 2.22). The purpose of the test is to assess the ease and degree of reflux, and examine the ability of the esophagus to clear the refluxed barium. Once reflux has been induced, primary peristalsis should be used to assess clearance, by asking the patient to swallow once every 15 to 20 seconds. A few patients clear the esophagus completely with a single dry swallow, while others are unable to clear any barium with several swallows, or have their primary peristalsis interrupted or replaced by nonperistaltic activity. The water siphon test has not been standardized, but is an effective way of inducing reflux of acidified barium and observing its effect on clearance.

Globus Hystericus

Many patients with globus have gastroesophageal reflux. Others have minor variations in movement of the pharynx. Yet others, on close questioning, turn out not to have globus but pharyngeal dysphagia. With such diverse causes, the symptom of globus requires more than a

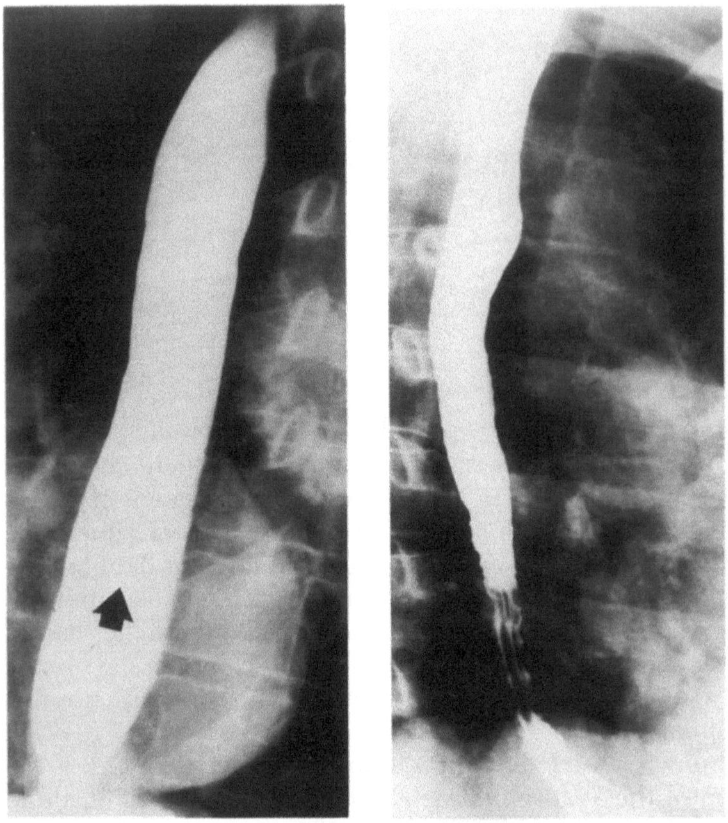

Fig. 2.22. Reflux (*arrow*) induced by water siphon test (**A**) with associated esophagitis (**B**). Mucosal relief films are sensitive method for diagnosing moderate or severe esophagitis, and occasionally reveal disease not apparent on double-contrast views.

routine examination. The examination should begin with a very brief fluoroscopy of the pharynx to exclude a large and obvious lesion, and then continue with the routine study and the maneuvers described for reflux. At the end, the pharynx should be examined in detail. This will include anteroposterior (AP) and lateral views of the barium-coated oropharynx at rest (Fig. 2.23), and an additional lateral view with the patient saying "eeeee" (Fig. 2.24), or doing a Valsalva maneuver, both of which move the larynx forward, open the valleculae, and show the epiglottis more clearly. Lateral and AP video recordings are made of pharyngeal swallowing of liquid barium, and here it is sometimes worth using a 50 : 50 dilution of the standard high-density barium to show webs more readily. If an abnormality is seen on video, two- to four-per-second, 100-mm spot films are a convenient way of obtaining a film of the lesion if this equipment is available.

Dysphagia

The examination for dysphagia is designed to detect motor disorders and obstructing lesions. The initial first swallow should be a small sip,

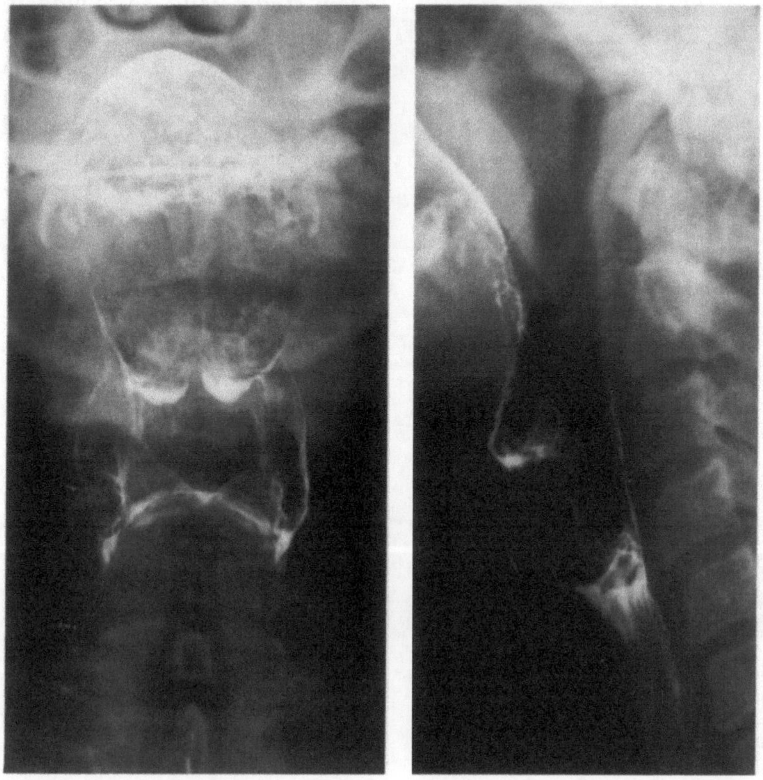

A B

Fig. 2.23. Anteroposterior (AP) (**A**) and lateral (**B**) views of oropharynx in resting state.

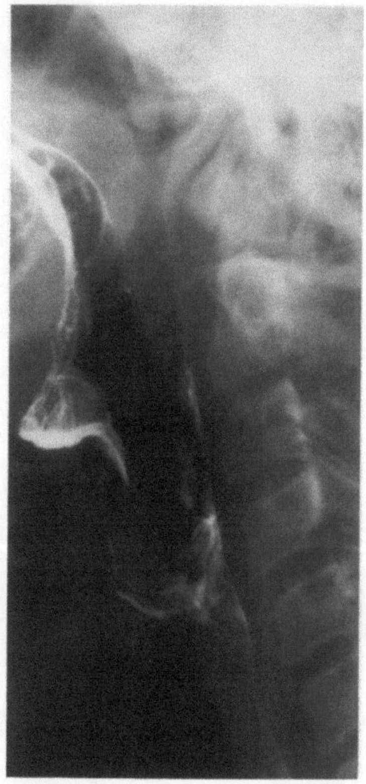

Fig. 2.24. Oropharynx during phonation.

to be sure there is no major or high obstruction, because the gas granules and barium may severely distress such patients and may be dangerous, causing massive aspiration or even perforation [12]. If no lesion is seen with the first sip, a routine examination is then performed, including prone oblique views of the lower end of the esophagus. If this is negative, or does not fully explain the patient's symptoms, a solid bolus swallow is helpful. By far the best bolus is a marshmallow (marshmallow study), which will maintain a globular shape as a bolus, but will dissolve within 5 or 10 minutes [27,28]. The table is brought erect, and the patient is asked to swallow a small marshmallow (1-cm diameter) without chewing it, washing it down with some barium. If this passes freely into the stomach, half a large marshmallow is given (2.5-cm diameter) and swallowed in the same manner. Many patients think they cannot swallow this larger bolus, but more than 90% can do so with a little encouragement after a few attempts. If the problem is believed to be pharyngeal, the marshmallow swallow should be performed in the lateral projection with careful videofluoroscopy as the attempt to swallow is made. The bolus may arrest on a web, cricopharyngeal bar, or other lesion. For minimal lower esophageal lesions, very rarely a whole marshmallow may be required (3-cm diameter), but many patients cannot swallow this size of bolus. A positive test usually shows arrest of the marshmallow and reproduction of the patient's symptoms (Figs. 2.25 and 2.26).

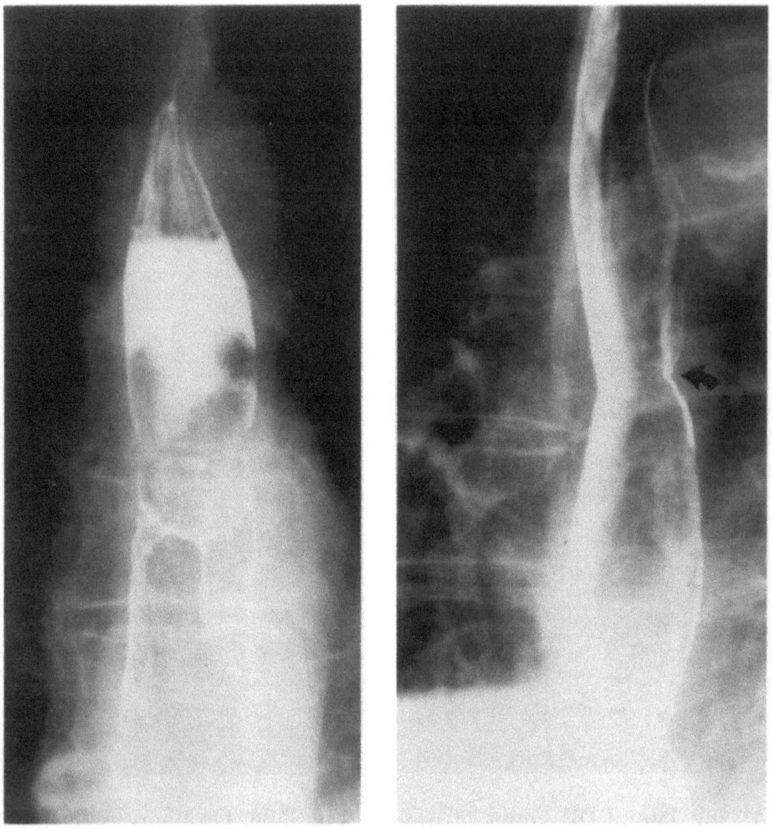

A B

Fig. 2.25. Positive marshmallow study. Mild narrowing in midesophagus in patient with occasional mild dysphagia (**B**). Marshmallow arrested in stenosis (**A**) and reproduced symptoms, confirming that this was relevant lesion. It represented squamocolumnar junction in Barrett's esophagus (*arrow*).

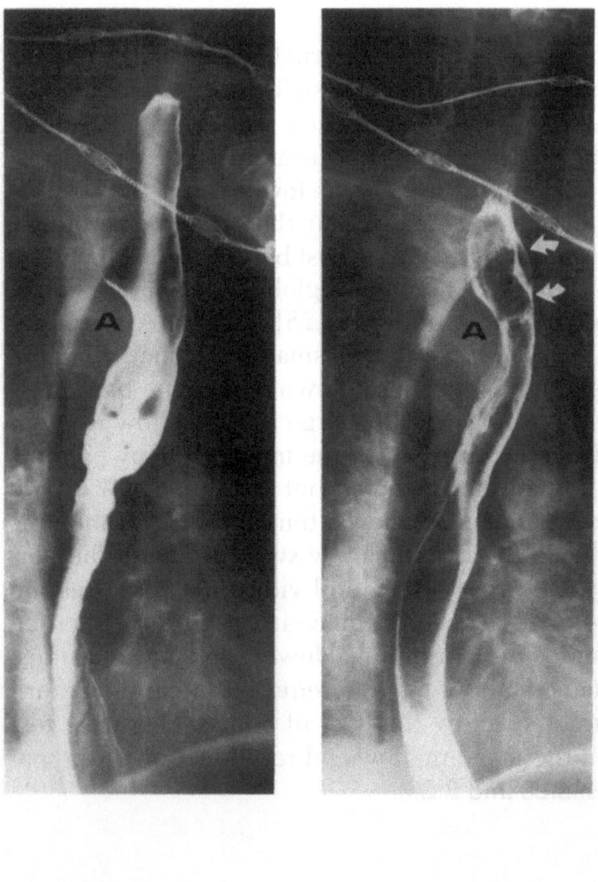

A B

Fig. 2.26. Marshmallow (*arrows*) arresting above right-sided aortic arch (A) in elderly patient with dysphagia. No other lesion was present.

Esophageal motility can also be studied by measuring capsule transit time [29]. In this test the patient swallows a small, barium-filled, hard gelatine capsule [30] and is placed in the supine position. The capsule is observed under fluoroscopic control and the time needed for the capsule to enter the stomach is recorded. The normal transit time is 15 seconds or less, and the test is valid only if the patient is supine. Isotopes can also be used to study esophageal transit [26].

Chest Pain

When the esophagus is considered as a source of chest pain, the three main causes to be evaluated are reflux disease, a motor disorder under the broad heading of spasm, or acute esophagitis caused by, for example, herpes infection or an arrested antibiotic tablet that has been swallowed without water. In most cases an esophageal cause is not found. The radiological examination should include an attempt to provoke the esophagus into producing the pain.

A thorough radiological examination of the esophagus in such a patient might be as follows. The examination includes the routine views, and the standard assessment of reflux as previously described. The stomach and duodenum should be examined, but suboptimally without glucagon or Buscopan. Esophageal motility is then examined in detail. Three to five primary peristaltic waves are observed following single swallows at 20-second intervals, with the patient horizontal; be absolutely sure that the patient does not double-swallow. Three half-marshmallows are then swallowed consecutively to assess the response to distention. Three swallows of ice-cold barium (the cold increases esophageal caliber, and may provoke the pain) are followed by three swallows of acidified barium at pH 1.6.

Acidified barium is prepared by mixing barium with hydrochloric acid. The amount of acid depends on the buffering capability of the barium used. We use our hospital pharmacists to prepare barium at the exact pH. This test is being used less often, mostly because of the Bernstein test, which is double blind and avoids bias; thus, this test is easier to standarize and control.

Pharmacological induction of abnormal esophageal motility may also be attempted. Tensilon (edrophonium chloride) at a dose of 80 micrograms(μg) per kilogram may be injected slowly intravenously, and will act within 30 to 60 seconds for 5 to 10 minutes. During this time further swallows of barium are given to see if abnormal motility has been provoked. Tensilon is a cholinesterase inhibitor, and may provoke nausea, vomiting, and bradycardia in some patients, so that atropine should be on hand to reverse the effects if necessary. Resuscitation equipment should also be available. Tensilon is a safer drug to use for provocative testing than bethanechol or ergonovine, whose use should probably be restricted to units in which the staff are prepared to deal immediately with sudden cardiac arrhythmias. The clinical utility of these various maneuvers is debatable, both in the motility laboratory and in the x-ray department [31]. In difficult clinical cases, it may be worthwhile trying a variety of methods to reproduce the pain or motility disturbance.

Acute Total Dysphagia

Acute total dysphagia is usually caused by food impaction, and endoscopy is often required for disimpaction. Frequently, there is an underlying problem that may need biopsy, most commonly a Schatzki ring. Barium sulfate destroys the endoscopic view of the obstructed esophagus for days, and can clog the endoscope. If a contrast swallow is requested, it should be done with a water-soluble agent, but remembering that large quantities of Gastrografin aspirated into the lungs may lead to pulmonary edema. Gastrografin may be used in very small amounts, to act as a guide to endoscopy. Isotonic metrizamide and nonionic contrast media should probably be the agents of choice for acute total obstruction, at least for the initial few swallows, despite their cost.

Perforation

When esophageal perforation is suspected, a plain chest radiograph may reveal air in the neck, mediastinum, or left inferior pulmonary ligament, and there may be a pleural effusion. Barium in the mediastinum is difficult to clear and should probably be avoided, although the evidence that it is dangerous is not convincing [32]. Gastrografin is the agent of choice unless a bronchoesophageal fistula is suspected or aspiration is likely, as the hypertonic Gastrografin is irritating to the lungs. In these patients, an isotonic, nonionic contrast agent is probably safest, at least for the initial few swallows. In most patients the examination can be started with Gastrografin, and the patient should be examined supine and in both obliquities so as not to miss small leaks (Fig. 2.27). If the study is negative, barium should then be given, because small perforations overlooked with Gastrografin may be visualized following large volume swallows of barium.

Tube Esophagram

Indications

To delineate suspected mucosal abnormalities in the distal esophagus when conventional double-contrast examination is suboptimal because patient cannot swallow large mouthfuls of barium, noncompliance of the patient, or retching [33]. The value of this examination can be debated. If a tube is to be introduced into the esophagus for better morphological assessment, then perhaps this tube should be an endoscope.

Contraindications and Precautions

Caution is taken during introduction of a nasogastric tube to prevent traumatization of the nasopharynx and possible epistaxis. The possibility of accidental intubation of the bronchial tree should be remem-

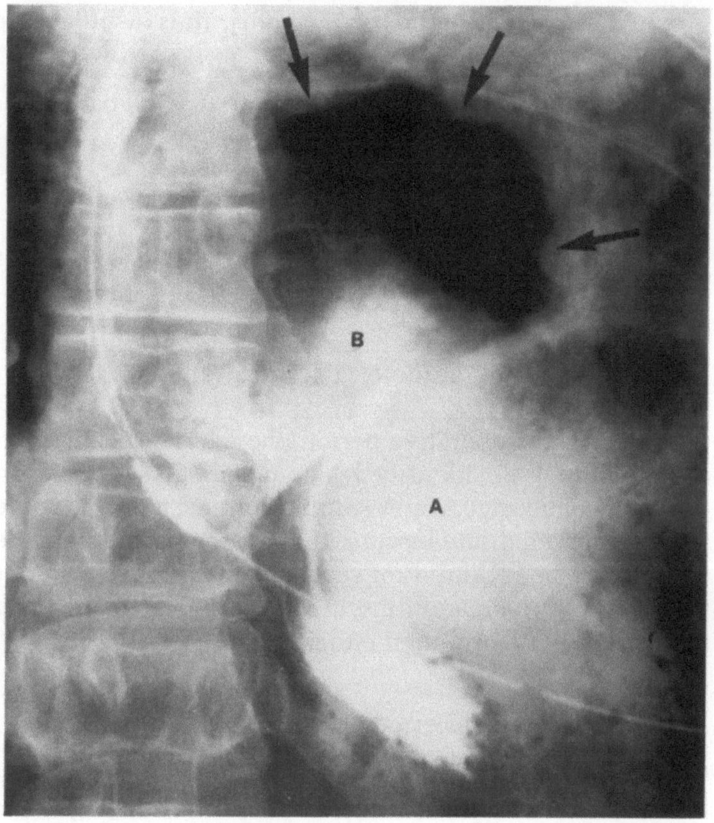

Fig. 2.27. Patient with Boerhave's syndrome; water-soluble contrast has been injected down nasogastric tube. Contrast and air have both leaked below diaphragm (A) into subphrenic space, and above diaphragm (B) into inferior pulmonary ligament (*arrows*).

bered and avoided. Local freezing of the oropharynx for this study should be used judiciously, because this could suppress the gag reflex and increase the risk of aspiration.

Materials

1. 10 or 12 French nasogastric tube, attached to a 50-cc syringe or air bulb
2. High-density barium suspension as per upper GI study (page 4)

Patient Preparation

The preparation is the same as for a routine upper GI study (page 5), because this study is not performed by itself but as an adjunct study to the barium meal.

□ *Procedure*

1. The nasogastric tube is introduced through the nose gently and into the stomach, with the patient sitting.
2. The patient is placed in the upright, left posterior oblique position on the fluoroscopic table and the catheter is withdrawn to the level of the midesophagus.

3. The patient is given high-density barium suspension to swallow (per os). After passage of the barium bolus, air is insufflated to distend the esophagus.
4. The patient is asked to take small sips of barium as needed to maintain optimal mucosal coating.
5. Spot films are taken as necessary.

Postoperative Examination

Indications and Choice of Technique [34]

In the early postoperative period, the main indication for radiological examination is to identify leaks and to assess for obstruction. For exclusion of leakage, water-soluble contrast medium is preferable, and for obstruction, dilute barium. In the late postoperative period, examination may be required for recurrent symptoms, or for assessment of vomiting or severe reflux symptoms. Recurrent ulcer, gastritis, and tumor should be excluded endoscopically.

Early Postoperative Period

Gastrografin is the contrast agent of choice when looking for anastomotic leaks. Patients should be turned into the right and left supine oblique positions, because Gastrografin runs through the anastomotic areas and gastric emptying should be confirmed (Fig. 2.28A). If no leak is seen, barium should be substituted because it allows for better definition (Fig. 2.28B). Initial films should be taken with a small amount of contrast medium with careful positioning for maximum detail. This is particularly important in patients who have had gastric partitioning or stapling operations, because the details of position and direction of leak will be obscured by a large amount of contrast.

Late Postoperative Period

A small amount of barium should be given initially while the surgical anatomy is determined. Once the anatomy of the anastomosis is understood, a larger amount of barium should be given to wash the residual gastric mucus and resting fluid from the stomach. Gas granules are then given in full amount and are used to drive most of the barium into the small intestine so that double-contrast films of the stomach and duodenum can be obtained (Fig. 2.29). A hypotonic agent is essential in the postoperative stomach. With a Billroth II anastomosis, it is usually possible to obtain double-contrast hypotonic duodenal films [35] by maneuvering barium around the afferent loop to the duodenal stump.

In summary the examination is performed in stages: a small amount of contrast to establish the anatomy; and a large amount of contrast to clean the stomach. Gas granules are used to distend the stomach and drive barium on into the intestine. A hypotonic agent helps to ob-

Fig. 2.28. Early postoperative esophagus. Gastrografin is used first in this fifth-day-postop swallow to exclude major leak (A). When this is normal, barium is given to further exclude small leak and assess rapidity of transit (B).

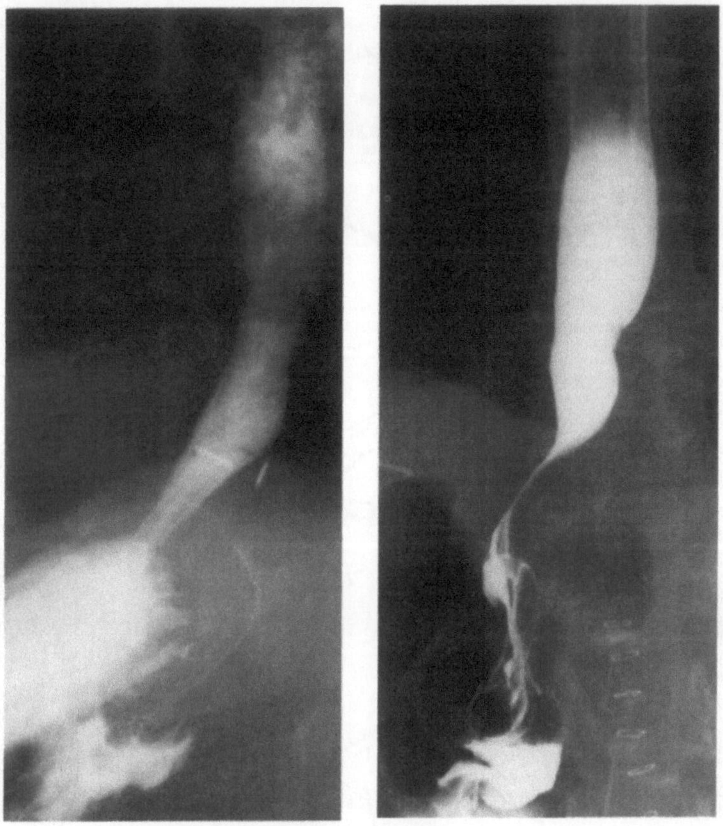

A B

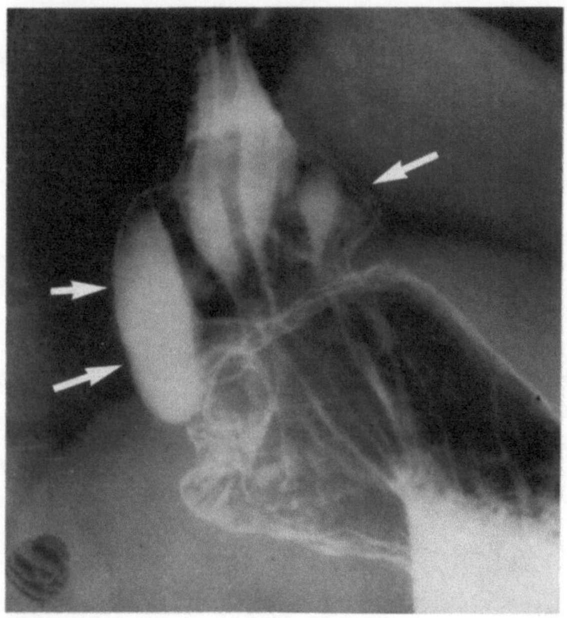

Fig. 2.29. Nissen fundoplication has become disrupted; the whole wrap has slipped up into chest (*arrows*). Gastric rugal folds can be seen running up within wrap, so that the fundus is now loosely wrapped around stomach rather than around esophagus.

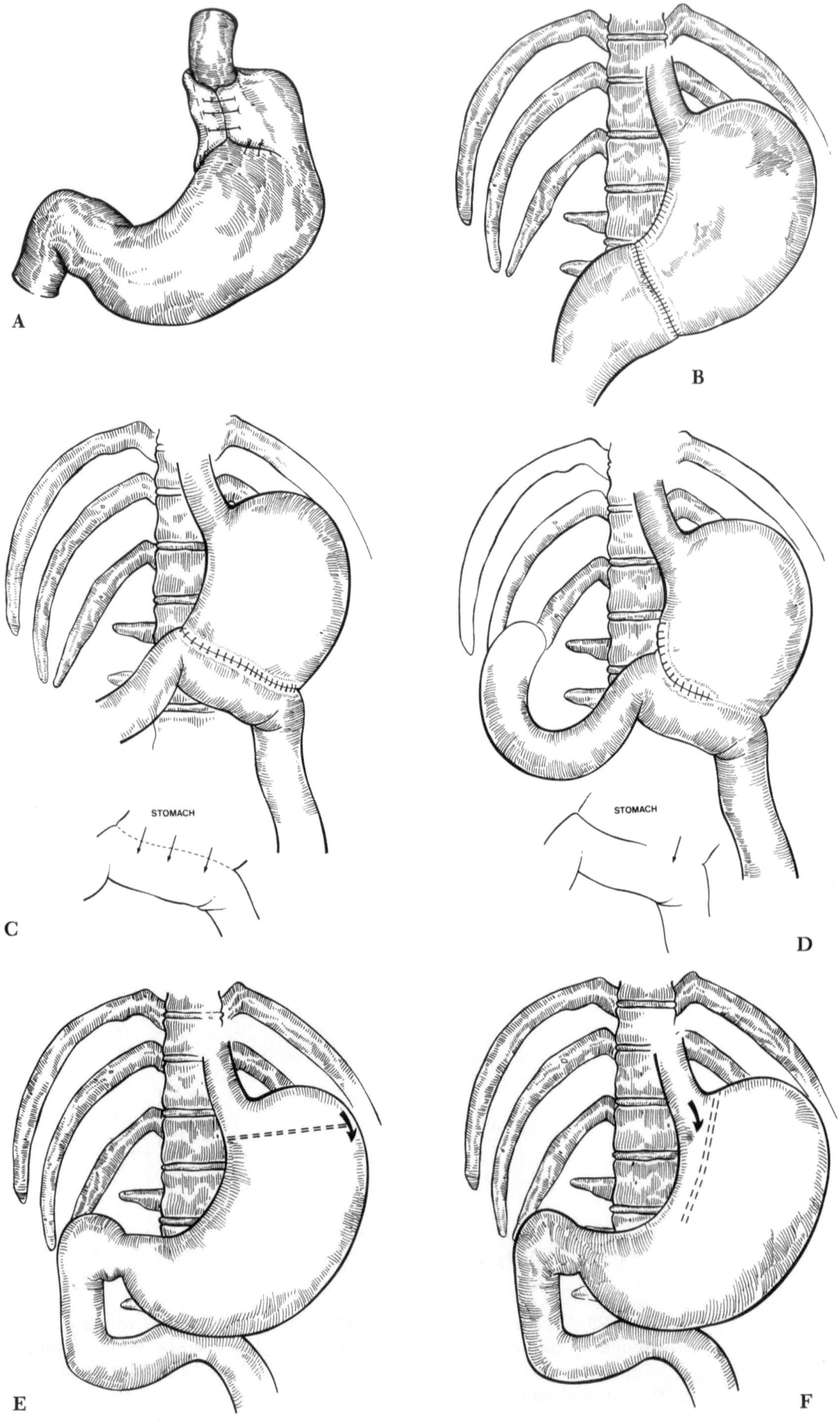
A
B
STOMACH
C
STOMACH
D
E
F

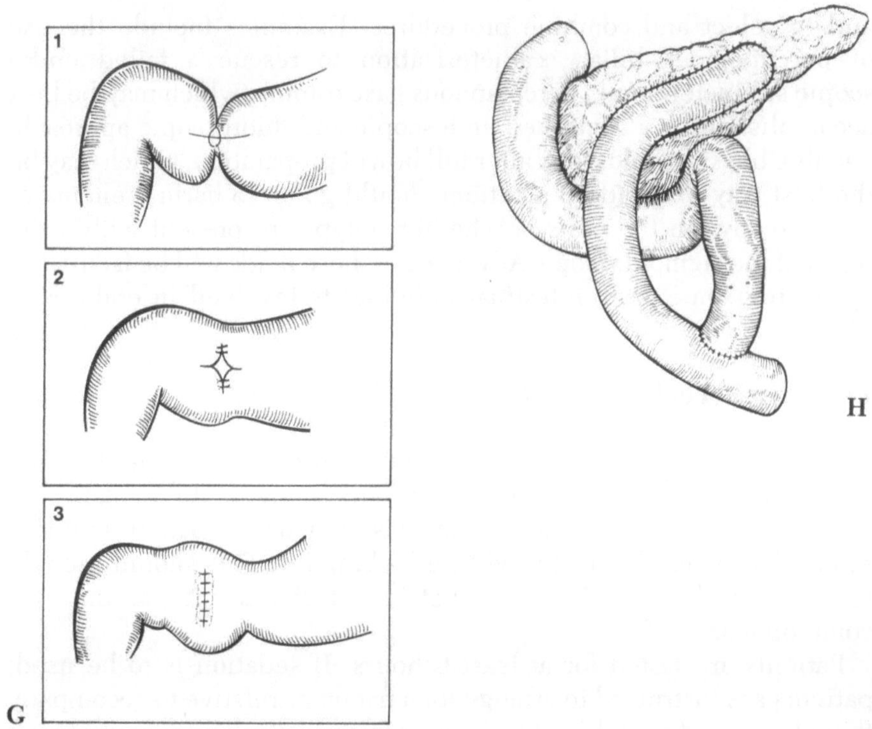

Fig. 2.30. **A.** Nissen fundoplication. Fundus has been brought up behind esophagus and wrapped around distal portion. **B.** Billroth I. Partial gastrectomy with gastroduodenostomy. **C.** Billroth II. Partial gastrectomy with gastrojejunostomy. Full section of gastric pouch can be used at anastomosis (Polya). **D.** Billroth II. Partial gastrectomy with gastrojejunostomy performed with resection and closure of lesser curvature (Hofmeister). **E.** Gastroplasty with horizontal rows of staples. **F.** Gastroplasty with vertical rows of staples (*arrow* signifies new narrowed lumen of stomach). **G.** Heinecke–Mikulicz pyeloplasty. Vertical incision (1) is made and closed transversely (2), giving characteristic deformity (3). **H.** Roux-en-y loop. Pancreatojejunostomy.

tain adequate distention. Finally, double-contrast films of stomach, duodenum, and anastomosis are obtained.

The following illustrations outline many of the frequently encountered stomach and duodenal surgical procedures (Fig. 2.30A–H). Knowledge of the postoperative anatomy is imperative for proper performance of the barium examination.

Technique of Upper Gastrointestinal Endoscopy

Radiologists and Endoscopy

Radiologists who wish to maintain a major interest in the alimentary tract will probably find it increasingly difficult to do so without becoming directly involved in endoscopy, because endoscopy has in many clinical settings now replaced barium radiology. Endoscopy enhances the understanding of barium appearances, and having radiologists involved in the provision of endoscopic services makes it easier to transfer patients from endoscopy suite to fluoroscopy room or vice versa, and to select and combine procedures. Examples include the use of percutaneous biliary catheterization to rescue a failed endoscopic sphincterotomy, percutaneous gastrostomy, which may be best accomplished by a combined endoscopic and fluoroscopic approach, and flexible sigmoidoscopy after full bowel preparation, which may be the best way to decide if a patient should go on to barium enema or colonoscopy, on the basis of whether polyps are present within the reach of the sigmoidoscope. Advances in these fields will be facilitated by having some gastrointestinal radiologists involved in endoscopy [36].

Diagnostic Technique [37]

Many patients are apprehensive about endoscopy, and therefore the first step in upper gastrointestinal endoscopy is to explain the procedure to the patient, with emphasis on what the patient will feel rather than what the doctor will be looking for. This should include reassurance that breathing will not be interfered with, as this is a common fear.

Patients are fasted for at least 6 hours. If sedation is to be used, patients are instructed to arrange for a friend or relative to accompany them home and are told not to drive or operate machinery for 12 hours after the procedure.

Premedication is usually unnecessary. Most endoscopists will give patients oral simethicone to reduce bubbles, and also spray the throat with a Xylocaine-based spray. The taste of the spray is for many patients the most disagreeable part of an endoscopic examination, and it may be omitted if sedation is used. Most units use intravenous sedation such as diazepam (Diazemuls), midazolam, or pethidine. Fentanyl, 100 μg (0.1 mg), is an excellent sedation for routine endoscopies, and for longer procedures a mixture of diazepam and pethidine is satisfactory.

The respiratory depression induced by diazepam has not been reversible until now; 5 mg may be a fatal dose for a patient with severe chronic lung disease, and as little as 2.5 mg may produce severe respiratory depression in such patients. A new drug, Flumazenil, which reverses the respiratory depression of diazepam, is just becoming available. Diazepam is a drug to use with very great caution in the elderly and in those with chronic lung disease. With fentanyl, 100 μg is a convenient dose up to the age of about 75, after which 50 μg is usually sufficient. Both fentanyl and pethidine cause respiratory depression, which is reversible with naloxone, 0.4 mg.

A very small (25-gauge) needle may be used routinely, and a butterfly needle can be inserted if a prolonged procedure is anticipated so that extra, "top-up" doses of medication can be given later. A few centers use no sedation to save the expense of recovery facilities, but this is unkind as a routine practice. A number of patients prefer not to have sedation for routine upper GI endoscopy so that they can return to work immediately. They are best examined with small endoscopes, and usually require thorough local analgesia with Xylocaine spray. The degree of hypoxia associated with endoscopy is proportional to both the amount of sedation and the diameter of the endoscope shaft, another reason for using a pediatric endoscope in elderly patients with chronic obstructive airways disease.

Intubation [38]

There are several methods of intubation. The first is now almost obsolete, and involves the examiner's left fingers being placed deeply into the patient's mouth while the endoscope tip is guided down the throat. Either of two other methods is satisfactory. The commonest is for the examiner to hold the controls in the left hand and the shaft of the endoscope at the 35-cm mark with the right hand. The endoscope tip is introduced blindly and the examiner's left thumb controls flexion of the endoscope tip, which is initially angled down to pass from mouth to pharynx, and then slightly up, which keeps it posteriorly and away from the larynx. With smaller endoscopes, a third method is becoming more popular; the instrument is introduced and passed through the pharynx under direct vision, the endoscopist looking through the endoscope to check the pharynx during insertion and directing the instrument tip directly behind the arytenoids into the upper sphincter.

A few patients, especially those with gastroesophageal reflux and a prominent cricopharyngeus, have great difficulty swallowing the endoscope. This can often be overcome by one of the three following methods. First, the endoscopist can resort to passing the fingers of the left hand into the patient's throat to guide the instrument down (with danger of being bitten). The second technique is to position the instrument just above the sphincter and instill a small amount of water to induce a swallow (often ineffective and may cause aspiration); the third is to pass a soft catheter such as an old endoscopic retrograde cholangiopancreatography (ERCP) cannula through the sphincter under direct vision, and to use this as a guide over which to gently advance the endoscope.

Once the endoscope has been introduced, a careful detailed examination of the esophagus, stomach, and duodenum is performed as far as the second part of the duodenum, and in bleeding patients, to the fourth part if necessary. Retroflexion of modern instruments has allowed elimination of what used to be considered blind spots, at least in normal subjects. The text by Blackstone describes detailed techniques and appearances at endoscopy [39].

Withdrawal

On withdrawal of the instrument the lower esophagus and gastroesophageal junction are again carefully examined. The endoscope is slowly removed, and particular care is taken to examine the proximal 5 cm of the esophagus and the mucosa of the upper sphincter and oropharynx. With the new smaller endoscopes the following structures can be checked routinely as the endoscope is removed: both pyriform fossae, the arytenoids, vocal cords, and supraglottic region, the epiglottis and ariepiglottic folds, and the valleculae.

When removing the endoscope at the end of the examination it is important to remember to unlock the controls, and not to remove the instrument with a 90° bend at the tip.

After the procedure, patients appreciated being given some idea of the findings (although they may not remember), and the endoscopist must ensure that appropriate follow-up has been arranged. This is particularly important if the examination has been performed by an endoscopist who is not clinically responsible for the patient's further care.

Provision of an Endoscopy Service

Most endoscopic services have been set up by gastroenterologists or surgeons, although a few have been developed by radiologists. Family physicians have been recruited in several units and can provide an integral part of the service. In some countries the problems of arranging for different disciplines to work together have led to the development of competing endoscopy units within a single hospital.

Therapeutic endoscopy has advanced just as rapidly as interventional radiology, but is beyond the scope of this manual. However, there are good texts on the subject [40].

Evaluation of Swallowing Function and the Palate

Evaluation of Swallowing Function

Feeding can be a long-term problem in patients who have suffered a stroke or have had a severe head injury and are left with a swallowing disability. In the short term they can be fed parentally or through a nasogastric tube. However, eventually a decision has to be made as to whether the patient should be fed indefinitely in this manner or given a permanent feeding gastrostomy. Before this decision is made, the patient should have a modified barium swallow [41,42,43]. This allows assessment of any particular consistencies of food that the patient can swallow. The examination may also allow you to see if there is any position in which swallowing is easier.

The examination consists of studying the process of swallowing in the erect position in the lateral and AP projections. As most of these patients are unable to stand, we have them sitting in a wheelchair that is attached to the tabletop of a remote control fluoroscopy unit. By attaching the chair to the tabletop we can move the patient from the console. The examination is recorded on a Sony 5800 Umatic recorder, which provides good still forward and reverse playback facilities.

The patient is first given liquid barium to drink. The swallowing mechanism is observed, and a note made if there is any aspiration. If there is aspiration, its cause is determined if possible. About 5 ml of contrast is given. The bolus is given with a spoon, or a Toomey irrigation syringe if the latter is easier for the patient. If this is tolerated, then 10–15 ml can be given at a time as a bolus. The next bolus should have the consistency of puree. We use apple sauce that has been opacified with barium. This is given in 5-ml boluses, and again the swallowing mechanism is studied. Finally, the patient is given cookie crumbs that have been opacified with barium.

The whole examination concentrates on the mouth and pharynx. The esophagus is only briefly examined to exclude an obstruction. During the examination, you may observe that the patient is unable to form a bolus and hence unable to transport the contrast medium into the pharynx. If this occurs try to place the bolus further at the back of the mouth and see if the bolus passes easier once it is in the pharynx. You may also find that the patient has difficulty swallowing liquids but may not have any problems with either of the other two consistencies. Therefore you should not abandon the procedure if you see problems with the first consistency that you use but should proceed to try all three.

Occasionally the patient may have paralysis of the pharynx that is worse on one side than the other. During this pharyngeal assessment you can then make a recommendation that the patient be fed the appropriate consistency with the head turned to the position in which oral feeding is possible. Asymmetrical paralysis may also be observed to advantage in the AP view, and again the appropriate recommendation regarding feeding can be made.

These assessments of swallowing should be made in cooperation with a speech pathologist [44]. Speech pathologists can provide useful information about the disability as they are actively engaged in the rehabilitation of these patients. This information can help in tailoring the examination and making a recommendation on feeding.

Examination of the palate is discussed in Chapter 5, page 117.

References

1. Cotton PB, Shorvon PJ (1984). Analysis of endoscopy and radiography in the diagnosis, follow-up and treatment of peptic ulcer disease. Clin Gastroenterol 13:383–403.
2. Ott DJ, Dodds WJ, Wu WC (1982). Current status of radiology in evaluating gastroesophageal reflux disease. J Clin Gastroenterol 4:365–375.
3. Ott DJ, Chen YM, Wu WC, Gelfand DW, Munitz HA (1986). Radiographic and endoscopic sensitivity in detecting lower esophageal mucosal ring. AJR 147:261–265.
4. Farivar M, Perotto JL (1979). Evaluation of dysphagia-esophagoscopy vs. x-ray. Gastrointest Endosc 25:39 (Abstr).
5. Laufer I, Mullens JE, Hamilton J (1975). The diagnostic accuracy of barium studies of the stomach and duodenum—correlation with endoscopy. Radiology 115:569–573.
6. Thompson G, Somers S, Stevenson GW (1983). Benign gastric ulcer: a reliable radiologic diagnosis? AJR 141:331–333.
7. Max MH, West B, Knutson CO (1979). Evaluation of postoperative gastroduodenal symptoms: endoscopy or upper gastrointestinal roentgenography? Surgery 86:578–582.
8. Janower ML (1986). Hypersensitivity reactions after barium studies of the upper and lower gastrointestinal tract. Radiology 161:139–140.
9. Hoyt TS, Peet GJ (1985). Allergic reaction during double-contrast upper GI series. AJR 145:653–654.
10. Obata WG (1972). A double-contrast technique for examination of the stomach using barium sulfate with simethicone. AJR 115:275–280.
11. Rubesin SE, Herlinger H (1986). The effect of barium suspension viscosity on the delineation of areae gastricae. AJR 146:35–38.

12. Rohrmann CA, Acheson MB (1985). Esophageal perforation during double-contrast esophagram. AJR 145:283–284.
13. Herlinger H, Grossman R, Laufer I, Kressel HY, Ochs RH (1980). The gastric cardia in double-contrast study: its dynamic study. AJR 135:21–29.
14. Kikuchi Y, Levine MS, Laufer I, Herlinger H (1986). Value of flow technique for double-contrast examination of the stomach. AJR 147:1183–1184.
15. Gardiner GA, Racker DR (1985). Cephalic angled views for detection of occult lesser curvature ulcers. Gastrointest Radiol 10:153–155.
16. Jacquemet P, Liotta D, Mallet-Guy P (1965). The Early Radiological Diagnosis of Diseases of the Pancreas and Ampulla of Vater. Springfield, IL: Charles C. Thomas.
17. Heron CW, Lynn AH, Marshall JH, Mason RR (1985). A comparison of paralysing agents in double-contrast barium meal examinations. Clin Radiol 36:391–393.
18. Stevenson GW, Somers S (1980). Routine double contrast barium meal: appearance of the normal duodenal papillae. Diagn Imag 49:6–14.
19. Ott DJ, Kelly RJ, Gelfand DW (1981). Radiographic effects of cold barium suspensions on esophageal motility. Radiology 140:830–833.
20. Cassel DM, Anderson MF, Zboralske FF (1981). Double-contrast esophagrams: the prone technique. Radiology 139:737–739.
21. Brombart M (1973). Roentgenology of the esophagus. In: Margulis AR, Burhenne HW (eds), Alimentary Tract Roentgenology, 2d Ed. St. Louis: Mosby, p. 347.
22. Wiljasalo M, Rissanen P (1966). A new double-contrast method in esophageal roentgenology. Ann Med Intern Fenn 55:77–80.
23. Gohel VK, Kressel HY, Laufer I (1978). Double-contrast artifacts. Gastrointest Radiol 3:139–146.
24. Hogan WJ, Dodds WJ, Hoke SE, Reid DP, Kalkhoff RK, Arndorfer RC (1975). Effect of glucagon on esophageal motor function. Gastroenterology 69:160–165.
25. Linsman JF (1965). Gastroesophageal reflux elicited while drinking water (water siphonage test): its clinical correlation with pyrosis. AJR 94:325–332.
26. Stevenson G, Robinson PJ (1988). The normal oesophagus: methods of examination. Hiatus hernia, gastroesophageal reflux and other motility disorders. In: Royal College of Radiologists, A Textbook of Radiological Diagnosis, Vol. 4. London: HK Lewis & Co. Ltd, pp. 52–105.
27. McNally EF, Del Gaudio W (1967). The radiopaque esophageal marshmallow bolus. AJR 101:485–489.
28. Somers S, Stevenson GW, Thompson G (1986). Comparison of endoscopy and barium swallow with marshmallow in dysphagia. J Can Assoc Radiol 37:73–75.
29. Channer KS, Virjee JP (1985). Oesophageal function tests: are they of value? Clin Radiol 36:493–496.
30. Danielson KS, Hunter TB (1985). Barium capsules. AJR 144:414.
31. Benjamin SB, Castell DO (1983). Esophageal causes of chest pain. In: Castell DO, Johnson LF (eds), Esophageal Function in Health and Disease. New York: Elsevier Biomedical, pp. 85–98.
32. Vessal K, Montal RJ, Larson SM, Chaffee V, James AE (1975). Evaluation of barium and gastrografin as contrast media for the diagnosis of esophageal rupture or perforations. AJR 123:307–319.
33. Levine MS, Kressel HY, Laufer I, Herlinger H, Goren R (1984). The tube esophagram: a technique for obtaining a detailed double-contrast examination of the esophagus. AJR 142:293–298.
34. Stevenson GW (1983). Technique of examination. In: Margulis AR, Burhenne HJ (eds), Alimentary Tract Radiology, 3d Ed, Vol 2. St. Louis: C.V. Mosby, pp. 1699–1719.

35. Op den Orth JO (1977). Tubeless hypotonic examination of the afferent loop of the Billroth II stomach. Gastrointest Radiol 2:1–5.
36. Shorvon P, Stevenson GW (1986). Should radiologists perform endoscopy? AJR 147:1078–1081.
37. Rozen P, Fireman Z, Gilat T (1982). The causes of hypoxemia in position of elderly patients during endoscopy. Gastrointest Endosc 28:243–246.
38. Cotton PB, Williams CB (1982). Practical Gastrointestinal Endoscopy, 2d Ed. Oxford: Blackwell Scientific.
39. Blackstone MO (1984). Endoscopic Interpretation. New York: Raven Press.
40. Silvis SE (1985). Therapeutic Gastrointestinal Endoscopy. New York: Igaku Shoin.
41. Siebens AA, Linden P (1985). Dynamic imaging for swallowing reeducation. Gastrointest Radiol 10:251–253.
42. Jones B, Kramer SS, Donner MW (1985). Dynamic imaging of the pharynx. Gastrointest Radiol 10:213–224.
43. Logemann J (1983). Evaluation and Treatment of Swallowing Disorders. San Diego: College Hill Press.
44. Sorin R, Somers S, Austin W, Bester S (1988). The influence of videofluoroscopy on the management of the dysphagic patient. Dysphagia 2:127–135.

CHAPTER 3

Small Bowel

Small Bowel Meal

Indications

1. Unexplained abdominal pain
2. Inflammatory bowel disease
3. Suspected intermittent partial small bowel obstruction
4. Steatorrhea
5. Diarrhea
6. Unexplained gastrointestinal bleed
7. Suspected small bowel fistula

It is difficult to perform a small bowel meal study after a double-contrast examination of the upper gastrointestinal tract (see follow-through study). This study is therefore performed as a *specific* small bowel examination. With meticulous supervision, fluoroscopy, and palpation, this study is as sensitive as the small bowel enema for most common diseases [1]. The advantages of the small bowel meal over small bowel enema are patient tolerance, less fluoroscopic time because there is no need for tube placement, and ease of performance of the test [2].

Contraindications and Precautions

1. Suspected perforated viscus
2. Complete obstruction

Materials

Barium recipe: 1350 g Ultra R is added to 1500 ml of distilled water. This combination is hand mixed and then refrigerated until the study is performed.

Patient Preparation

On the day before the examination, a strong laxative may be given to empty the cecum. Some radiologists feel that this improves the quality of the examination and accelerates the transit time.* One bottle of citromag with a full glass of water is quite effective. No solid foods are taken until the examination. Patients are encouraged, however, to drink one glass of water per hour until 3 hours before the study, after which time the patient is kept NPO.

□ *Procedure*

Step 1. A preliminary film of the abdomen is usually not necessary. One may be taken if the patient has had a recent barium study, to ensure that the bowel is clear.
Step 2. If the stomach and duodenum have not been previously examined, it is convenient to give a small amount of barium initially and perform a limited single-contrast study of these organs with compression (see Chapter 2, page 23)
Step 3. The patient drinks 400 ml of the dilute chilled barium in the sitting position and then is allowed to lie on the right side. There is a strong clinical impression that chilled barium causes less nausea and improves examination quality. Cold barium leaves the stomach faster and passes through the small intestine more rapidly, therefore decreasing transit time [4,5,6].
Step 4. The first film is obtained 5 minutes after administration of contrast medium to assess the rate of transit (Fig. 3.1). This film can be taken in the prone or supine position. The prone position usually gives better separation of the small bowel loops.
Step 5. If transit is occurring rapidly, a second film is taken at 15 minutes (Fig. 3.2). At this point, thorough palpation and compression of all the proximal small bowel loops is carried out.
Step 6. A further film (Fig. 3.3) is taken at 25 minutes. This usually shows contrast within the large bowel. Palpation and compression of the distal small bowel is carried out with spot films of the terminal ileum (Fig. 3.4) and extra films if any abnormal lesions are observed (Figs. 3.5, and 3.6). If adequate visualization of the terminal ileum was not obtained despite change in patient position and compression, a peroral pneumocolon is then performed (page 56) [7].

Some patients have multiple small bowel loops in the lower pelvis, and these loops may be difficult to separate with normal compression or palpation. Separation can sometimes be obtained by the patient lying prone with the compression paddle (deflated) positioned under the patient's pelvis. In this position, inflation of the paddle can displace these low-lying loops out of the pelvis. If tube angling is available in a remote unit, the pelvic loops can be visualized by having the patient lie prone with the tube angled 35–45° toward the feet. This can also be done with an overhead tube [8].

Note: Once the examination is started, the stomach is kept full until the barium reaches the large bowel. A full stomach ensures more rapid transit, and the examination seldom takes more than 45 minutes.

---

*A recent study on this [3] showed that colon cleansing does not decrease transit time to the cecum and does not affect the examination quality. We have found similar findings in our own institution.

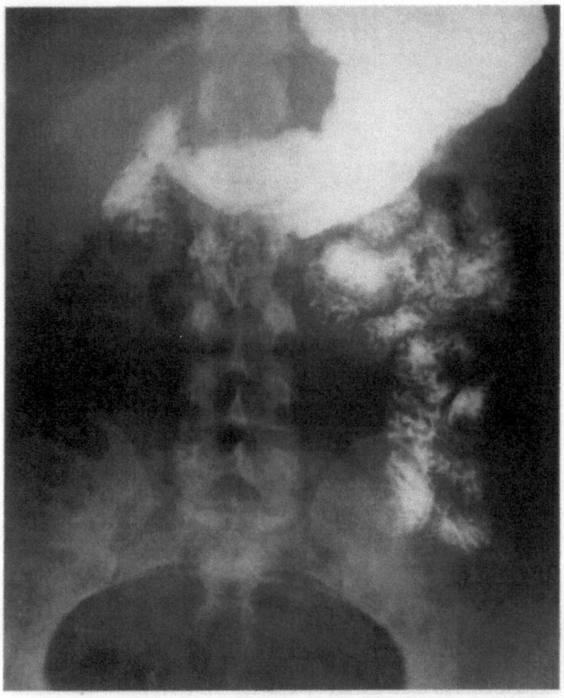

Fig. 3.1. Initial 5-minute film of abdomen allows assessment of transit time.

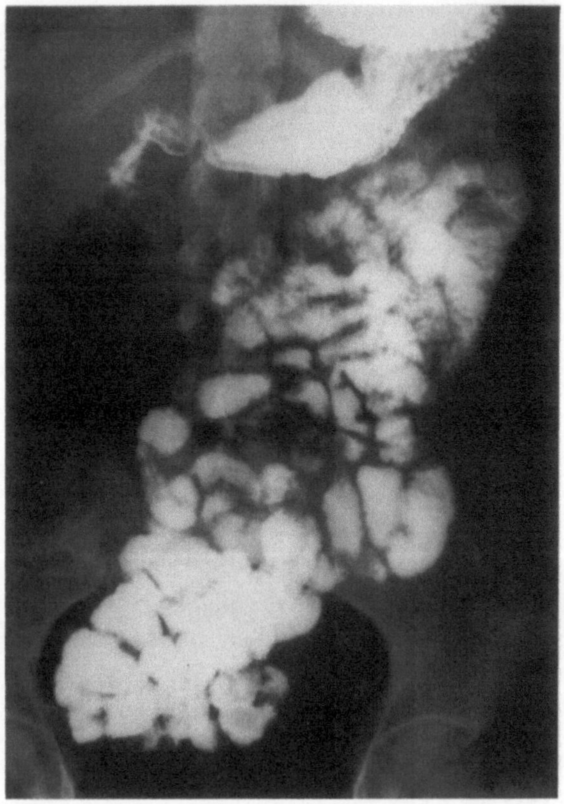

Fig. 3.2. A 15-minute film shows opacified loops of jejunum and proximal ileum.

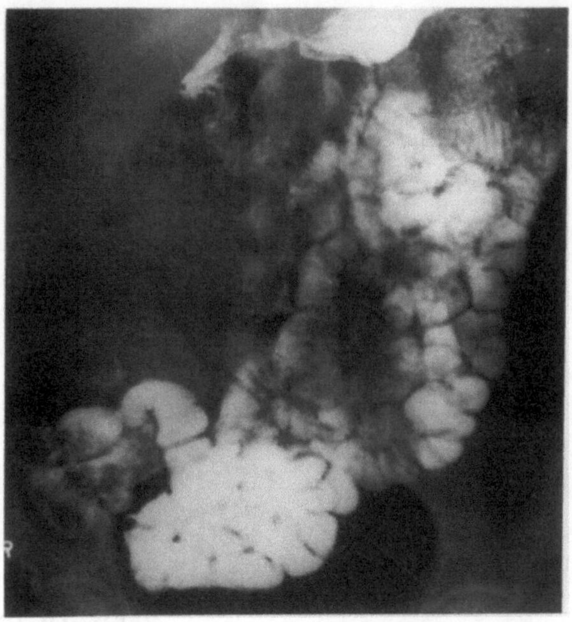

Fig. 3.3. A 25-minute film shows contrast within cecum. It is essential to keep stomach topped up with additional barium if it appears almost empty on early film, to maintain good rate of flow.

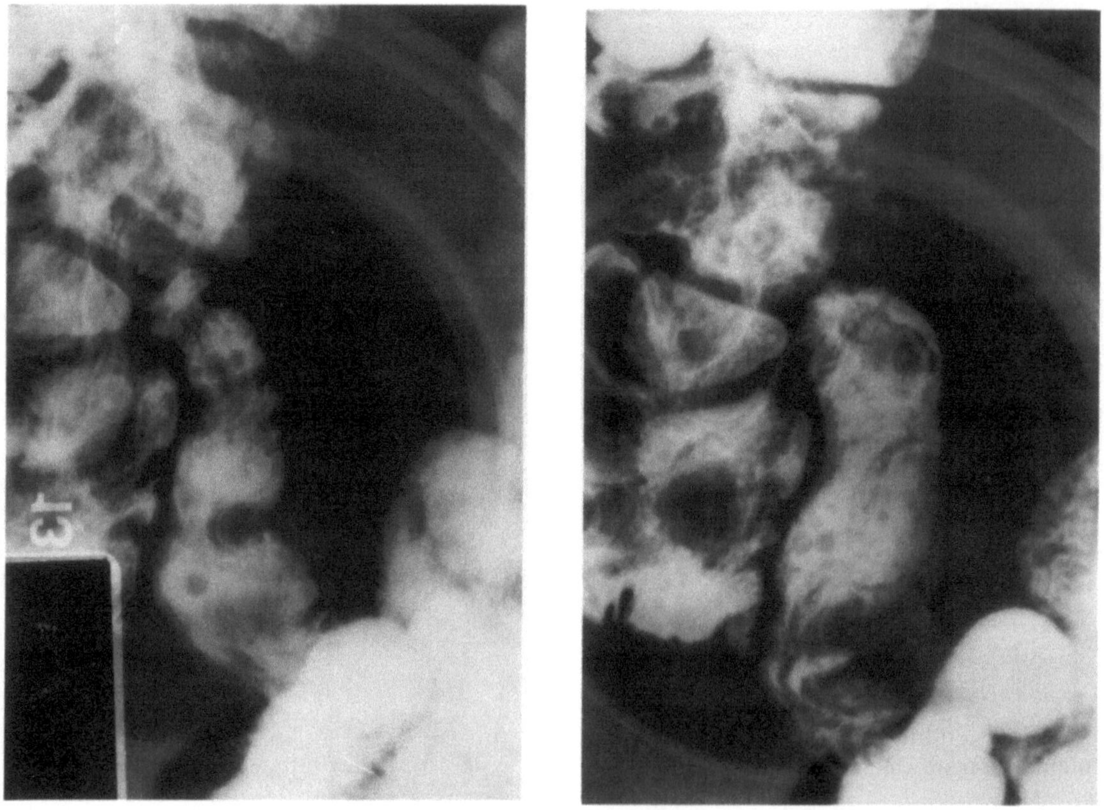

A B

Fig. 3.4. Supine (**A**) and supine oblique (**B**) spot films of terminal ileum.

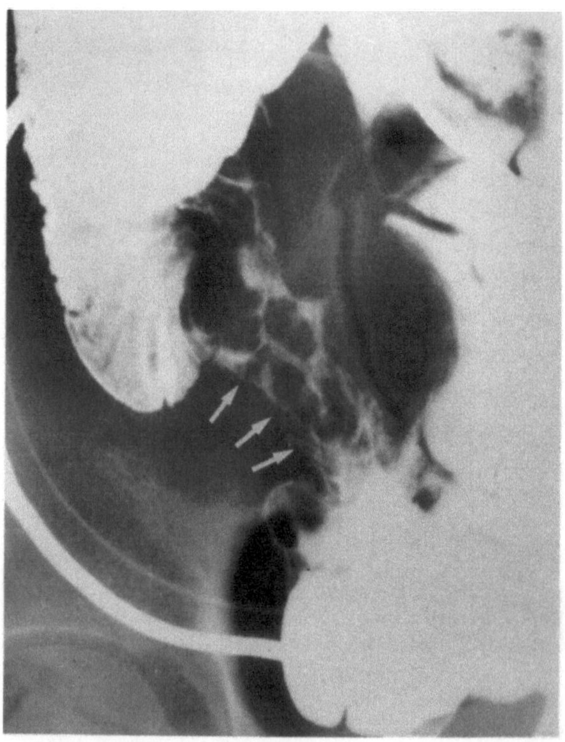

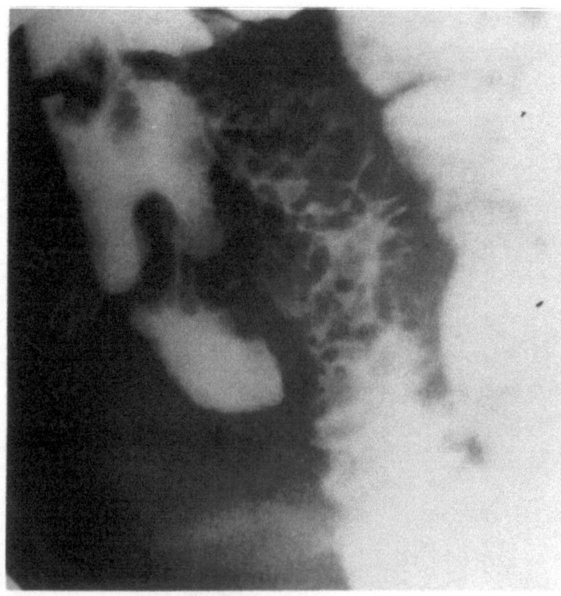

Fig. 3.6. Yersinea ileitis.

Fig. 3.5. Patient with Crohn's disease. Spot film reveals wall thickening, nodular mucosa, and fistula from terminal ileum to lower pole of cecum (*arrows*).

Double-Contrast Small Bowel Examination

This examination is performed initially the same as routine small bowel meal (page 43). After barium has reached the large bowel, the patient is given enough gas granules orally to generate a liter of gas (usually two to three packages of E-Z Gas) [9]. To allow this gas to enter the small bowel, the patient lies in the left-side-down position. The filling of the small bowel with gas is observed intermittently under fluoroscopic control. Radiographs are obtained with the patient in the prone or supine position, using compression to separate any overlapping loops. Spot films with compression are taken if an abnormality is observed. The gas generates considerable peristalsis, and occasionally confirms normality of a segment that appears narrow or deformed.

Small Bowel Enema (Enteroclysis)

Indications

The prime indications for enteroclysis are

1. Intermittent partial small bowel obstruction
2. Unexplained gastrointestinal bleed
3. Assessment of extent of inflammatory bowel disease

Less common indications are

4. Diarrhea
5. Steatorrhea
6. Unexplained abdominal pain
7. Suspected small bowel fistula.

Since its introduction [10], there has been considerable controversy as to the role of the small bowel enema. In some hospitals it is believed to be the only acceptable form of radiological examination of the small bowel. In others, it is believed that the small bowel meal provides acceptable accuracy for most common diseases at considerably less cost, radiation exposure, and physician time. At present, the three major indications given are our guidelines for the use of small bowel enema, but the best indications are probably intermittent small bowel obstruction, when looking for adhesions or a short stricture, and unexplained gastrointestinal hemorrhage, when looking for a small tumor. The very accurate demonstration of aphthous ulceration in Crohn's disease is of less importance, although the accurate demonstration of the number and length of strictures may be useful before surgery, and for this the small bowel enema is the most satisfactory method.

Contraindications and Precautions

1. Suspected perforated viscus
2. Complete obstruction
3. Bleeding dyscrasias (possibility of bleeding from nasal intubation technique).

Patients should be told to expect diarrhea from the large fluid volumes used. Caution: Perforation of a viscus can occur with guide wire manipulation.

Materials

1. Catheter, 12 or 14 French, with end hole; 150-cm length with guide wire (Cook Inc). Put a 45° bend on the guide wire about 3 cm from its tip (Nolan and Herlinger modification of Bilbao–Dotter tube). This bend will give torque control to the direction of catheter advancement when turning the knob on the end of the guide wire.
2. Maglinte tube, 200-ml Polibar (four 50-ml syringes)
3. Methylcellulose solution, 0.5%, 1–1.5 liter
4. Fentanyl
5. Maxeran
6. Xylocaine, 1% spray
7. Electric pump

Liquid Polibar may be substituted by Enterobar (E-Z-Em). The methylcellulose solution is available from E-Z-Em (MC E-Z-Em or Enterocel).

Patient Preparation

1. 2 ounces of castor oil at 4:00 P.M. on day before examination.
2. NPO after 10:00 P.M. on evening before examination.

□ *Procedure*

Step 1. Before the small bowel intubation, the patient may be premedicated with 0.05–0.1 mg fentanyl I.V. (Fentanyl is a narcotic and should not be used if the patient is driving after the procedure; see Chapter 8). The intubation may be carried out using the oral or nasal approach. Depending on the approach, either the oropharynx or nasopharynx is anesthetized with 1% Xylocaine spray (usually four to five sprays during 2-to 3-minute period are sufficient). Most patients find intubation easier by the oral route, but find the catheter less troublesome once it is in position, if it has been introduced by the nasal route.

Step 2(a). Oral approach. The guide wire is withdrawn approximately 10–15 cm. In the sitting or supine position, the patient is asked to swallow the tip of the catheter.

Step 2(b). Nasal approach. In the sitting position, the patient is given ice chips to suck on. While the patient is swallowing the liquid from the melting ice the catheter is inserted into the esophagus through the nose. The guide wire is withdrawn within the catheter to minimize the risk of traumatizing the nasal mucosa.

Step 3. After the catheter has advanced into the esophagus, the patient is put into the supine position and the catheter is advanced into the stomach (Fig. 3.7A). The guide wire is now pushed to the end of the catheter. IMPORTANT: Always advance the guide wire and catheter under fluoroscopic control.

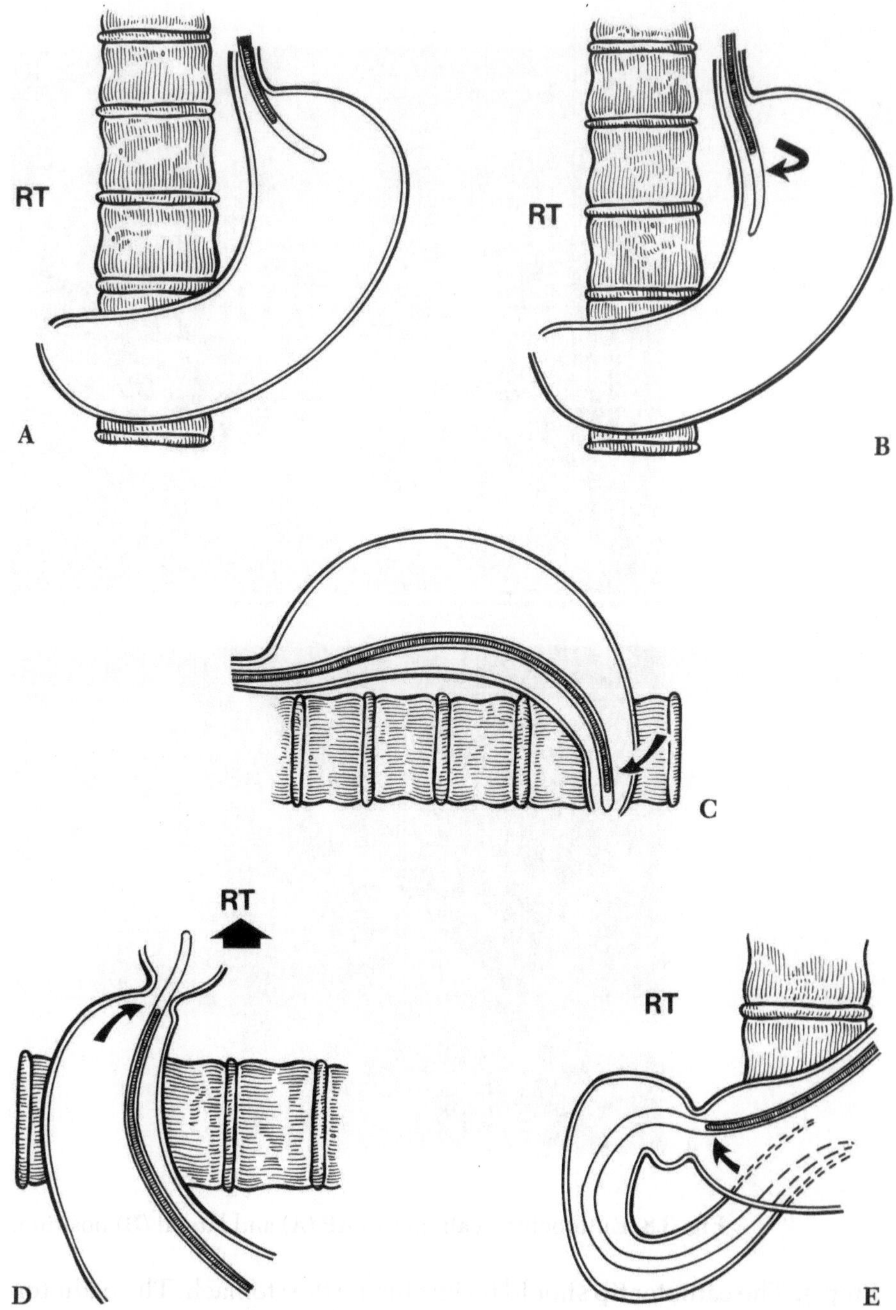

Fig. 3.7. Small bowel intubation. **A.** Enteroclysis catheter is advanced into region of cardia. **B.** Catheter is rotated (*arrow*) so that tip is directed inferiorly and toward antrum. **C.** With patient lying on right side, catheter is advanced into the antrum. Gravity helps catheter drop into most dependent portion (*arrow*) of stomach and antrum. **D.** Duodenal cap is distended by rising air as patient lies on left side. Catheter tip is advanced into duodenum. The guide wire tip (*arrow*) remains in the antrum. **E.** Catheter is advanced past ligament of Treitz with tip of guide wire always remaining at level of pylorus.

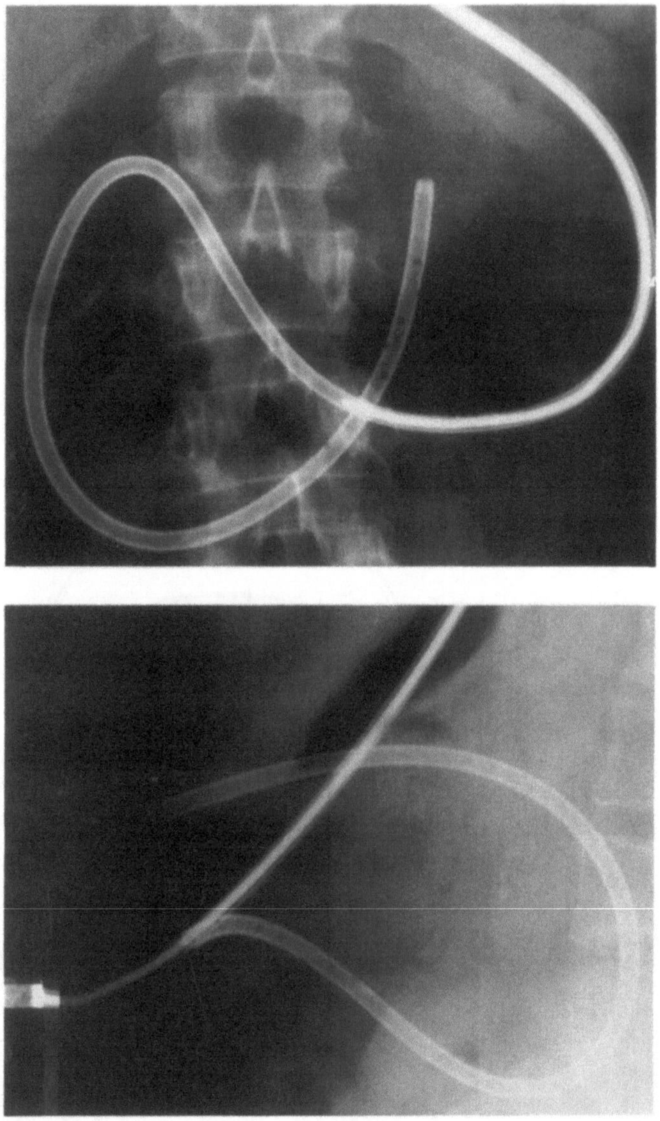

A

B

Fig. 3.8. Enteroclysis catheter in AP (**A**) and lateral (**B**) position.

Step 4. The catheter tip should be just inside the stomach. The catheter is advanced with a slight clockwise twist on the guide wire knob to turn the tip of the catheter anteriorly away from the fundus (Fig. 3.7B). The patient is now turned on the right side. As the catheter is advanced, the tip will pass down the anterior wall of the stomach and the catheter will fall into the antrum and pyloric canal (Fig. 3.7C). The patient is then turned supine to confirm the catheter position.

Step 5. By turning the patient onto the left side, gas in the stomach will fill the duodenum and distend it (Fig. 3.7D). The duodenum can also be distended by air insufflation. (The guide would have to be removed for this.) The catheter is pushed forward into the duodenum. As the catheter advances into the duodenum, the guide wire is withdrawn so that it is not advanced past the pylorus. The guide wire tends to coil into the fundus of the stomach.

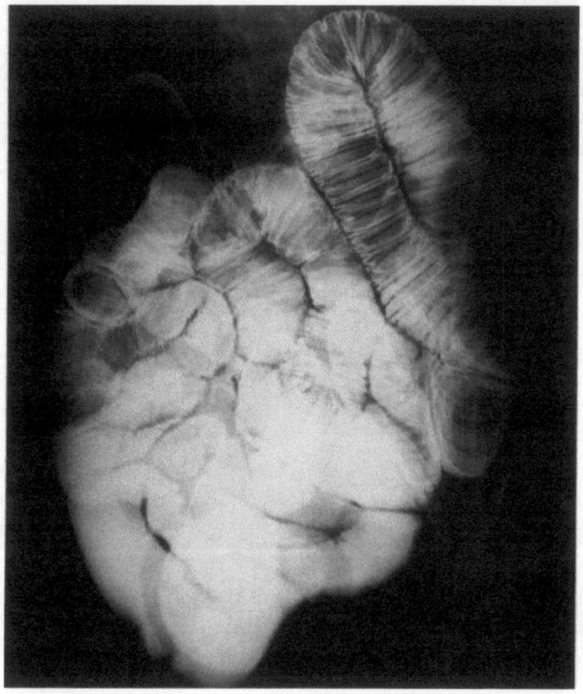

Fig. 3.9. Loops of jejunum show characteristic folds (valvulae conniventes).

Step 6. The catheter is advanced past the ligament of Treitz by slowly advancing the catheter tip and withdrawing the guide wire (Fig. 3.7E). If holdup of the catheter occurs within the duodenum, deep inspirations, coughing, air insufflation, compression with a paddle, or I.V. Maxeran can facilitate passage of the catheter. Temporary holdup of the catheter tip in the third part of the duodenum is most readily overcome by turning the patient prone. The catheter tip will pass the ligament of Treitz and advance into the jejunum if the patient lies on the right side, because the air within the duodenum then rises to the ligament of Treitz, opening up the angle between the fourth part of the duodenum and the proximal jejunum.
Step 7. Once the enteroclysis catheter tip has passed the ligament of Treitz, the guide wire is carefully removed (Fig. 3.8). Pay attention to not withdraw the catheter tip as well and to not leave a loop in the stomach. If an excessive amount of fluid is present within the small bowel, this can be aspirated before introduction of barium.
Step 8. The catheter is secured with tape around the patient's mouth or nose.
Step 9. The barium (200 ml) is injected with the electric pump into the small bowel followed by 0.5% methylcellulose solution at 75–80 ml/min [11]. The barium and methylcellulose can also be injected with a manually operated rotary pump; however, it is difficult to control the flow rate with this method. The electric motor-driven pump has been found to be the most effective method of infusion [12].
Step 10. As the methylcellulose advances it pushes the Polibar forward, coating the walls of the small bowel and giving a double-contrast study. Spot films are obtained of proximal loops of jejunum (Fig. 3.9). If

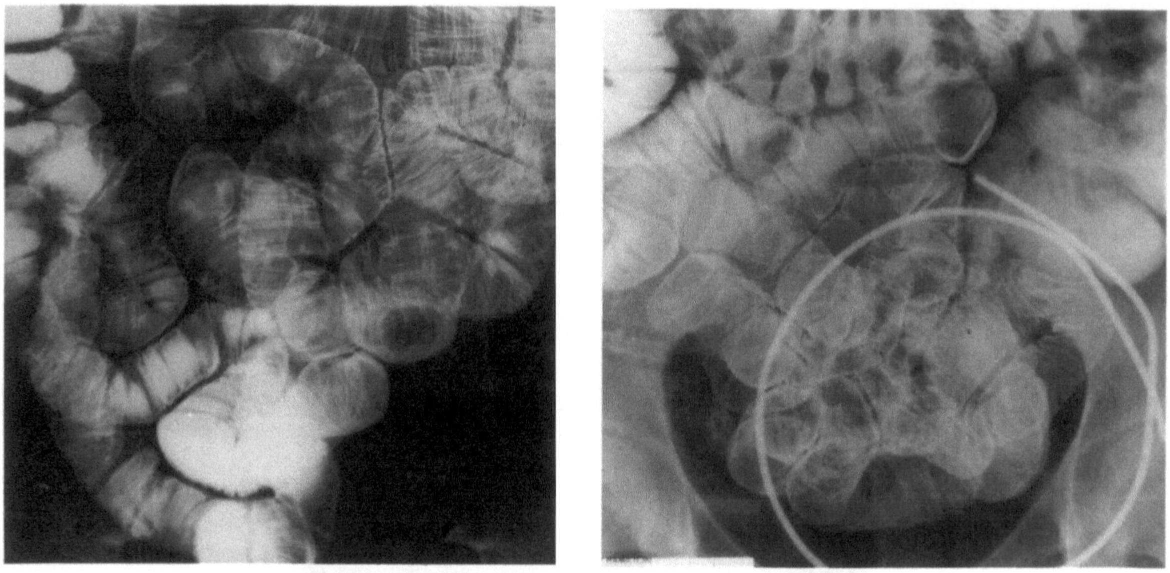

A B

Fig. 3.10. Examples of normal ileal loops. A and B. There is good transradiance but careful fluoroscopy and palpation are required to see all pathology. One cannot rely on the films alone with small bowel enema examination.

the patient is kept in the same prone position without moving too much, better double-contrast coating is obtained. If transit is very slow, it may be necessary to move the patient so that gravity can help advance barium, but this will impair the quality of the double-contrast films.

Step 11. Spot film of loops of ileum (Fig. 3.10).

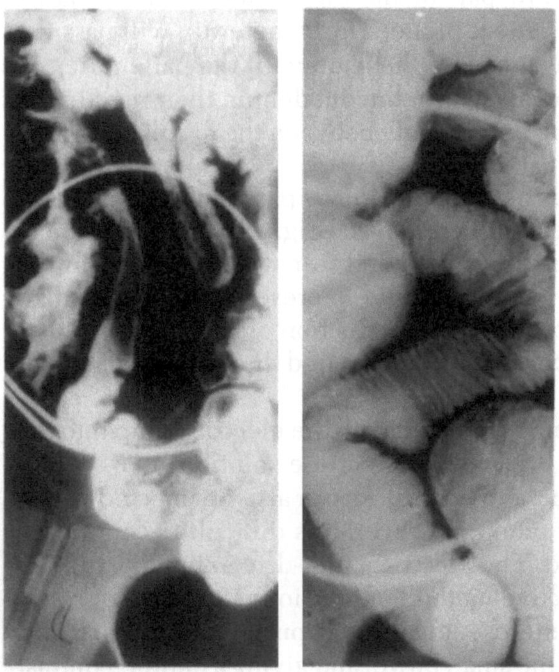

A B

Fig. 3.11. Spot films of terminal ileum. Note appearance on early film is misleading (A) before adequate distension has been achieved (B).

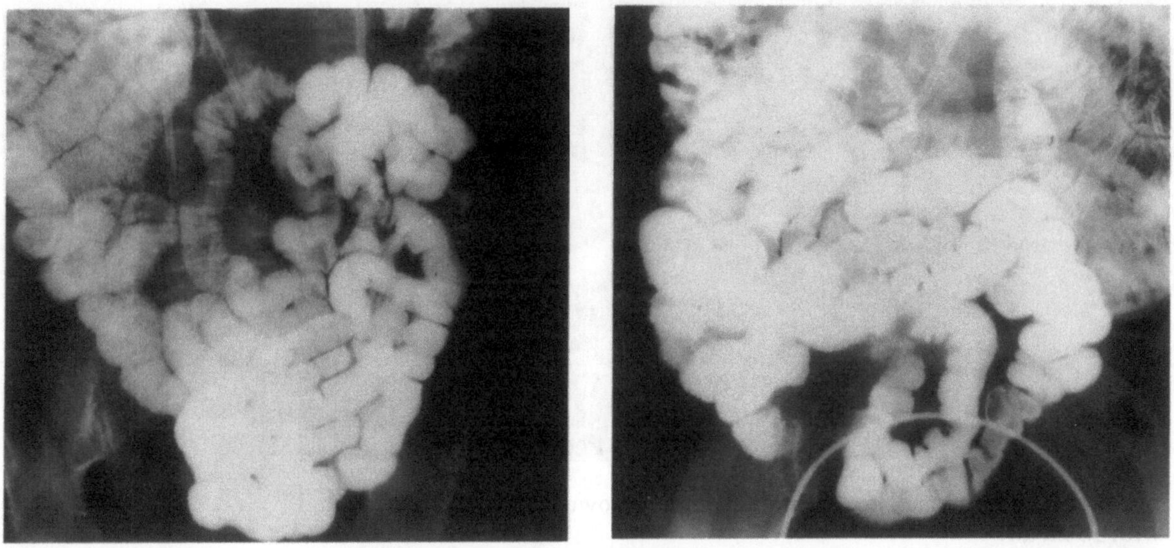

Fig. 3.12. In some patients, ileal loops cluster in pelvis (**A**). Using paddle balloon with patient prone may elevate loops into abdomen and permit their separation and demonstration (**B**).

Step 12. Two split spot films of terminal ileum in supine and prone positions. Use compression if needed (Fig. 3.11).
Step 13. If difficulty arises in visualizing the terminal ileum, visualization can be improved by passing a rectal tube and insufflating the large bowel with air (peroral pneumocolon) [12] (see page 56).
Step 14. The catheter is now ready for removal. The most proximal jejunum and duodenum can be visualized before removing the catheter by injecting Polibar while withdrawing the catheter slowly. Without this step, it is possible to overlook major pathology around the duodenojejunal flexure.
Step 15. It is important to inspect the whole length of the small bowel by using a paddle to palpate loops one after the other so that the entire length is observed inch by inch. Overlapped pelvic loops of bowel can be separated by having the patient lie prone on an inflatable paddle positioned just above the symphysis. The paddle is then inflated, separating the loops (Fig. 3.12). Reliance on only the overhead films does not allow optimal observance of details.
Step 16. **Variations**
Maglinte [2] has described a modification of the small bowel enema that may give consistently superior results. The following paragraphs summarize what appear to the authors to be the essentials of his techniques.

The patient is given intravenous Diazepam (Diazemuls) immediately before the procedure; 5 mg is an adequate dose for most adults, but caution is required in elderly patients or those with respiratory disease. Metoclopramide, 20 mg I.V., is also given to aid peristalsis and maintain small bowel tone. Zylocaine (viscous), 3 ml, is injected into the selected nostril with a syringe and the patient is asked to sniff. The

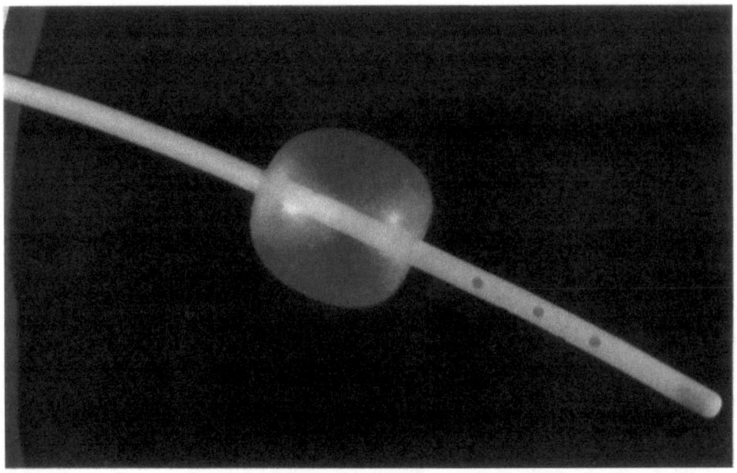

Fig. 3.13. Maglinte small bowel enema catheter shown with its balloon inflated with 15 ml air.

Maglinte balloon catheter (Cook or E-Z-Em) (Fig. 3.13) is introduced with the tip of the guide wire withdrawn about 12 in. from the tip of the catheter. When the catheter reaches the lower esophagus, the patient is turned on the right side. The tube is advanced; the tip will curl in the fundus while a loop forms in the stomach. Maglinte calls this the double-back maneuver. The tube is then withdrawn under fluoroscopy while the guide wire advances down the stomach, which takes the tip out of the fundus to the midbody so that the tip points distally. The tube is then advanced with the patient on the right side; the tone and peristalsis produced by the metoclopramide usually ensure rapid advance of the tube around the duodenal loop, to the distal duodenum or proximal jejunum. The balloon is then inflated with 15 ml of air or water, or, occasionally, up to 20 ml.

Contrast medium such as Enterobar is infused initially at 75 ml per minute. Precise control of the flow rate is important: flow that is too fast produces jejunal atony, and a rate too slow gives a poor column. When barium reaches the distal ileum the flow rate is gradually increased, and after the 300 ml of Enterobar has been finished, methylcellulose Enterocel is started. When the colon starts to fill, the flow rate is further increased to 95 ml per minute, and as Enterocel starts to approach the lower ileum the flow rate is further increased to 125, 150, or even 175 ml per minute. This produces dilatation, resulting in small bowel paralysis with the double-contrast effect throughout the small bowel (Fig. 3.14). The flow can be turned off, the balloon deflated and the tube removed at this point. There will be several minutes of atony with distension and double-contrast effect during which films can be taken of the various loops at leisure. A pump with accurate flow rate measurement is a great asset for this technique [12]. Increasing the rate too early results in paralysis before the double-contrast effect is present throughout the ileum, and prolongs the examination. The balloon is very helpful in preventing backflow and in allowing the high flow rates recommended. Caution should be exercised in patients with suspected obstruction.

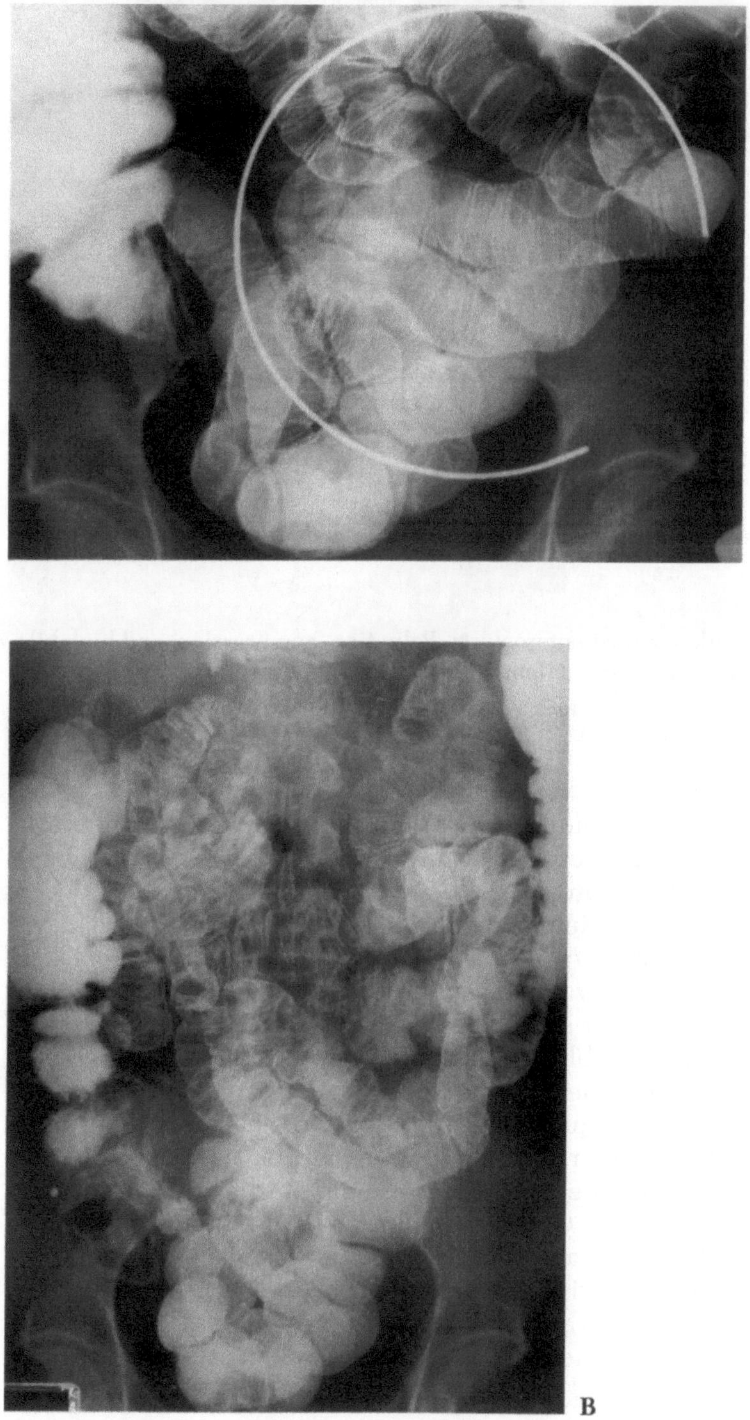

A

B

Fig. 3.14. Spot film (**A**) and overview (**B**) show improved ileal films obtainable with Maglinte technique.

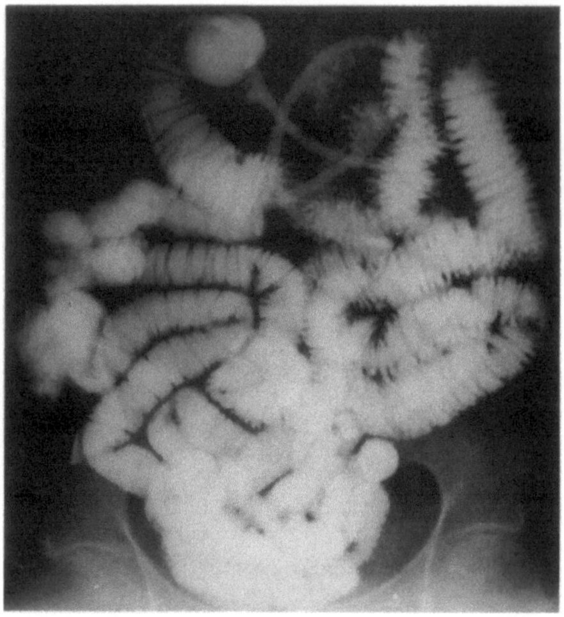

Fig. 3.15. Single-contrast enteroclysis. Palpation, compression, and high kilovolts (kV) are even more important with this type of enema, and contrast density is crucial. In this patient, pelvic loops must be lifted into abdomen, either by compression or by inflating rectum with air.

Single-contrast technique using dilute barium can give good results, and some authors advocate using air or water instead of methylcellulose for the double-contrast effect. In the single-contrast method [13], weaker mixtures of barium are infused (28% w/v for asthenic, 345 w/v for average, and 42% w/v for obese patients) (Fig. 3.15). Compression again is important in evaluating and separating small bowel loops. In the air double-contrast study [14], air is introduced after a 60% w/v barium infusion. Double contrast can also be obtained by infusing 600 ml of water after the barium [15].

A very rapid technique using dilute barium has been found to be effective in some centers (injecting dilute barium approximately 50% w/v at 240 ml per minute [16]. This will complete the procedure within 6 minutes, on average. Others would argue that the rapid technique results in gastric filling and vomiting in an unacceptable proportion of patients and does not give as good detail as the double-contrast techniques. There are clearly many ways to perform the small bowel enema, and at present there is no general agreement on the optimal technique.

Peroral Pneumocolon

Peroral pneumocolon is performed if visualization of the terminal ileum was inadequate after a small bowel meal, despite the use of compression. A rectal tube is introduced and air or carbon dioxide is insufflated. Intravenous glucagon may be given to faciliatate reflux of the air into the terminal ileum. If the patient lies on the left side, air

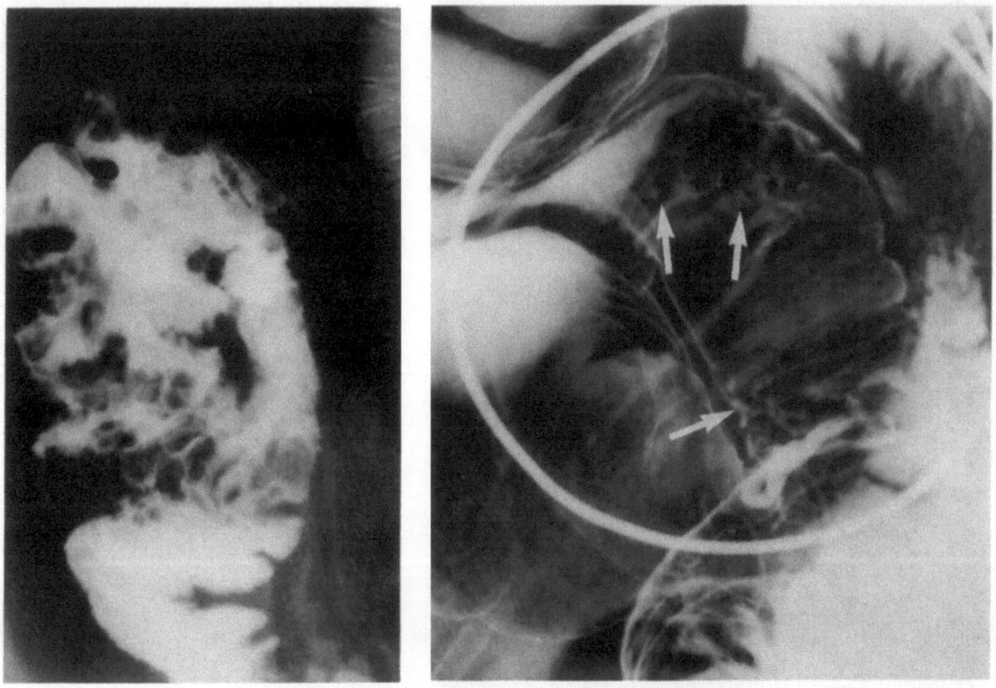
A B

Fig. 3.16. Peroral pneumocolon; spot films of terminal ileum. Note single-contrast uncompressed image (**A**) gives only slight suggestion of mucosal irregularity. Double-contrast study (**B**) shows clearly small clusters of aphthous ulcers (*arrows*). Dilute single contrast with compression can also show such lesions, but less clearly.

will rise into the right colon. After reflux has occurred, the terminal ileum is palpated and compressed. Spot films are taken (Fig. 3.16) [7, 17, 18, 19].

Small Bowel Follow-Through

A barium follow-through may be obtained after a single-contrast barium meal, but after a double-contrast meal the follow-through is usually of lesser quality because of the high density of the barium that is used for the gastric and duodenal examination. Furthermore, follow-through examinations performed in the middle of a busy barium meal examination schedule are seldom given the frequent attention with palpation of the loops because of the number of other patients being examined. Ideally, the patient should be examined every 15–20 minutes (Fig. 3.17) with palpation of the accessible loops of small bowel, followed by palpation and spot films of the distal and terminal ileum when the large bowel has been reached. Frequent fluoroscopy and compression can improve the accuracy of this study [20].

Reflux Small Bowel Enema

In this method, the small bowel is examined in the retrograde manner [21]. The colon is filled with dilute barium (20% w/v), usually 2 liter

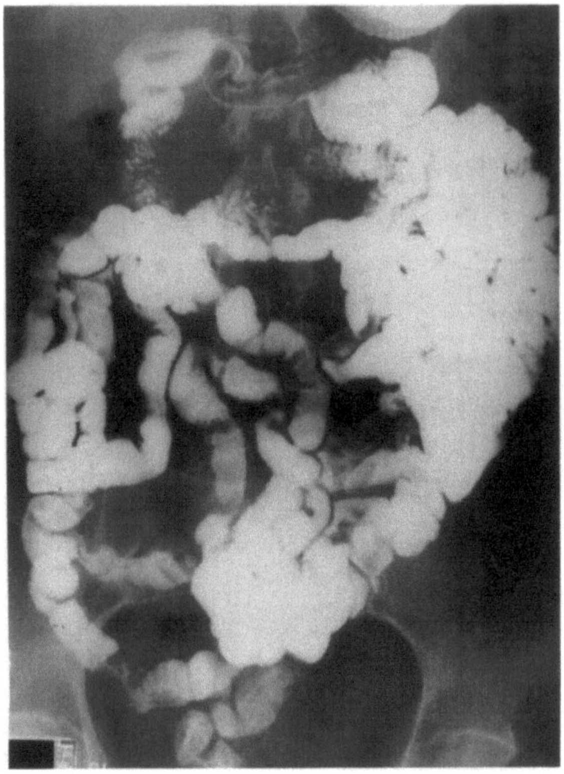

Fig. 3.17. Follow-through study at 15 minutes. Note high-density barium makes it difficult to see good mucosal detail with single contrast.

followed by 2.5 liter of water (Fig. 3.18). If spontaneous reflux does not occur, this can be facilitated by intravenous use of glugaon, which increases the reflux rate into the terminal ileum from 45% to 75% during barium enema [22].

Postoperative Small Bowel

A patient with an ileocolic anastomosis can be examined in either antegrade (per oral) or retrograde (per rectum) manner. The selection of the proper approach depends on the clinical problem. If the small bowel surgery was performed because of inflammatory bowel disease, the examination is performed antegrade in the same way as the standard small bowel meal (page 43). Smooth muscle relaxants are used to ensure that the anastomotic site is properly visualized. No washouts are given before the study because water refluxing into the small bowel will prevent proper mucosal coating with barium. In patients with prior surgery for bowel carcinoma, the standard bowel preparation is given (page 62) and examination is in the retrograde manner. Usually adequate double contrast can be achieved. Buscopan or glucagon is used to optimize distension at the anastomotic site.

In a patient with an ileostomy, the small bowel can also be examined either antegrade or retrograde. The antegrade procedure is the same as described above. The retrograde study requires introduction of a Foley catheter into the ileostomy stoma (Fig. 3.19). The balloon is not insufflated because of risk of perforation. Methods of preventing backflow of barium around the catheter are described in chapter 4 (page

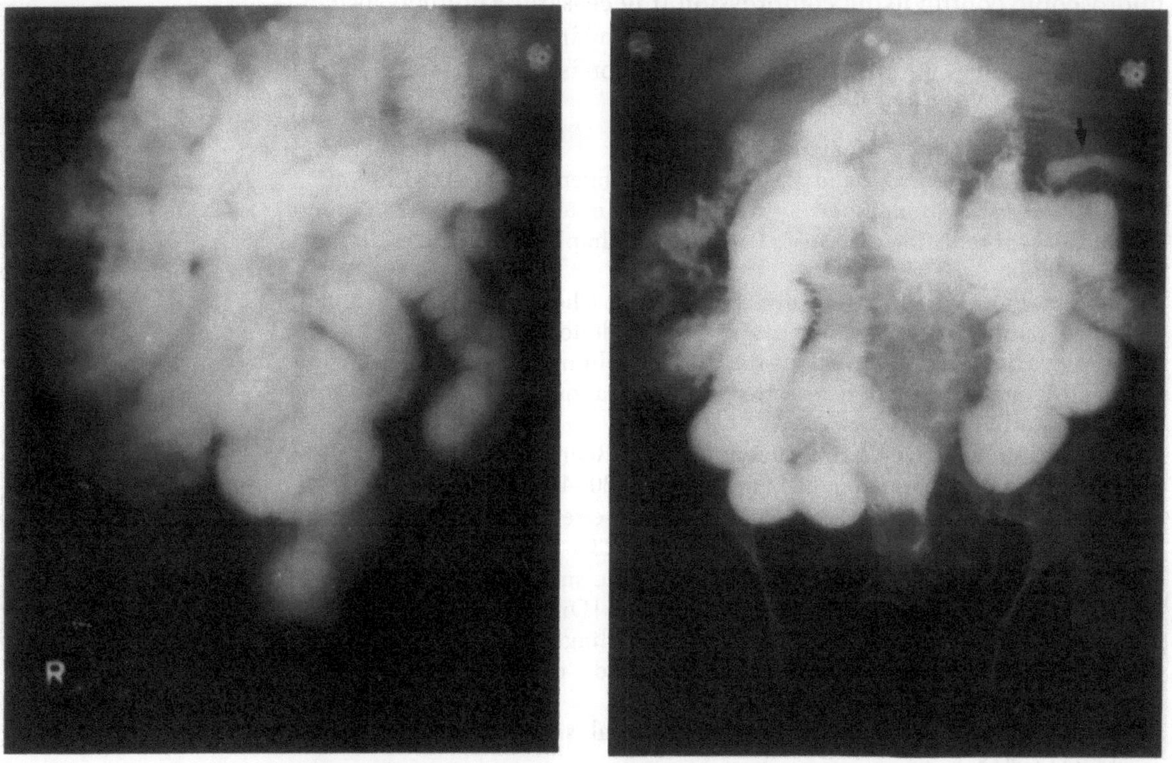

A B

Fig. 3.18. Reflux small bowel enema was performed for repeated cramping pain in patient with recent abdominal trauma. First film (**A**) shows large and small bowel opacified with refluxed dilute barium, but volume of contrast obscures diagnosis. Postevacuation film (**B**) reveals jejunal stricture (*arrow*) that was ischemic and cause of patient's symptoms. Postevacuation films are seldom helpful after double-contrast studies, but are frequently useful with single-contrast examinations.

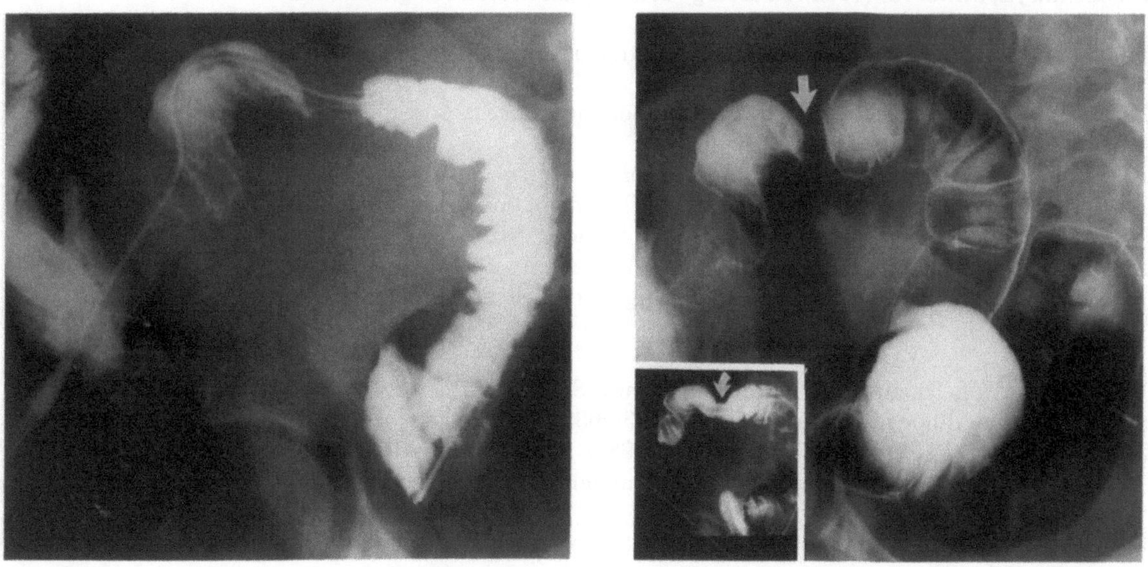

A B

Fig. 3.19. Retrograde small bowel study, postoperative. Single-contrast approach with high-density enema barium (**A**) is followed with air insufflation (**B**), giving good double-contrast examination. Variable narrowing (*arrows*) is often seen where ileum exits the peritoneum.

102). After the barium is introduced the small bowel is examined under fluoroscopic control using compression if necessary. Enteroclysis can also be performed in patients with an ileostomy in either the antegrade or retrograde manner; the retrograde intubation is better tolerated [23].

References

1. Ott DJ, Chen YM, Gelfand DW, Van Swearingen F, Munitz HA (1985). Detailed per-oral small bowel examination vs enteroclysis. Part I. Expenditures and radiation exposure. Part II. Radiographic accuracy. Radiology 155:29–34.
2. Maglinte DDT, Lappas JC, Kelvin FM, Rex D, Chernish SM (1987). Small bowel radiography: how, when, and why? Radiology 163:297–305.
3. Garvey CJ, DeLacey G, Wilkins RA (1985). Preliminary colon cleansing for small-bowel examinations: results and implications of a prospective survey. Clin Radiol 36:503–506.
4. Weltz GA (1937). Der kranke Duenndarm im Roentgenbild. Fortschr Geb Rontgenstr Nuklearmed Erganzungsband 55:20–40.
5. Gershon-Cohen J, Shay H, Fels SS (1940). The relation of meal temperature to gastric motility and secretion. AJR 43:237–242.
6. Brun B, Hegedus V (1980). Radiography of the small intestine with large amounts of cold contrast medium. Acta Radiol [Diagn] 21:(Stockh)65–70.
7. Kressel HY, Evers KA, Glick SN, Laufer I, Herlinger H (1982). The peroral pneumocolon examination: technique and indications. Radiology 144:414–416.
8. Fisher JK (1982). Angled view of the distal small bowel. Radiology 144:417–418.
9. Fraser GM, Preston PG (1983). The small bowel barium follow-through enhanced with an oral effervescent agent. Clin Radiol 34:673–679.
10. Schatzki R (1943). Small intestinal enema. AJR 50:743–751.
11. Oudkirk M (1981). Infusion rate in enteroclysis examination. Thesis. Leiden, The Netherlands: Leiden University.
12. Maglinte DDT, Miller RE (1984). A comparison of pumps used for enteroclysis. Radiology 152:815.
13. Sellink JL, Miller RE (1982). Radiology of the Small Bowel. Hingham, MA: Kluwer-Nijhoff.
14. Ekberg O (1977). Double contrast examination of the small bowel. Gastrointest Radiol 1:349–353.
15. Sellink JL (1976). Radiological Atlas of Common Diseases of the Small Bowel. Leiden: H.E. Stenfort.
16. Personal communication, Dr. C. Lu, University of Iowa Hospital.
17. Kellett MJ, Zboralske FF, Margulis A (1977). Per oral pneumocolon examination of the ileocecal region. Gastrointest Radiol 1:361–365.
18. Wolf K-J, Goldberg HI, Wall SD, Rieth T, Walter EA (1985) Feasibility of the peroral pneumocolon in evaluating the ileocecal region. AJR 145:1019–1024.
19. Fitzgerald EJ, Thompson GT, Somers S, Franic SF (1985). Pneumocolon as an aid to small-bowel studies. Clin Radiol 36:633–637.
20. Maglinte DDT, Burney BT, Miller RE (1982). Lesions missed on small bowel follow-through: analysis and recommendations. Radiology 144:737–739.
21. Miller RE (1965). Complete reflux examination of the small bowel. Radiology 84:457–462.
22. Monsein LH, Halport RD, Harris ED, Feczko PJ (1986). Retrograde ileography: value of glucagon. Radiology 161:558–559.
23. Zagoria RJ, Gelfand DW, Ott DJ (1986). Retrograde examination of the small bowel in patients with an ileostomy. Gastrointest Radiol 11:97–101.

CHAPTER 4

Large Bowel

The barium enema examination still retains a central role in the detection and prevention of colorectal carcinoma and in the demonstration of polyps. Controversy exists as to the role of single- and double-contrast examinations. Most radiologists now regard double contrast as the routine procedure of choice. Single contrast, however, when properly performed for appropriate indications, remains a useful and accurate examination [1].

Double-Contrast Barium Enema

Indications

The primary indications for barium enema examination are (a) abnormal bowel habit, especially change of previously stable bowel pattern; (b) rectal bleeding, with negative upper GI examination; (c) abdominal pain; (d) strong predisposing factors for colonic carcinoma; and (e) delineating and following course of inflammatory bowel disease.

Double-contrast examination should be attempted unless there are contraindications or the patient is too frail.

Contraindications and Precautions

1. Toxic megacolon
2. Perforation
3. Acute abdomen

Caution should always be taken with insertion of the enema tube tip to avoid the possibility of rectal perforation [2]. Perforation can also occur with over-insufflation of the enema tip cuff, and instructions concerning insufflation should be carefully followed [3,4]. The balloon should never be insufflated in patients with a low rectal carcinoma or acute ulcerative colitis, and only with extreme caution in patients with previous pelvic therapeutic irradiation.

Materials

1. 1/2-in. catheter tubing
2. Miller air tip, green, with or without inflatable cuff

3. High-density barium. E-Z-Em, liquid Polibar, or E-Z-Em liquid Polibar plus are all good. Our current preference is for Polibar plus, which flows quickly and provides excellent coating.
4. Air or carbon dioxide insufflation equipment
5. Glucagon, 0.5 mg I.V.
6. Buscopan, 20 mg I.V.

Patient Preparation

Until recently, preparation for barium enema has required dietary restriction for 1 to 2 days, encouragement of additional fluids, strong laxatives on the day before the examination, and 2-liter, tap water enemas shortly before the barium enema. Although some centers achieve satisfactory results without washouts [5], comparative studies have shown repeatedly that washouts are essential for a reliably clean colon [6].

In recent years materials have become available for an oral purge that is quite acceptable to patients [7–11]. Four such preparations (Golytely, Colyte, Lyteprep, and Kleanprep) are already on the market and others are likely to follow. The principle is a combination of a large molecular weight substance that is not absorbed, with a balanced electrolyte solution. As much as 4 liters of this preparation may need to be consumed, but the advantages are that it can be taken at home the evening before the procedure without previous dietary restriction, and washouts are not necessary. For colonoscopy, this method is even more satisfactory as the patient can consume the liquid between 7 A.M. and 9 A.M. and be ready for colonoscopy by 10 A.M. without previous dietary restriction, although Dulcolax the previous night to move the cecal contents seems to make the consumption of the large volume of fluid a little more tolerable.

The role of routinely performed preliminary abdominal films for barium enema examination is uncertain. In one study they were found to add significant diagnostic information in 8.4% of all cases [12]. Another study, however, found preliminary films to be not helpful in identifying clinically significant abnormalities and plain films to be misleading in the assessment of residual fecal material [13].

Standard Preparation

1. No solid food for 2 days before examination. Fluids encouraged, at least 3 liter (5 pints) each day.
2. 60 ml of castor oil, 6:00 P.M. on day before examination.
3. Four Dulcolax (bisacodyl) tablets with 300 ml of water, 10:00 P.M. on evening before examination.
4. No fluids for 4 hours before examination.

Washouts are performed by nurse or technician 2 hours before the examination.

Polyethylene Glycol Preparation

The last complete meal is taken at lunchtime the day before the examination. After lunch, four Dulcolax tablets are taken. In the evening the patient takes 10 mg of metoclopramide to reduce nausea, and then starts drinking the chilled polyethylene glycol solution at 200 ml every 10 minutes. Bowel movements usually begin within about 45 minutes. The patient continues drinking until the bowel movements consist of only completely clear fluid or until the four liter have been consumed, whichever is first. After this the patient may drink further clear fluids if desired until retiring to bed for the night, but subsequently fasting until the barium enema examination is finished.

□ *Procedure (Examination of the Rectosigmoid Colon)*

The examination is started with the patient on the left side. Each patient undergoes a rectal examination before insertion of the rectal tube. The purpose of the rectal examination is mainly to assess anal tone, which helps in deciding whether a rectal tube with an inflatable cuff is required. With the rectal tube in position the patient is turned prone. Barium is allowed to run into the bowel until the splenic flexure is reached; usually 300–400 ml is sufficient.

If the patient has difficulty holding the barium despite good anal tone, the standard Miller tube is removed, and a Miller tip with an inflatable balloon (cuff) is introduced into the rectum. One complete emptying of the inflator will distend the balloon to the recommended safe dimension. The rectal tube can be further secured by taping the tube to the buttocks. If readily available these tubes can be inserted in all patients, with the balloon inflated only if necessary.

Barium enema is still used in the diagnosis of colorectal disease and can have a high sensitivity [14]. The majority of diagnostic errors occur in the sigmoid colon, and result from perceptive misses, poor technique, diverticular disease, spasm, and poor bowel preparation [15]. The standard approach to the barium enema is to run barium in to the midtransverse colon before draining the rectum of excess barium with

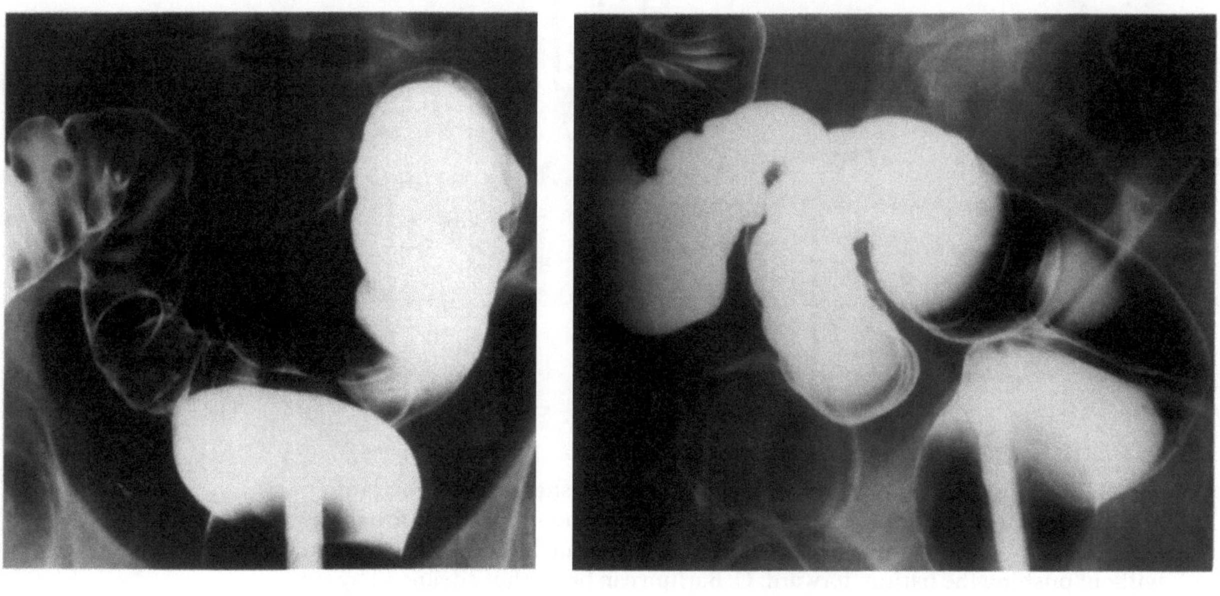

A B

Fig. 4.1. Routine DCBE examination. Spot films of sigmoid colon (**A,B**) show segments obscured by barium in one projection seen in double contrast on other projections.

the patient prone or erect. Air is then insufflated. For the sigmoid colon, a set of double-contrast films is obtained, with enough views that segments full of barium in one projection are shown in double contrast on another film (Fig. 4.1). There are two major pitfalls to this method: (1) overlapping loops may hide crucial segments, and (2) because the cecum and ileum have filled with barium, they may obscure the sigmoid colon.

An alternative approach of examining the sigmoid colon in double contrast with no residual barium pools remaining in the sigmoid is described next.

Theoretical Concept

Problem:

How do you clear the sigmoid colon of all barium puddles?

Answer:

1. With air insufflation. Air will drive a column of barium along a tubular structure (pipe or colon) only if the barium column forms a solid interface with the air. The air will then push the barium like a piston (Fig. 4.2A).

When this solid air–barium interface is broken because of a curve in the pipe or colon, the air will bubble ahead of the barium (Fig. 4.2B).

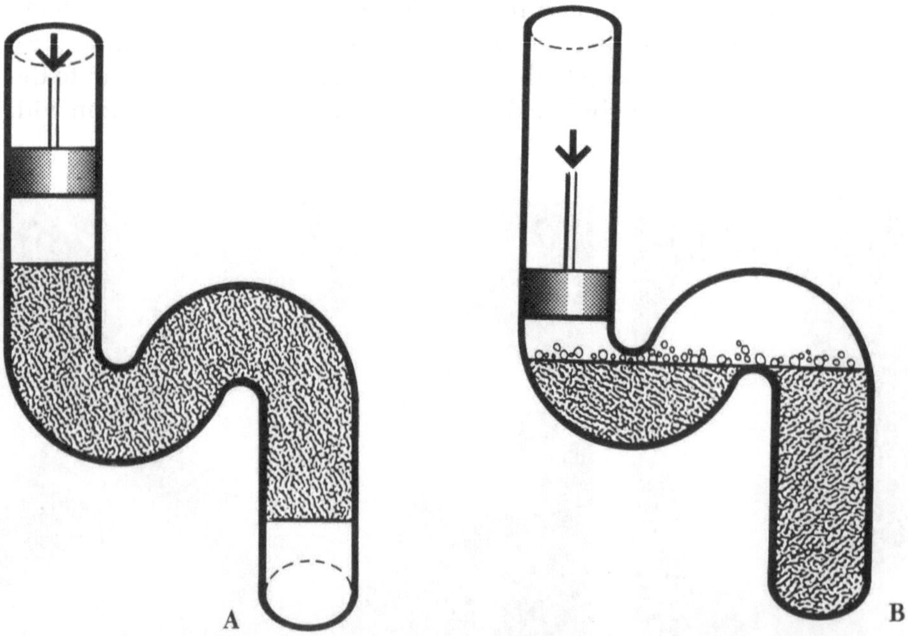

Fig. 4.2. Theoretical concept. **A.** The piston (air) pushes barium forward so long as air–barium interface remains in vertical segment. **B.** When the interface has been pushed out of the vertical segment, air bubbles past barium without pushing the barium forward. **C.** Barium can be further advanced by air (*arrow*) by changing patient's position and creating a new vertical air–barium interface.

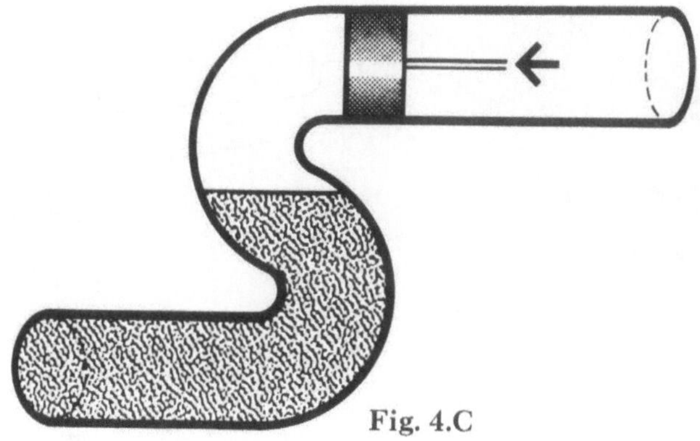

Fig. 4.C

Further addition of air will no longer advance the barium and is unnecessary.

2. With gravity. To achieve further progress in advancing the barium, the patient or pipe is turned into a lateral position. (If the curve is directed to the left, turning is into the left lateral position.) Gravity will now move barium onward in this segment (Fig. 4.2C). A new air–barium interface will also be formed and again air insufflation will drive the barium column forward.

Normal Anatomy

There is considerable variability in the configuration of the normal sigmoid colon. In a recent review of 106 consecutive patients in Ontario, Canada, undergoing barium colon examination, we were able to establish three basic configurations of the sigmoid colon.

Type 1, Standard, 65%

Two curved segments are present (Fig. 4.3). The first curved segment (A–B) starts posteriorly from the rectosigmoid junction (point A) and

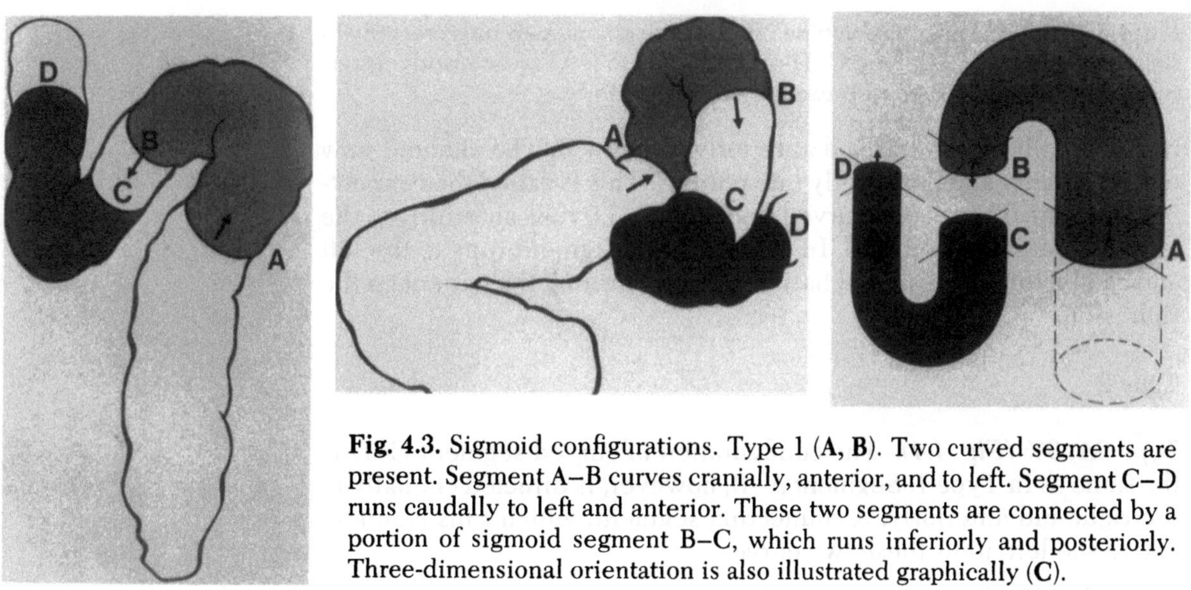

A

B,C

Fig. 4.3. Sigmoid configurations. Type 1 (**A, B**). Two curved segments are present. Segment A–B curves cranially, anterior, and to left. Segment C–D runs caudally to left and anterior. These two segments are connected by a portion of sigmoid segment B–C, which runs inferiorly and posteriorly. Three-dimensional orientation is also illustrated graphically (**C**).

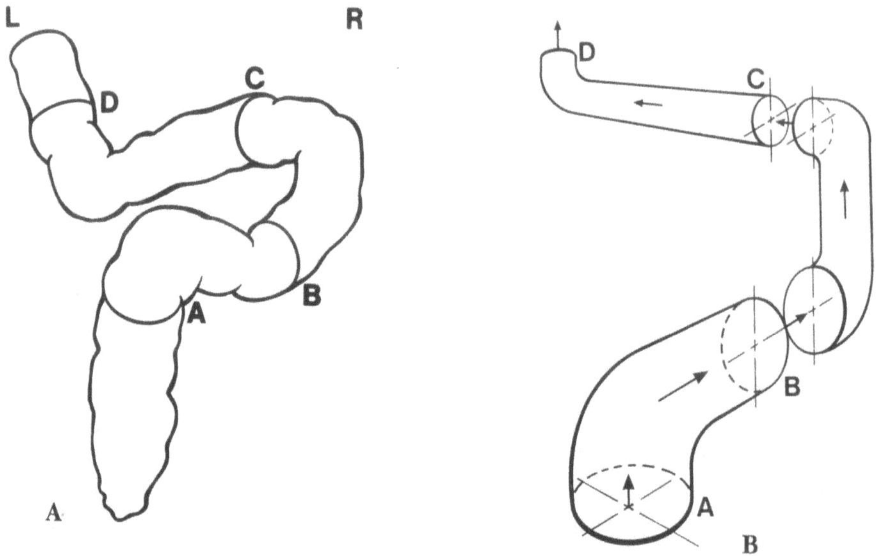

Fig. 4.4. Sigmoid configuration type 2A (**A, B**). Segment A–B runs cranially to right and anteriorly; segment C–D runs caudally to left and anterior. They are joined by connecting section running cranially and to left.

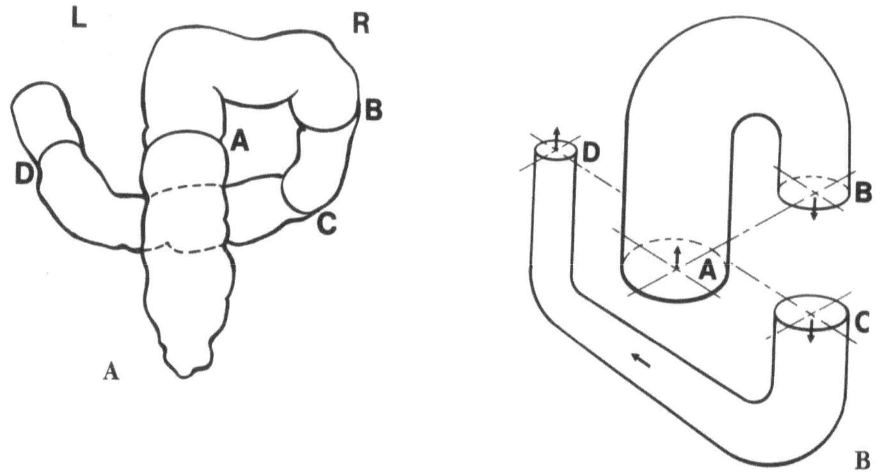

Fig. 4.5. Sigmoid configuration type 2B (**A, B**). Segment A–B runs cranially to right and anteriorly. Segment C–D runs caudally to left and anteriorly. Interconnecting Segment B–C runs caudally and posteriorly.

runs cranially to the left and anteriorly to point B. The sigmoid now drops caudally and posteriorly into point C. This is called the connecting segment. The second curved segment (C–D) runs anteriorly to the left and cranially (point D). In summary, the sigmoid runs to the left and can be totally cleared of barium without turning the patient on the right side.

Type 2

Type 2A, 9% (Fig. 4.4). The configuration of curved segment C–D is the same as in Type 1. Segment A–B, however, is directed cranially to the right and anteriorly. A connecting segment, which runs cranially and to the left, joins these two curves.

Type 2B, 11% (Fig. 4.5). The configuration of curved segment C–D is

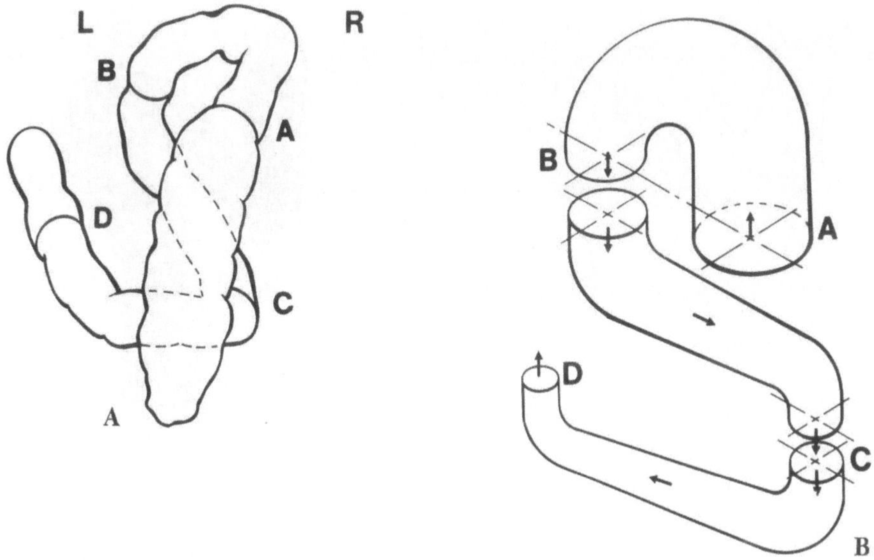

Fig. 4.6. Sigmoid configuration type 2C (**A, B**). Orientation of A–B and C–D segments is same as in type 1, but interconnecting segment runs caudally to right and posteriorly.

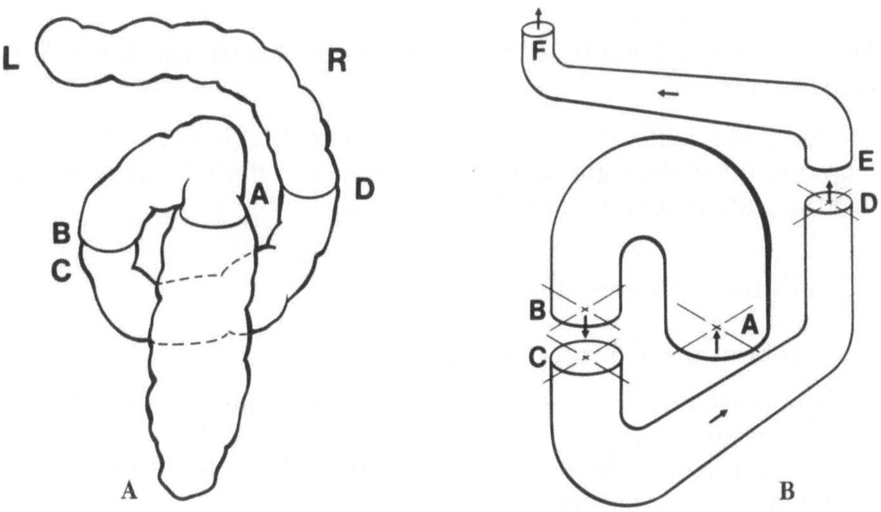

Fig. 4.7. Sigmoid configuration type 2D (**A, B**). Curved segment C–D runs caudally to right and anteriorly. From here, extra segment (E–F) runs cranially to left and anteriorly. A–B segment is the same as type 1.

the same as in Type 1. Segment A–B is the same as Type 2A, but the connecting segment runs caudally and posteriorly.

Type 2C, 4% (Fig. 4.6). The configuration of curved segment A–B and C–D is the same as Type 1, but the connecting segment runs caudally, posteriorly, and to the right so that point C is to the right of the midline. The sigmoid forms an S shape.

Type 2D, 5% (Fig. 4.7). Curved segment A–B is the same as Type 1. The second curved segment C–D runs caudally to the right and anteriorly. After crossing the midline, the sigmoid loops cranially to the left and anteriorly into the descending colon.

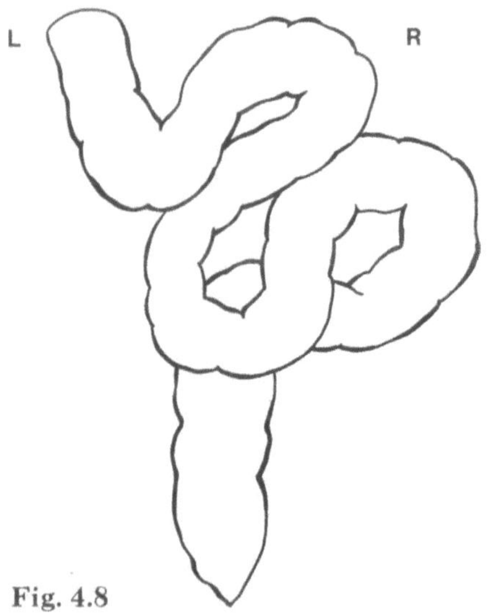

Fig. 4.8

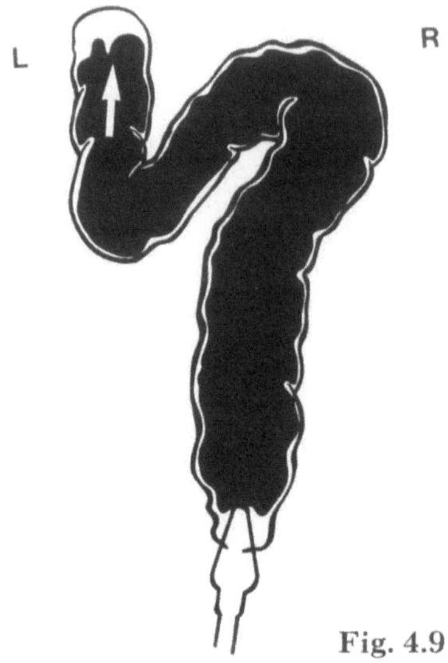

Fig. 4.9

Fig. 4.8. Sigmoid configuration type 3 complex. Multiple loops of sigmoid can be present in various orientations. Type 3 is usually associated with a very redundant sigmoid colon.

Fig. 4.9. Step 1. Introduction of barium (shown in *black*).

Type 3 Complex, 6% (Fig. 4.8). In this pattern, at least two right-sided loops are present.

Type 2 and 3 differ from Type 1 in that there is at least one sigmoid loop running to the right. Complete clearance of these loops requires that the patient be turned on the right side.

Technique of Examination

The performance of this technique requires:

1. An understanding of the spatial orientation of the two curved segments of sigmoid.
2. The advancing of the trailing end of barium from the rectosigmoid into the descending colon.

Step 1. All double-constrast barium enemas (DCBE) examinations are started with the patient prone with the rectal tube in position. Barium is allowed to run into the colon (Fig. 4.9). Usually less barium can be used with this technique (400 ml), because gravity and air is used to propel the barium onward leaving less barium to be drained from the rectum. The barium is run to the level of the splenic flexure. Under fluoroscopic control, the radiologist can identify the type of sigmoid configuration. The configuration can also be established from previous colon studies, if available. Type 1 (standard) configuration is discussed further. The salient feature of Type 1 is that the major curves are all to the left; the patient does not have to be turned on the right side to clear the sigmoid.

Step 2. Air or carbon dioxide [6] is introduced with an air bulb, and the air will push the barium onward so long as the air–barium interface remains intact (Fig. 4.10). Insufflation is stopped when air is seen

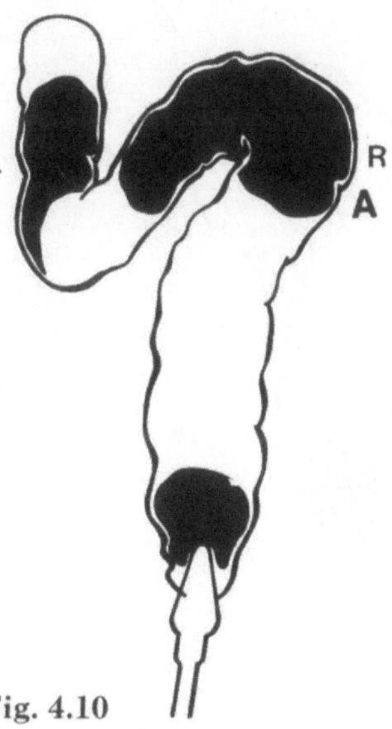

Fig. 4.10

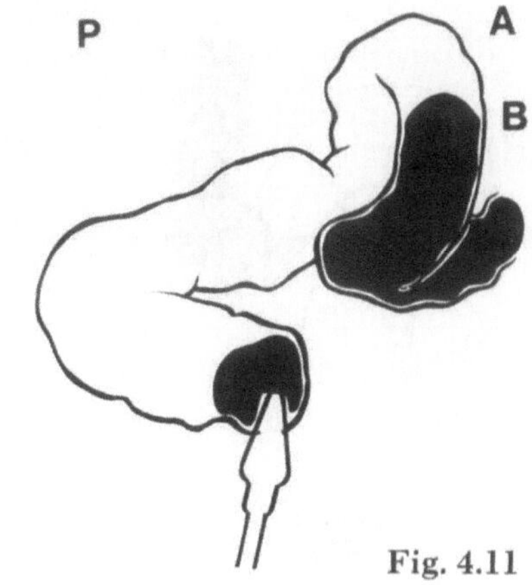

Fig. 4.11

Fig. 4.10. Step 2. Air insufflation. Air is introduced to propel barium (*black*) onward. Insufflation is stopped if air is seen bubbling into descending colon. Trailing end of barium is at point A.

Fig. 4.11. Step 3. Clearing of curved segment A–B. Turning patient on left side allows tail end of barium (*black*) to flow to point B, which now lies in dependent position.

bubbling into the descending colon (usually only three or four puffs are required) (see Fig. 4.2 A,B,C). Much, and sometimes all the barium in the rectum is pushed forward in this manner. Any barium left within the rectum is ignored at this time. The trailing end of the barium lies at point A (Fig. 4.10).

Step 3. The first curved segment A–B runs cranially to the left and anteriorly (Fig. 4,3A,B). To use gravity to advance the trailing end of barium to point B, the patient is turned onto the left side. A new air–barium interface is created, and further air may be insufflated (Fig. 4.11).

Step 4. The next area to be cleared is the connecting segment, which runs caudally and slightly posteriorly. To do this, the head of the table is raised 45° and the patient is turned supine (Fig. 4.12). The trailing end of barium is now at point C. The table is brought into the horizontal position.

Step 5. The second curved segment, which runs anteriorly to the left and cranially out of the pelvis, is cleared by turning the patient on the left side and prone (Fig. 4.13).

Step 6. If necessary, any residual rectal barium is now drained by elevating the head of the table 45° again with the patient still prone (Fig. 4.14). Drainage is performed under fluoroscopic control and with a steady slow air insufflation; do not allow the barium within the descending colon to refill the rectum. After the rectum is drained and the sigmoid is adequately distended with air, the table is returned to a horizontal position and the patient is turned supine oblique, right-side-forward. The rectosigmoid colon is now clear of all barium, and spot films are obtained.

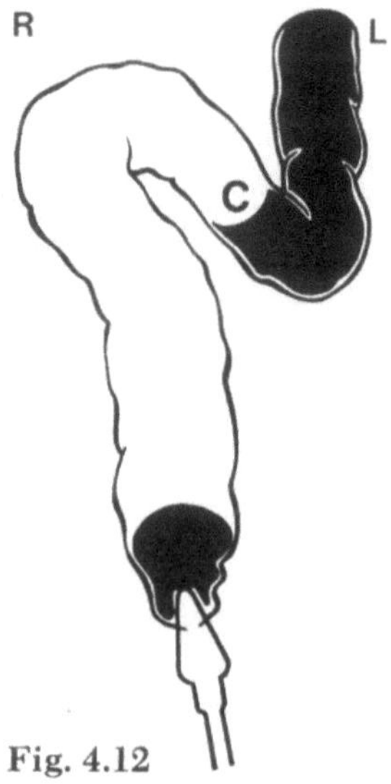

Fig. 4.12

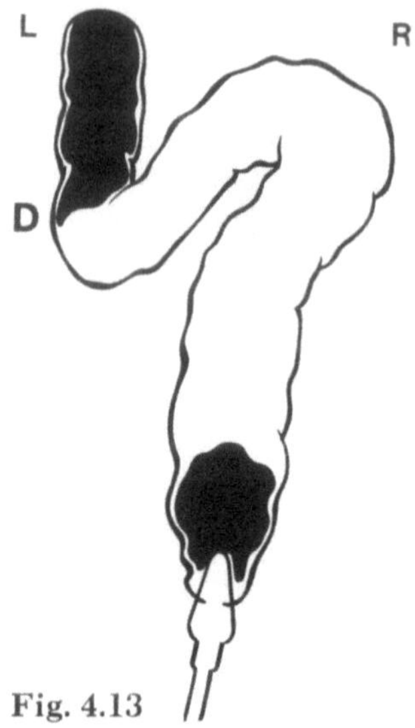

Fig. 4.13

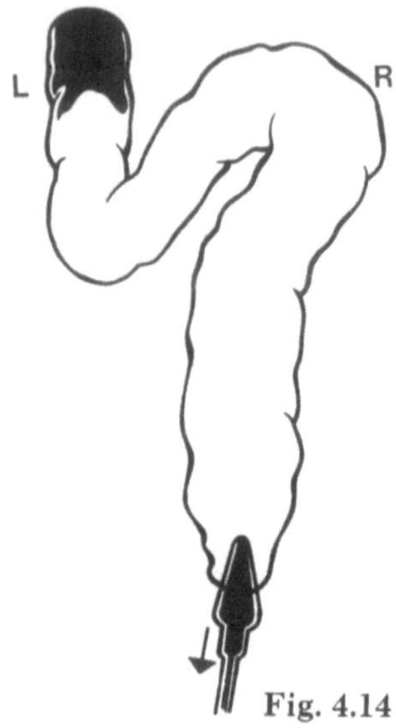

Fig. 4.14

Fig. 4.12. Step 4. To clear interconnecting segment B–C, head of table is elevated and patient turns supine. Trailing end of barium (*black*) is now at point C. Table is again lowered into horizontal position.

Fig. 4.13. Step 5. Clearing of segment C–D. Patient turns on left side and prone, allowing barium (*black*) to drain into descending colon.

Fig. 4.14. Step 6. Drainage of residual barium (black) from rectum is usually performed with patient prone, head of table elevated. After drainage, air is again insufflated to fully distend rectum and sigmoid colon.

If barium did flow back into the sigmoid curved segment C–D, step 4 is repeated after drainage of rectum is complete. Table 4.1 summarizes the foregoing steps.

Table 4.1. Steps to clearing of barium from type 1 sigmoid colon.

Step	Position	Procedure
1	Prone	Filling of colon with barium
2	Prone	Air/insufflation
3	Left lateral	Clearing of curved segment A–B
4	Elevate head of table supine	Clearing of connecting segment.
5	Left lateral to prone	Clearing of curved sgment C–D
6	Elevate head of table	Drainage of rectum

Spot Films

For the average colon, four films are sufficient and can be taken with one rotation of the patient from the supine oblique right-side-forward (Fig. 4.15A), left lateral (Fig. 4.15B), prone (Fig. 4.15C), and prone oblique left-side-up (Fig. 4.15D) positions.

Note that during the clearing of barium in the standard configuration of sigmoid, the patient is not required to lie or to turn on the right side; therefore, the cecum and ascending colon will still be free of barium.

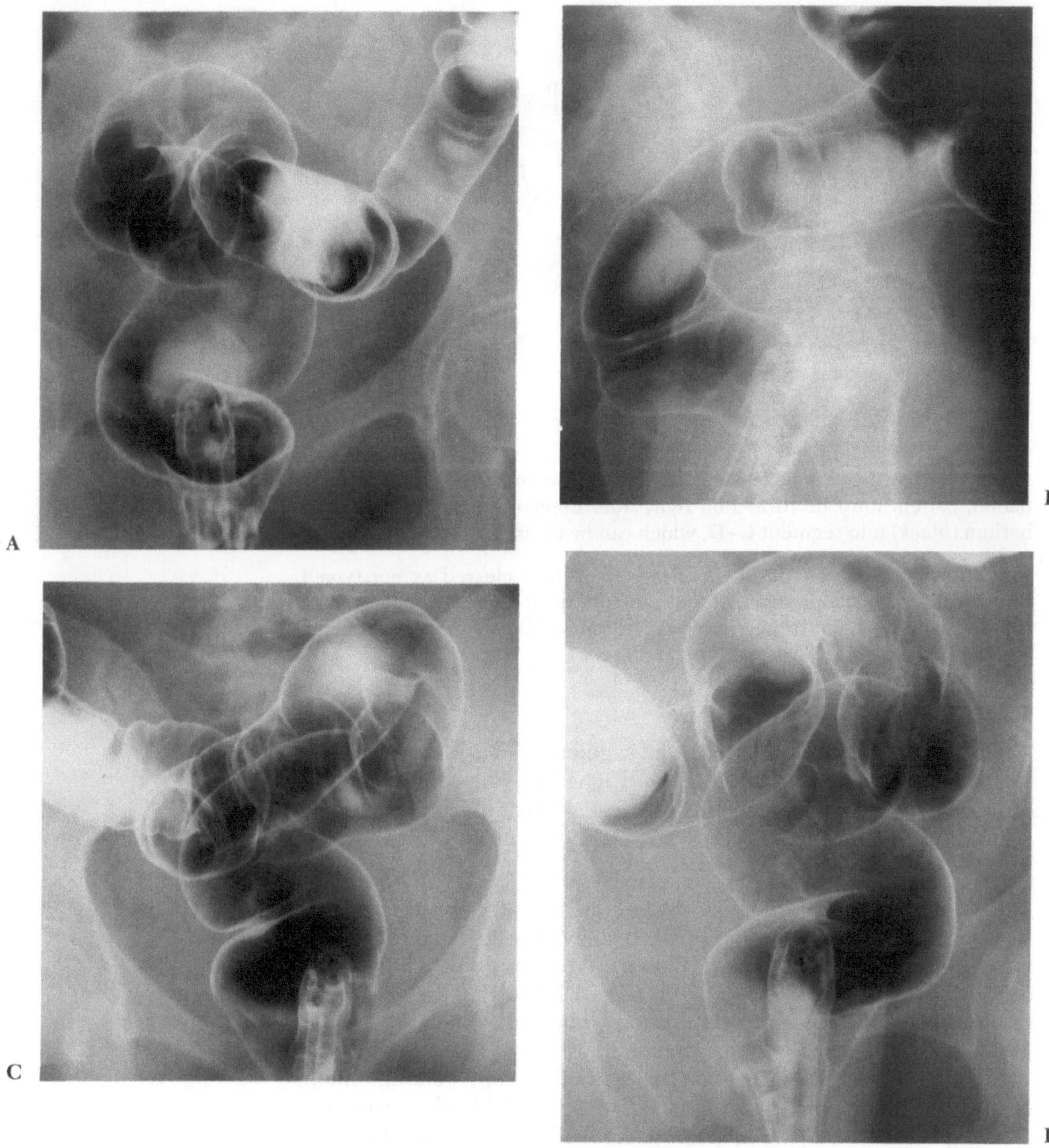

Fig. 4.15. Spot films. **A.** Supine right-side-forward oblique; B, left lateral; C, prone; D, prone left-side-forward oblique.

Application of Technique for Other Configurations

Type 2B

The main characteristic of Type 2 configurations is that there is at least one curve to the right, and the patient will have to be turned on the right side to achieve complete clearing of the sigmoid.

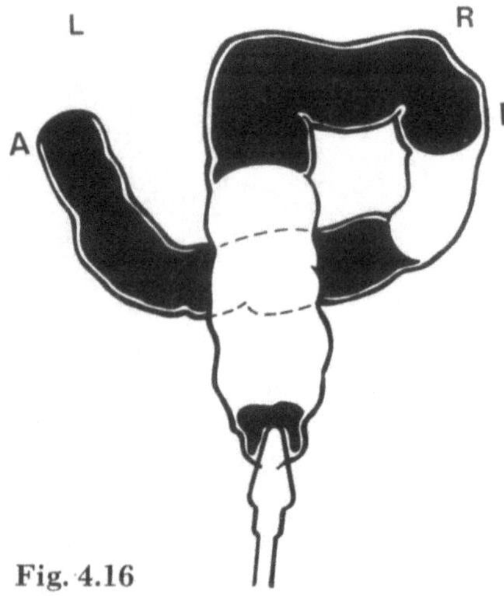

Fig. 4.16

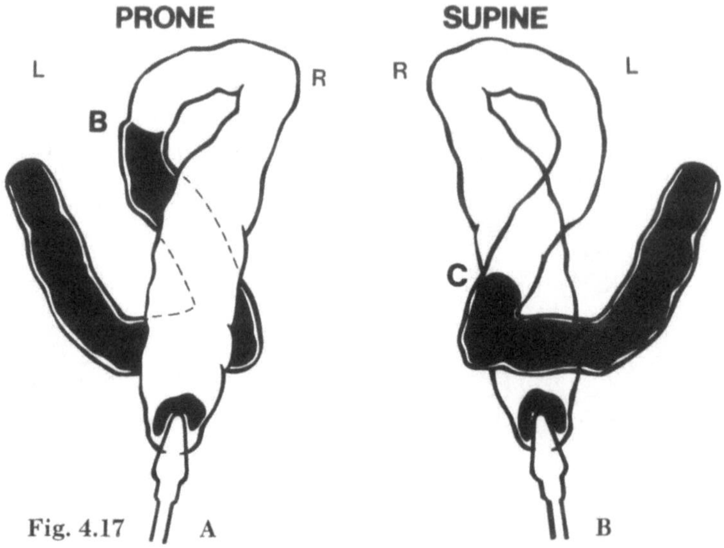

Fig. 4.17 A B

Fig. 4.16. Clearing of type 2B sigmoid. To drain segment A–B after air insufflation, patient must be turned on right side. Elevating head of table drops barium (*black*) into segment C–D, which can be cleared as in type 1.

Fig. 4.17. Clearing of type 2C. **A.** Segment A–B is cleared as per type 1. Because interconnecting segment runs caudally and to right side, head of table is elevated and patient turned into right lateral and then supine. **B.** Segment C–D can now be cleared as per type 1.

After initial air insufflation, curved segment A–B will be cleared by turning the patient on the right side (Fig. 4.16). The connecting segment will be cleared by elevating the head of the table and turning the patient supine. Segment C–D is cleared now as in Type 1.

Type 2C

Segment A–B is cleared as in Type 1. By elevating the head of the table and turning the patient supine (Fig. 4.17A) and on the right side, the barium will drain into segment C–D (Fig. 4.17B). With the head of the table still elevated, the patient is turned prone and on the left side. The table is now brought into the horizontal position.

After the technique has been mastered for the simpler configurations of sigmoid colon, the principles can be applied to allow complete clearing of more complex loops (Fig. 4.18) of sigmoid as well as other segments of colon.

Examination of Remainder of Colon

Step 1. After completion of the spot films of the sigmoid colon, the patient is turned right-side-down and air is insufflated again, using the piston principle to propel the barium from the transverse colon into the ascending colon.
Step 2. The patient is put into the supine position. The table is brought into the semierect position, which allows the barium to drop toward the cecum. The patient is now turned on the left side and prone, which

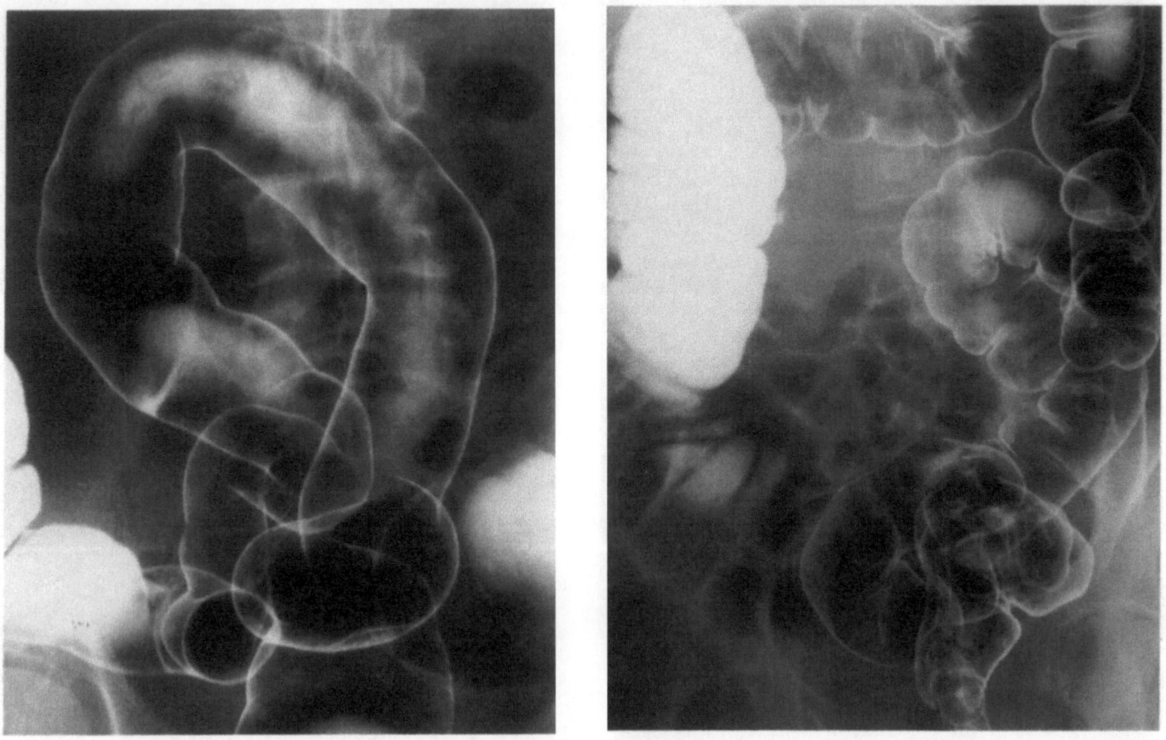

A B

Fig. 4.18. Complex loops. Complete clearing of complex loops of sigmoid (**A**) and entire left colon (**B**).

drops the barium fully into the cecum. At this point the hepatic flexure is poorly coated. To improve coating, the table is put horizontal with the patient prone, and the patient is rolled completely once or twice. Then with the patient supine, the table is brought erect.

Step 3. Film, 10 × 12 in. In the erect position, a left-side-forward spot film of splenic fixture is obtained (Fig. 4.19).

Step 4. Film, 10 × 12 in. Erect right-side-forward spot film of hepatic flexure (Fig. 4.20).

Step 5. The table is brought into the horizontal position with the patient left-side-down. When the table is horizontal, the patient is turned on the right side and the head of the table is lowered 5°–10°. This should empty the cecum of barium. Film, 10 × 12 in., two split. One film of cecum in supine right-side-down position (Fig. 4.21).

Step 6. The patient is now turned supine, then left-side-down, and finally to the prone position. Second exposure of split film from Step 5. Cecum in prone position. Insufflated paddle (page 80) may be beneficial for the prone examination in difficult patients (Fig. 4.22).

Step 7. Six overhead films [16] are now taken in the following positions (Fig. 4.23A–I) (see Chapter 7, page 213):

Supine
Prone
Prone angled view of sigmoid
Right lateral decubitus
Left lateral decubitus
Lateral film of rectum.

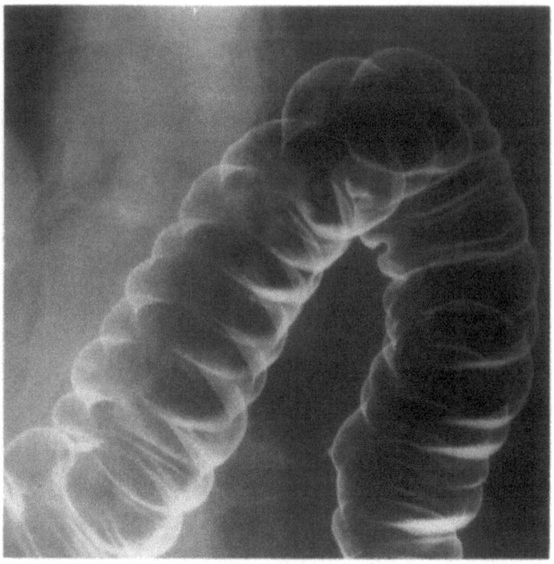

Fig. 4.19

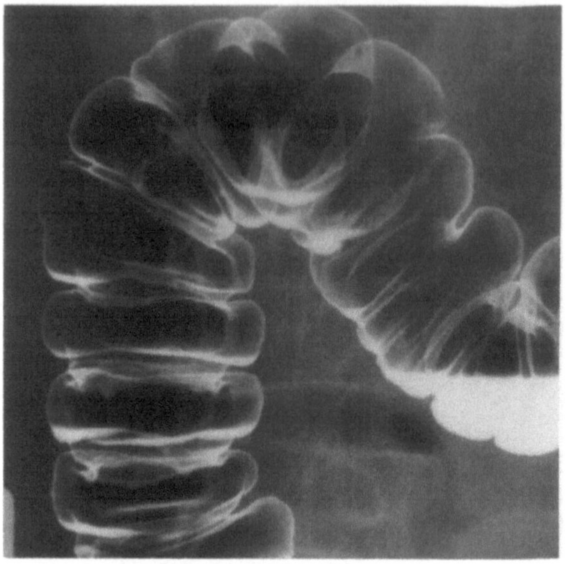

Fig. 4.20.

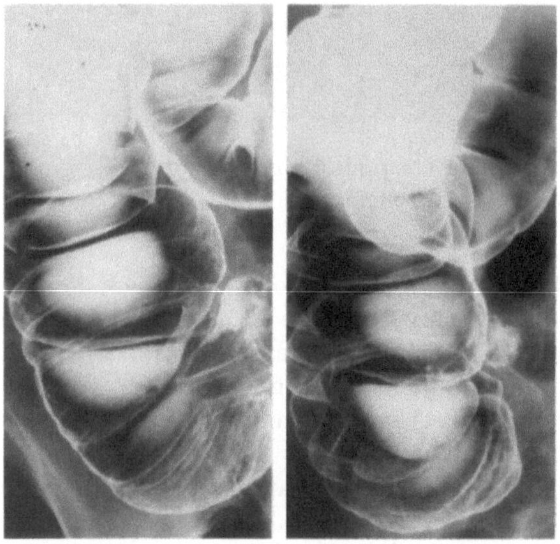

Fig. 4.21

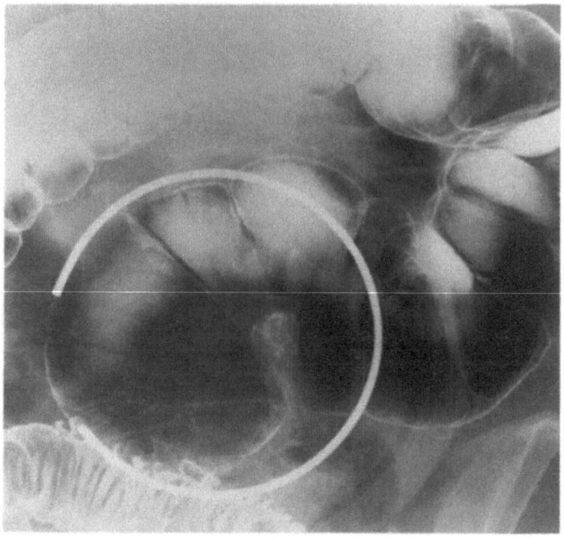

Fig. 4.22.

Fig. 4.19. Splenic flexure. In erect position, barium flows out of flexure, allowing double-contrast visualization. Positioning patient oblique left-side-forward usually separates ascending and descending portions of flexure, preventing obscuration of information from overlap.

Fig. 4.20. Hepatic flexure; best seen with patient oblique right-side-forward.

Fig. 4.21. Cecum supine. Spot films of cecum identify ileocecal valve. Note small amount of reflux into terminal ileum.

Fig. 4.22. Cecum prone. Insufflated balloon paddle is usually necessary to displace small bowel loops that obscure cecum in this position.

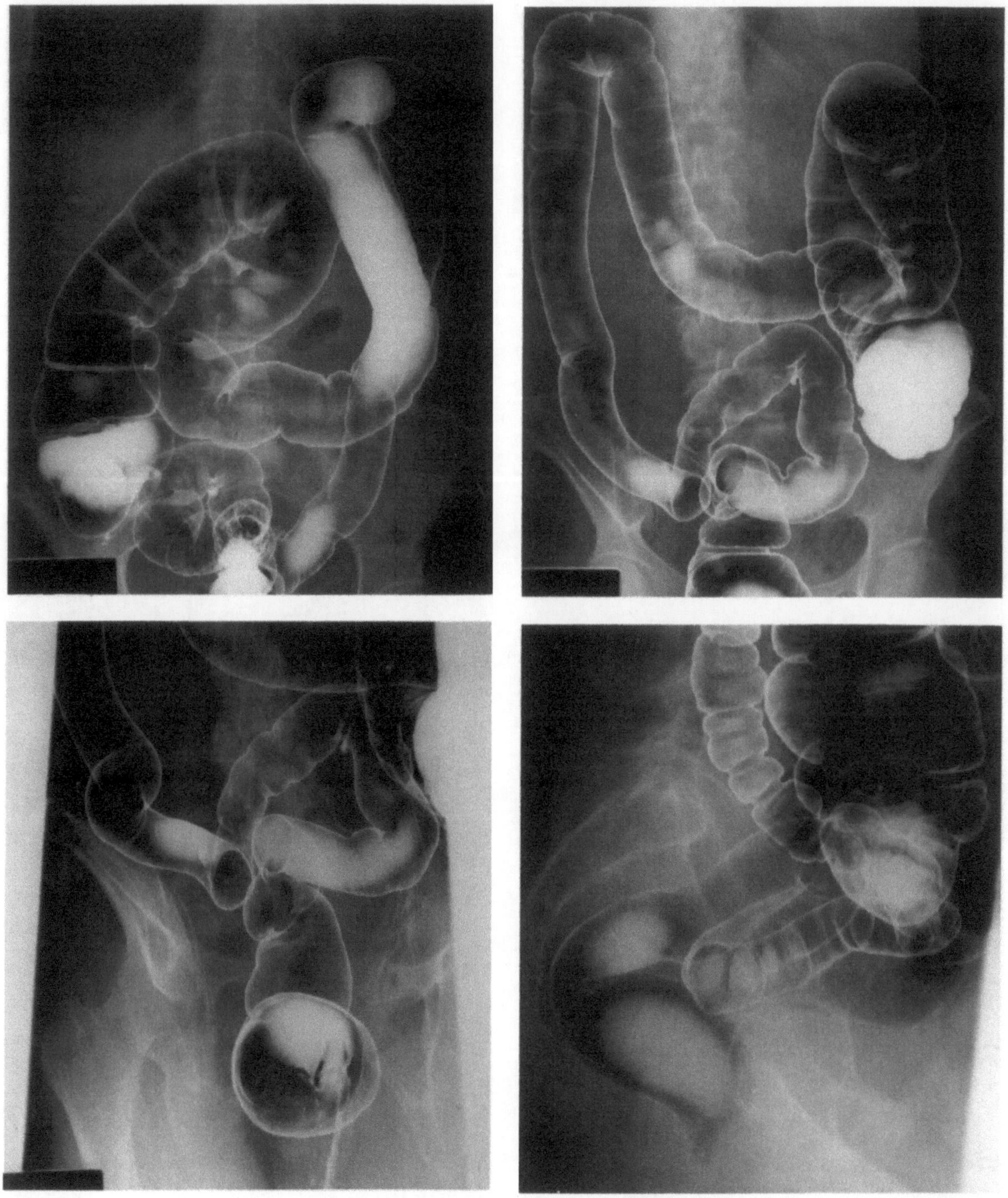

A B C D

Fig. 4.23. Overhead films. **A,** Supine; **B,** prone; **C,** prone angled; **D,** lateral. (*Continued.*)

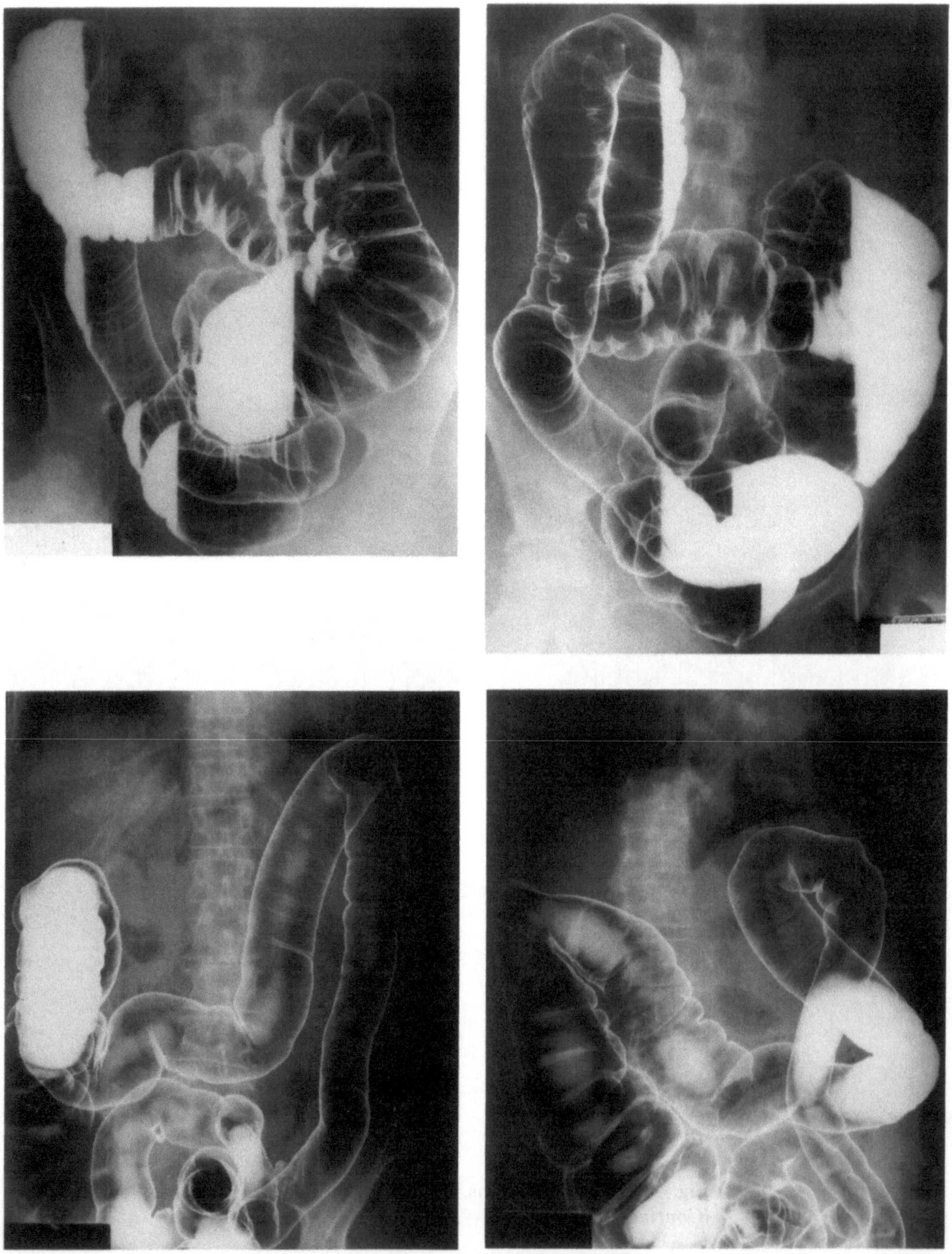

E F G H

Fig. 4.23. E, right lateral decubitus; **F,** left lateral decubitus; **G,** left oblique; **H,** right oblique; **I,** erect.

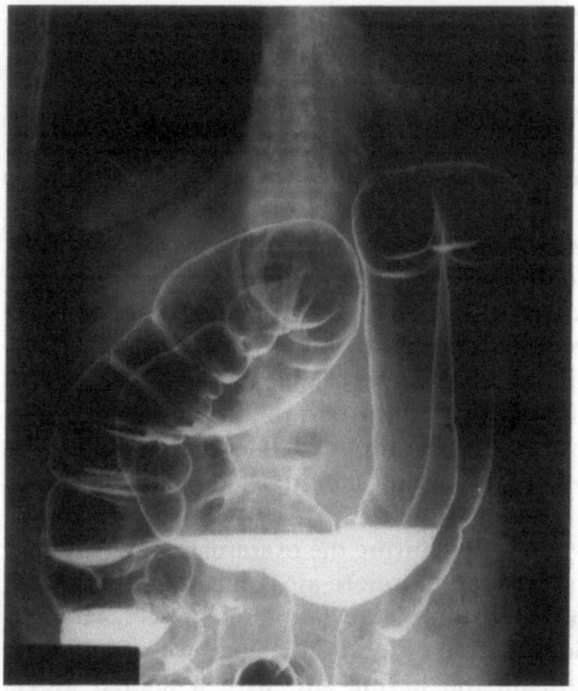

Fig 4.23 I

The sequence just described is appropriate for a conventional room with under-the-table tube for spot films and overhead tube for all the technician films. With a remote control table or a 100-mm camera, different sequencing may be used. The initial spot films of the rectum and sigmoid will be as described, but with a remote table the flexure spot films can be replaced by oblique 17 × 14 in., full-size films.

The ability to take 17 × 14 in. films with a remote unit, or 14 × 14 in. films on a conventional unit, allows an alternative to decubitus films that can save considerable time. After the sigmoid spot films have been completed, all the barium in the left colon can be moved to the right colon by placing the patient supine head down, and then turning to the right and prone while slowly instilling air. This moves the barium column into the left side of the transverse colon and anterior wall of the splenic flexure. Raising the head of the table 30° and turning the patient on the right side moves the column to the hepatic flexure, and then bringing the patient slightly back into the left-side-up supine oblique position permits a view of the left colon that may render the lateral decubitus films unnecessary in most patients (Fig. 4.23G).

Later, after the right colon has been well coated, a similar maneuver can be used to empty the right colon. The patient starts supine and the table is tipped 15° to 20°, head down. The patient is turned partly on the right side to run barium from the cecum into the ascending colon, and then supine again. The patient is then assisted to roll slowly to the left and prone, which moves the barium from ascending colon to the anterior wall of the hepatic flexure and the right side of the transverse colon. The table head is elevated 30° to run the column from hepatic flexure to midtransverse colon, and the patient turns on the left side. The table is brought flat, and the patient rolls slightly back to the right-side-up supine oblique position, allowing a film of the right colon

(Fig. 4.23H) that renders a right-side-up decubitus film unnecessary in about two-thirds of patients.

These head-down turning maneuvers require a technologist positioned at the head of the table, preferably with thyroid collar and lead glasses for corneal protection, and patients require encouragement and assistance. The savings of the 5–20 minutes that would otherwise be required for the decubitus films usually justifies the added inconvenience.

Many problems can arise in the performance of the DCBE examination. If the patient is allowed to turn on the right side or barium is run too far into the transverse colon before the sigmoid spot films are obtained, much of the sigmoid colon will be obscured with this barium. Slow flow of barium and unnecessary discomfort to the patient can be caused by air being left within the barium tubing at the start of the examination and the air being propelled into the colon by the advancing barium; therefore, the tubing should be completely cleared of air before the study.

If a herniated colon is identified during the examination, an attempt should be made at hernia reduction before air is insufflated [17]. Air insufflation can lead to distension of the herniated bowel, strangulation, or perforation. Reformation of the hernia can be prevented by applying steady pressure on the hernia site with a leaded glove. Knowledge of the principles of clearing of the rectosigmoid colon will also allow for correction of an "air block" through positioning of the patient [18]. An air block refers to insufflated air reaching the right colon before enough barium has flowed into that area.

The double-contrast barium enema examination is very difficult to perform in patients with spasm and diverticulitis, and diagnostic accuracy of the examination is enhanced in these patients with the use of intravenous glucagon or Buscopan [19,20]. Some patients complain of severe pain after leaving the X-Ray Department after having had DCBE. An evaluation of this at our hospital showed 7% of patients record this as severe pain and 28% as moderate. Carbon dioxide is absorbed from the colon 32 times more quickly than air, and it was logical, therefore, to suspect that there might be less pain following barium enema if carbon dioxide was used. Prospective evaluation confirmed this, with moderate pain being recorded in 11% of patients and severe pain in none [21]. A carbon dioxide delivery system for DCBE has been described [22] (Fig. 4.24). Carbon dioxide is, therefore, the gas contrast medium of choice when a radiologist is using a remote control table. With conventional tables, because the carbon dioxide is absorbed very quickly, it is necessary for the technologist to take the overhead films very rapidly if adequate distension is to be maintained. Alternatively, additional gas may have to be instilled while overhead films are being taken.

Single-Contrast Barium Enema

Indications

The principal indication for single-contrast barium enema is suspected large bowel obstruction, in which case it may be performed with no

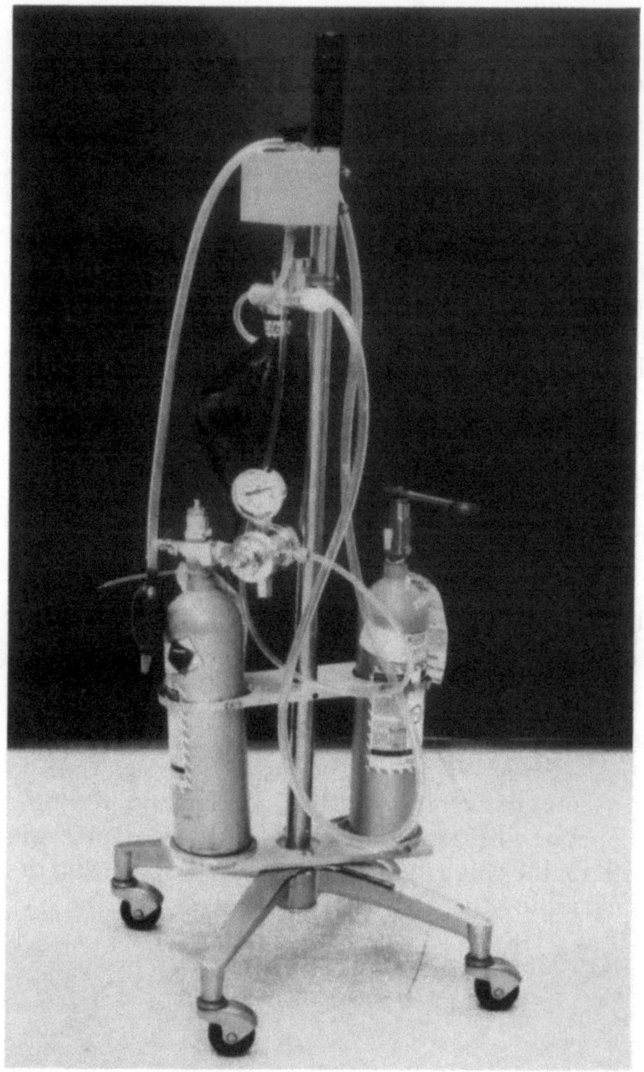

Fig. 4.24. Carbon dioxide delivery system includes carbon dioxide tanks.

bowel preparation. It is a suboptimal examination for patients with rectal bleeding, inflammatory bowel disease, or colorectal neoplasm, and should be employed only in those patients incapable of turning on the table sufficiently to allow a double-contrast examination to be performed. As an approximate guide, patients who cannot climb onto the table unaided and turn over on their stomach are not suitable for double-contrast examination. Single-contrast barium enema is appropriate in such patients for exclusion of large tumors, but if fine detail of the colonic mucosa is required, colonoscopy should be performed. In thin elderly patients, a high-quality colon examination can be obtained, with single contrast by extensive use of palpation and compression. However, this technique demands very good fluoroscopic skill and relies on fluoroscopy rather than films. It is, therefore, not checkable by later film review. This examination can also be useful and is safe in patients with suspected appendicitis [23,24].

Contraindications

1. Toxic megacolon
2. Perforation.

Contrast examination may be required in patients with recent perforation or diverticular abscess. For these patients, a water-soluble contrast is appropriate.

Materials

1. Miller air tip, brown
2. Regular $\frac{3}{8}$-in barium enema tubing
3. Barium Polibar Plus 400 ml or HD85 400 ml
4. Water, 1600 ml
5. Compression devices
6. Glucagon I.V., 0.5 mg
7. Buscopan I.V., 20 mg
8. Enema retention balloon.

Barium should be dilute so that you can see through it on the radiographs, between 18% and 30% w/v. High kilovolts, about 125 kV, should be used.

Compression Devices

Colon compression is unsatisfactory with the standard fluoroscopic table compression cone, or with a large balloon paddle. Compression devices that work well for the colon include the plastic F spoon and the wooden Mayo Clinic paddle (Fig. 4.25) [25].

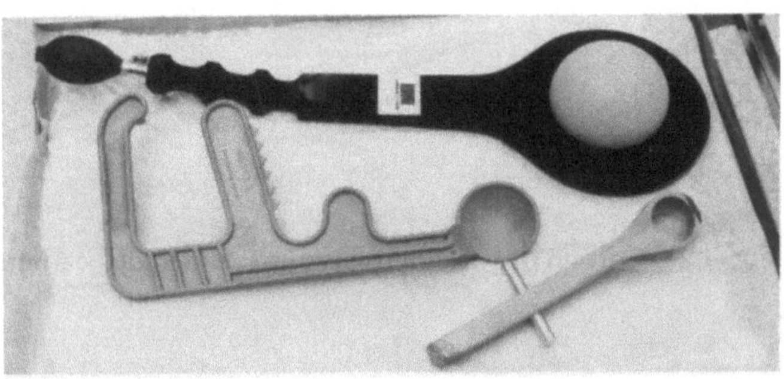

Fig. 4.25. Three useful compression devices: balloon paddle (New PX Imaging), F spoon [25], and Mayo Clinic spoon. Every fluoroscopy area should be equipped with at least two of these devices. Balloon paddle is particularly helpful for prone compression.

Patient Preparation

Preparation is just as important for a single-contrast examination as for a double-contrast examination. No preparation is used in patients suspected of obstruction. Otherwise, preparation is the same as for a double-contrast examination. In patients with poor anal tone in whom barium spillage is anticipated, it is wise to position an inflated enema ring under the patient's buttocks before the study to prevent unnecessary delays for x-ray table-top cleaning during the examination.

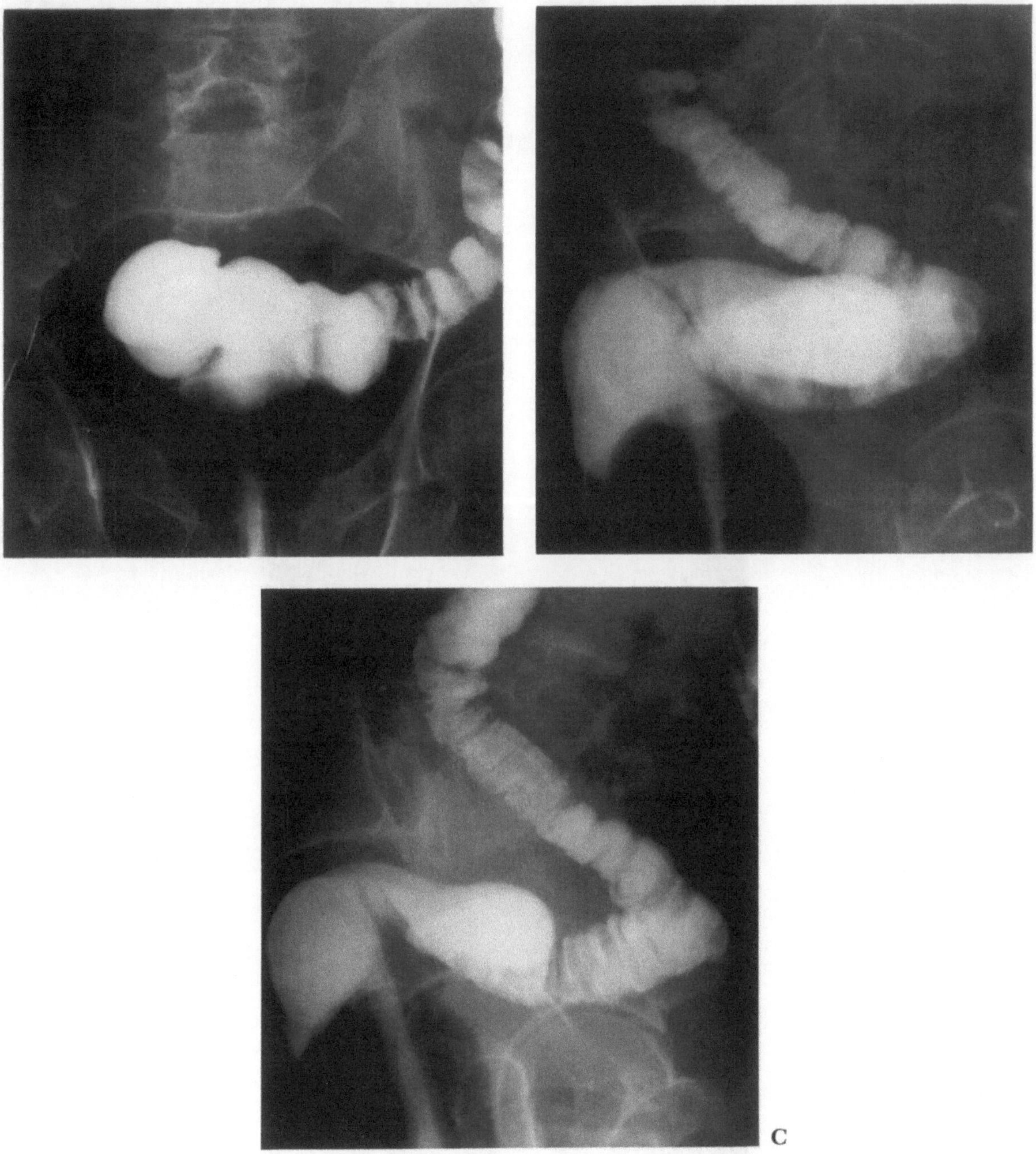

A B C

Fig. 4.26. Sigmoid colon. Spot films in supine left-side-forward oblique (**A**), supine (**B**), and lateral (**C**) positions.

□ *Procedure*

Step 1. The patient is on the left side. A rectal tube is inserted after digital examination.
Step 2. Dilute barium is now allowed to run into the bowel. The column of barium is followed carefully under fluoroscopic control. Spot films of the rectosigmoid are obtained (Fig. 4.26), initially with as little distension as possible so that polyps can be seen clearly before

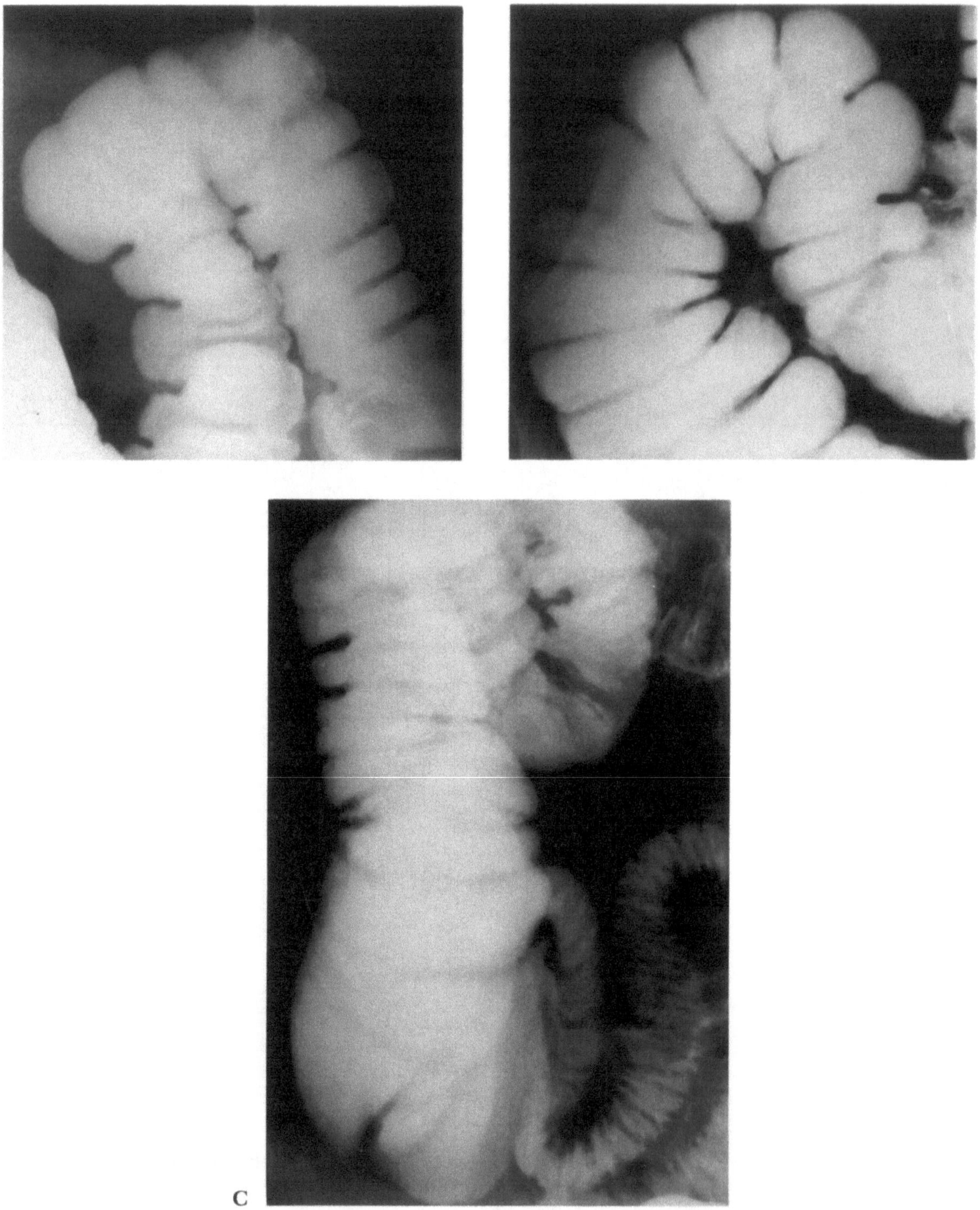

A B C

Fig. 4.27. Enough barium is allowed to flow to fully distend splenic (**A**), hepatic flexures (**B**), and cecum (**C**).

Fig. 4.28 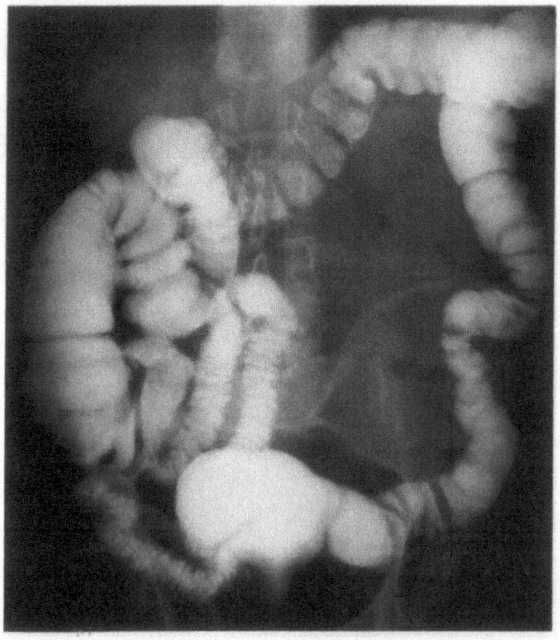 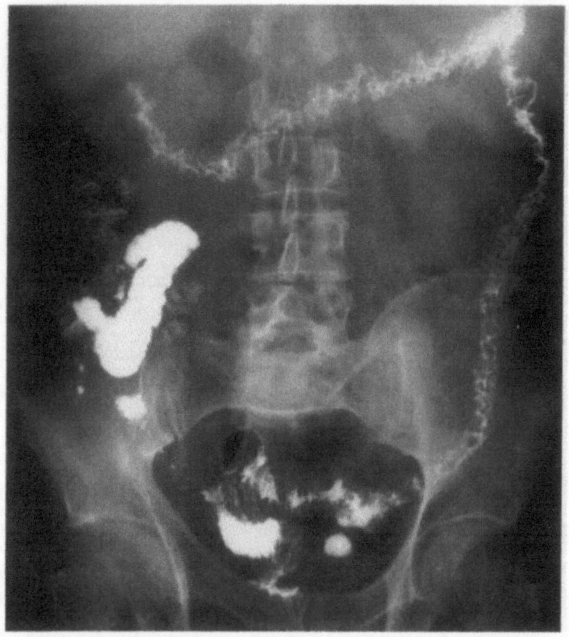 Fig. 4.29

Fig. 4.28. PA overhead film of entire colon.

Fig. 4.29. Postevacuation study shows almost complete emptying of barium from bowel.

they are obscured by full distension. Tube angling, if available, is ideal for separation of loops. Glucagon or Buscopan I.V. can be used in patients with spasm.

Step 3. The barium is allowed to flow into the descending colon. Compression may be used to facilitate flow of barium and delineate filling defects.

Step 4. When the barium has passed the splenic flexure into the transverse colon, positioning the patient on the right side will bring the barium into the hepatic flexure and ascending colon.

Step 5. Elevating the head of the table will now direct the barium into the cecum.

Step 6. Enough barium is introduced to keep the flexures and cecum opened wide. Spot films of the flexures and cecum are obtained (Fig. 4.27). Careful palpation with a gloved hand or paddle is then performed along the entire length of the accessible colon to look for filling detects. Additional spot films are taken if an abnormality is encountered.

Step 7. 14 × 17 in. film PA (AP in debilitated patients) (Fig. 4.28).

Step 8. Post evacuation (Fig. 4.29). Before allowing the patient to go to the washroom it may be wise to drain as much barium as possible out of the colon back into the bag. In single contrast, the postevacuation film is invaluable and may be the only film to show pathology (Fig. 4.30).

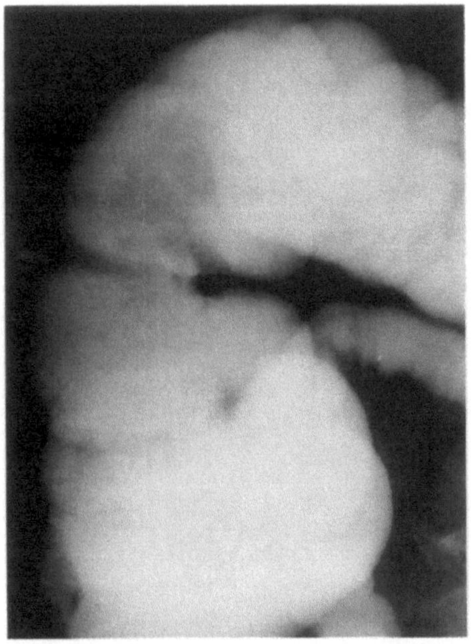

A

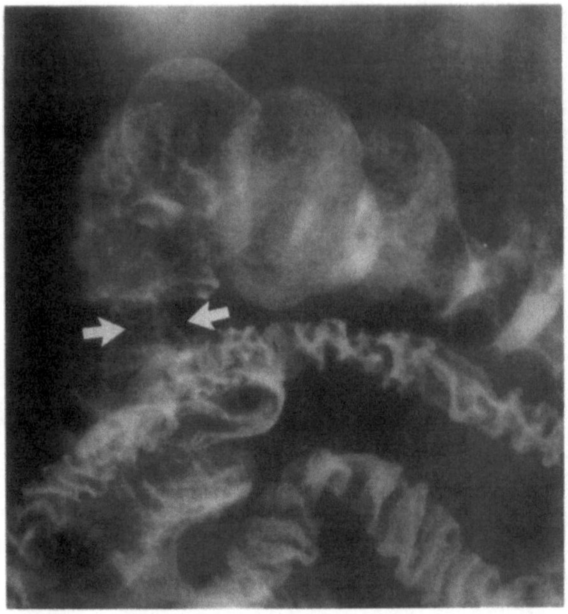

B

Fig. 4.30. Lesion not identified initially (**A**) is clearly visualized (*arrows*) on postevacuation film (**B**). Carcinoma was surgically proven.

Instant and Air/CO_2 Enemas

This examination is intended only for patients with known ulcerative colitis who previously had proctitis or proctosigmoiditis, and in whom sigmoidoscopy or plain abdominal films suggest further extension of disease [26,27].

Technique

A preliminary film is taken with no preparation, and will reveal the site of stool in colon or any abnormalities precluding the performance of this test (Fig. 4.31). Based on the principle that the diseased bowel is empty in active ulcerative colitis, an estimation can be made of the extent of the disease. Barium is then introduced and run in until stool is encountered. The rectum and distal sigmoid are then allowed to drain completely and air is introduced. Three films are usually taken: prone, left-side-up decubitus, and lateral rectum. These four films give a useful assessment of the degree of severity and extent of ulcerative colitis. It may become obsolete as the flexible sigmoidoscope comes into more general use.

Air Enema

In patients with acute inflammatory bowel disease, plain radiographs of the abdomen will often give sufficient information as to the extent and severity of disease. When a patient has acute disease but very little air in the colon, further information may be obtained, without introducing barium, by insufflating approximately 100 ml of air to produce

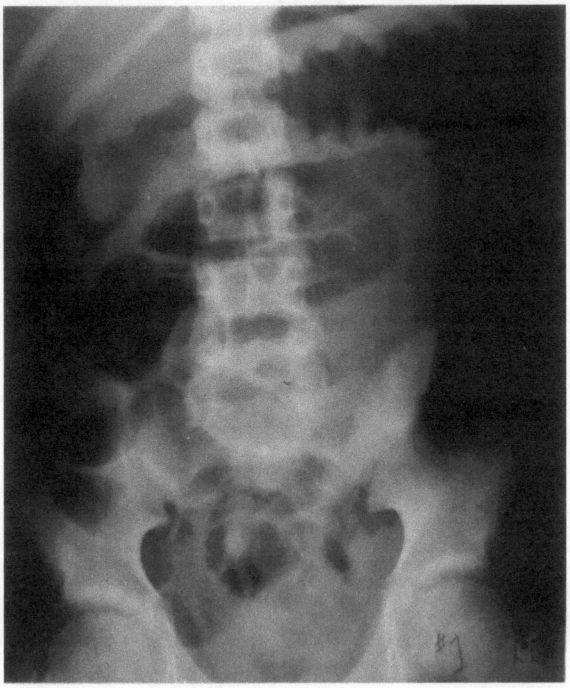

Fig. 4.31. Abdominal film in 12-year-old with acute ulcerative colitis shows dilatation with thumbprinting and pseudopolyposis with no stool in right colon. These findings indicate severe total Ulcerative Colitis (UC), and barium enema is completely contraindicated.

mild distension [28]. Prone, supine, and left-side-up decubitus films will then give considerable detail as to the presence of edema or pseudopolyposis and the extent of disease (Fig. 4.32). If carbon dioxide is used, rapid absorption will occur, and this procedure with air or carbon dioxide appears to be safe in these ill patients. The presence of toxic dilatation would be a contraindication, and decubitus plain films may provide further information in these patients.

Flexible Sigmoidoscopy

Most of the polyps and carcinomas missed by barium enema are in the sigmoid column. This part of the bowel is readily and safely examined by flexible sigmoidoscopy (FFS) [29]. Although FFS is traditionally carried out in the clinic after one or two Fleet enemas, it can also be carried out immediately before a barium enema study, saving the patient the discomfort of two separate bowel preparations. The combination of flexible sigmoidoscopy and barium enema is probably more sensitive for polyp detection than colonoscopy. Excess fluid present in the distal 60 cm of the colon can be removed by the sigmoidoscope, which will improve the coating, and the air introduced does not appear to be a problem.

Before the examination is started, it should be adequately explained to the patient and a consent form must be signed. The patient should

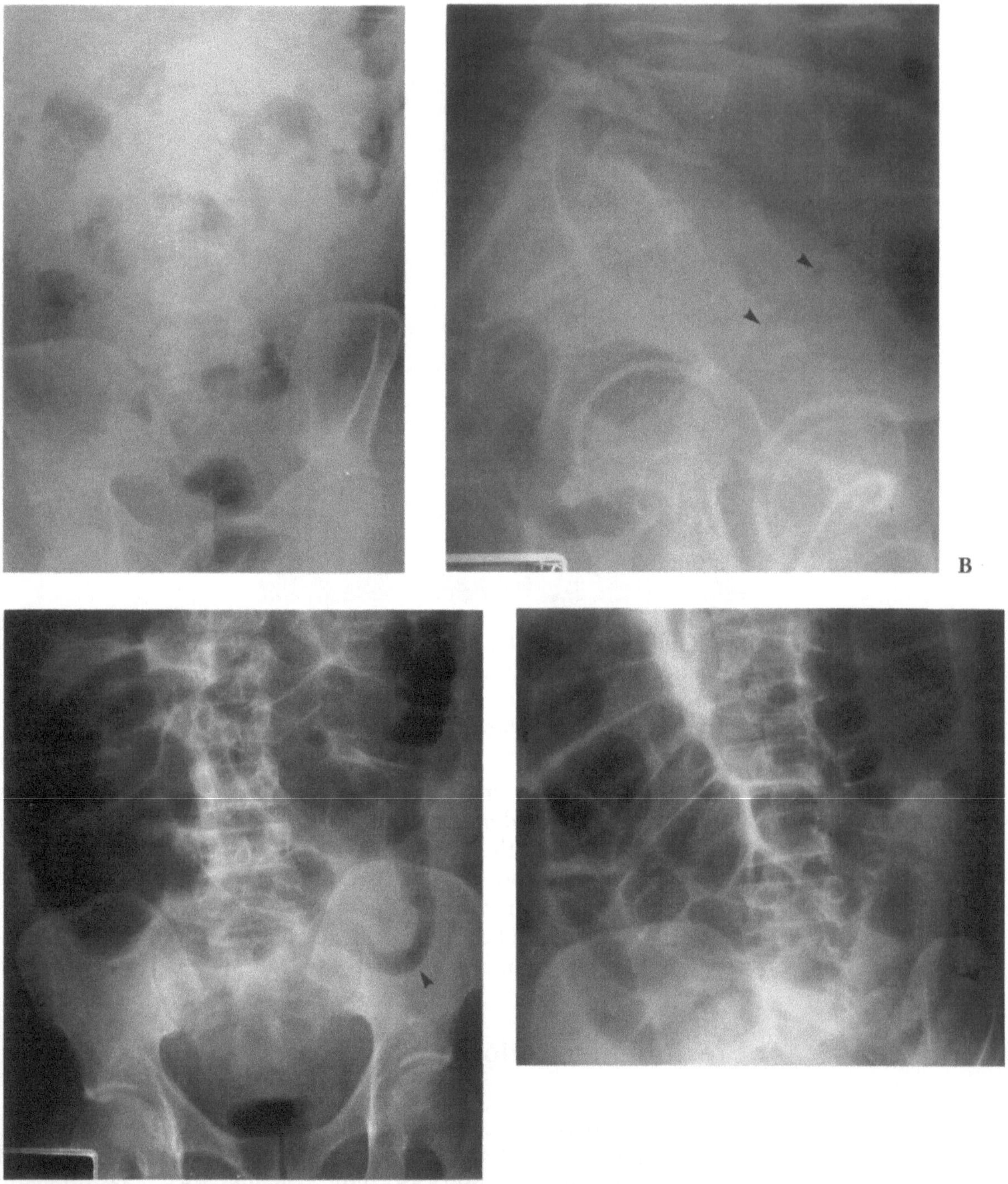

Fig. 4.32. **A.** Preliminary film before CO_2 enema. Note paucity of gas in distal descending and proximal sigmoid colon. **B.** Lateral film after introduction of CO_2 shows narrow irregular spastic sigmoid colon (*arrowheads*). **C.** CO_2 enema shows narrow ahaustral distal descending and sigmoid colon (*arrowhead*). Proximal colon is well distended and normal. **D.** Carbon dioxide enema. Proximal descending colon and sigmoid colon are normal. Distal descending and sigmoid colon are narrow, spastic, and ahaustral (*arrowheads*). Note abrupt change in middescending colon.

be told that the examination will be uncomfortable as air is introduced, but should not be painful, and that if any pain is experienced the patient should say so at once. The procedure is performed with the patient lying on the left side with the knees flexed. A rectal examination is performed to assess the anal canal and the instrument tip is then introduced. At first, the tip is slightly withdrawn as air is introduced so as to obtain a view of the rectal lumen, and then rectal fluid is aspirated. Once the direction of the next bend is seen, the scope tip is advanced to the bend and then angled in the direction of the bend. When the next straight segment is seen, the scope is again advanced. Into the sigmoid, advances may be made with short rotary twists, rapid clockwise advances, and slower anticlockwise withdrawals with the advances gaining over the withdrawals. This clockwise emphasis tends to prevent formation of a large sigmoid loop in most patients, but occasionally the opposite approach will be required. In general, the tip should never be advanced unless lumen can be seen, and if the luminal view is lost, withdrawal is necessary to reestablish it.

Full insertion to 60 cm without pain will be achieved in about 80% of patients and to 45 or 50 cm in most others. Patients with previous pelvic surgery, active small bowel Crohn's disease, and anal fissures may not be able to tolerate the full examination. At the end of the examination, surplus air can be removed, and this is most effective if the patient lies prone while air is aspirated from the rectum. Small biopsies (2.8-mm channel forceps) can probably safely be taken before a barium enema, certainly from polypoid lesions, but large biopsies (5-mm channel, or rigid sigmoidoscope forceps) require 1 week's delay before a barium enema is done [30,31,32].

Colonoscopy

Colonoscopy is performed mainly by surgeons and gastroenterologists, but there are many hospitals in which radiologists also carry out this procedure.

Indications

Indications include further evaluation of a lesion seen on a barium enema, resection of polyps seen at sigmoidoscopy or on barium enema, investigation of rectal bleeding, assessment of inflammatory bowel disease, especially for detection of dysplasia, and for follow-up of patients with previous resection of carcinoma or adenomatous polyps. Laser treatment of obstructing or bleeding tumors will probably soon be another indication.

Contraindications

Very acute inflammatory bowel disease, suspected perforation, and an uncorrected bleeding diathesis.

Preparation

Bowel preparation is the same as for barium enema, except that when a polyethylene glycol lavage is used, the Dulcolax is given the night before the examination, and the polyethylene glycol mixture is given on the morning of the colonoscopy.

Patient preparation includes an explanation of the procedure, the need for sedation with the consequence that the subject will not be able to drive home, and a discussion of polypectomy and its complications. Consent for polypectomy is obtained before all colonoscopies because unexpected polyps are often encountered. The remote risk of bleeding (1%) and of perforation (0.2%) [33] should be mentioned and accepted by the patient, together with the possibility of surgery to handle the problem, before colonoscopy is started.

☐ *Procedure*

After the endoscope has been recleaned and its function has been checked, its tip is introduced into the rectum with the patient lying in the left lateral position. Fluid is aspirated from the rectum, enough air (or carbon dioxide) is introduced to identify the lumen, and the tip is advanced into the rectosigmoid. The principles of tip advancement are as described for flexible sigmoidoscopy, with the scope being advanced only when the lumen is seen; once a corner is reached, the tip is angled into the corner in the direction of the next segment of the bowel. When the view is lost, the scope is withdrawn to refind the lumen and never blindly advanced.

Many techniques for colonoscopic intubation have been described during the past 15 years. Refinements have been made, and the need for fluoroscopy has declined as instrumentation and techniques have improved and more endoscopists have acquired personal expertise [34].

A greater awareness of the variations in the anatomy of the colon, and of the dynamics of endoscopy, has provided a rationale for the development of abdominal compression techniques. There are situations in which a loop will form, thus reducing control over the instrument tip and causing discomfort or pain to the patient. Compression is never used to try and straighten a looped instrument, but after reduction of a loop has been achieved by withdrawal and rotation, compression is used to maintain a straight segment so that when the colonoscope is advanced again tip advancement occurs rather than loop reformation.

There are only four basic compression techniques, which may be required singly or in combination (Fig. 4.33). They are used to prevent formation of a sigmoid loop, to pull the splenic flexure and descending colon medially, to prevent downward looping of the transverse colon, and to bring a low cecal pole up to the tip of the colonoscope. They are described in the sequence in which they are used during a colonoscopic examination.

Sigmoid Colon

Colonoscopy is started in the usual way with the patient lying in the left lateral position and the nurse/assistant behind the patient and to

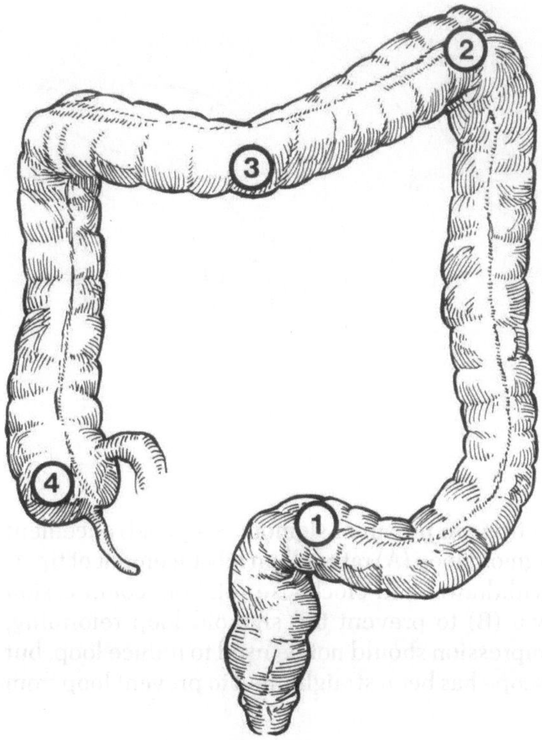

Fig. 4.33. Four main compression points. Sigmoid (1) is usually required; transverse (2) colon is often required; splenic flexure (3) and cecal (4) compression are only occasionally necessary.

the left of the colonoscopist. Passage through the sigmoid colon is achieved by careful steering and "straightening" of the sigmoid loops. This is achieved by constantly pulling back the instrument after each advance is made, so that the instrument is advanced only when there is a view of the lumen to the next bend, and the slide-by technique is avoided.

It is often possible to reach the descending colon without forming a sigmoid loop, and almost always without the need to apply abdominal compression, which may partially obstruct the lumen and make intubation more difficult if applied too early. If a sigmoid loop has been formed (Fig. 4.34A), it should be reduced once the upper descending colon is reached, usually by clockwise rotation and withdrawal. The particular benefits of compression applied to the sigmoid colon are in preventing the reformation fo a sigmoid loop, while intubation of the splenic flexure and transverse colon are undertaken. The patient should continue to lie in the left lateral position, which allows the nurse to apply compression with the heel of the left hand in the region of the umbilicus, pressing down into the left iliac fossa and compressing the anterior abdominal wall against the ala of the sacrum. The palm of the left hand is brought down over the left iliac fossa and the fingers compress the abdominal wall against the iliac crest (Fig. 4.34B), leaving a channel under the palm of the hand in which the straightened sigmoid colon is constrained. In this position, it is often possible for the nurse to sense the pressure of the colonoscope against the palm of the hand when a loop is either forming or reforming.

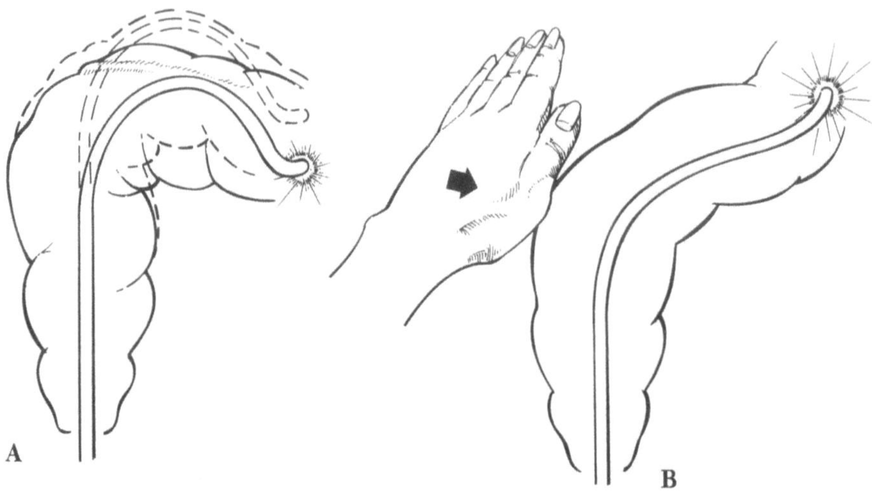

Fig. 4.34. A. When endoscope tip is in proximal sigmoid, scope advancement often produces an enlarging sigmoid loop (**A**) rather than advancement of tip. If loop is reduced, usually by withdrawal and clockwise rotation, compression can often be applied as shown (**B**) to prevent the sigmoid loop reforming, permitting tip to advance. Compression should not be used to reduce loop, but is only applied once the endoscope has been straightened to prevent loop from reforming.

Splenic Flexure

When the splenic flexure has been passed, it may not be necessary to maintain compression on the sigmoid loop. However, if progress through the transverse colon is slow or difficult, then reapplication of the sigmoid compression (after first restraightening the sigmoid) will often facilitate passage along the transverse colon by permitting the force of insertion to be transmitted to the distal tip of the colonoscope.

In patients who have a high splenic flexure, insertion into the transverse colon may be made easier by the nurse/assistant hooking the right hand around the patient's left loin and compressing medially (Fig. 4.35), thus pulling the descending colon and splenic flexure medially, while the colonoscopist makes repeated short advances and withdrawals with clockwise rotation.

Transverse Colon

Compression may be especially useful in the transverse colon. In patients who have a dependent U-shaped transverse colon descending into the pelvis, upward compression by the nurse/assistant, using the medial border of the right hand pressed into the patient's abdomen just above the umbilicus, will prevent the transverse colon from sagging into the pelvis (Fig. 4.36). This will often permit passage of the colonoscope to and around the hepatic flexure, and it may also be useful to apply this compression when in the ascending colon but having difficulty in reaching the pole of the cecum or entering the ileocecal valve. The usual techniques of withdrawal of the endoscope will often help to straighten the transverse colon, and compression can be used to maintain the straightened instrument.

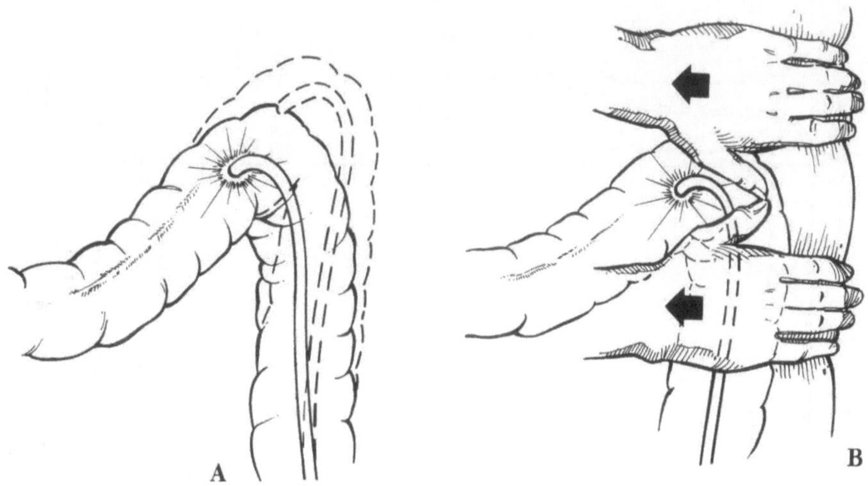

Fig. 4.35. A. Occasionally the endoscope tip will not advance around the splenic flexure into transverse colon, but simply rises higher under left diaphragm. (**B**) Pulling forward (*arrows*) on upper descending colon from flank often resolves this holdup, sometimes with simultaneous sigmoid compression to stop a sigmoid loop from forming again.

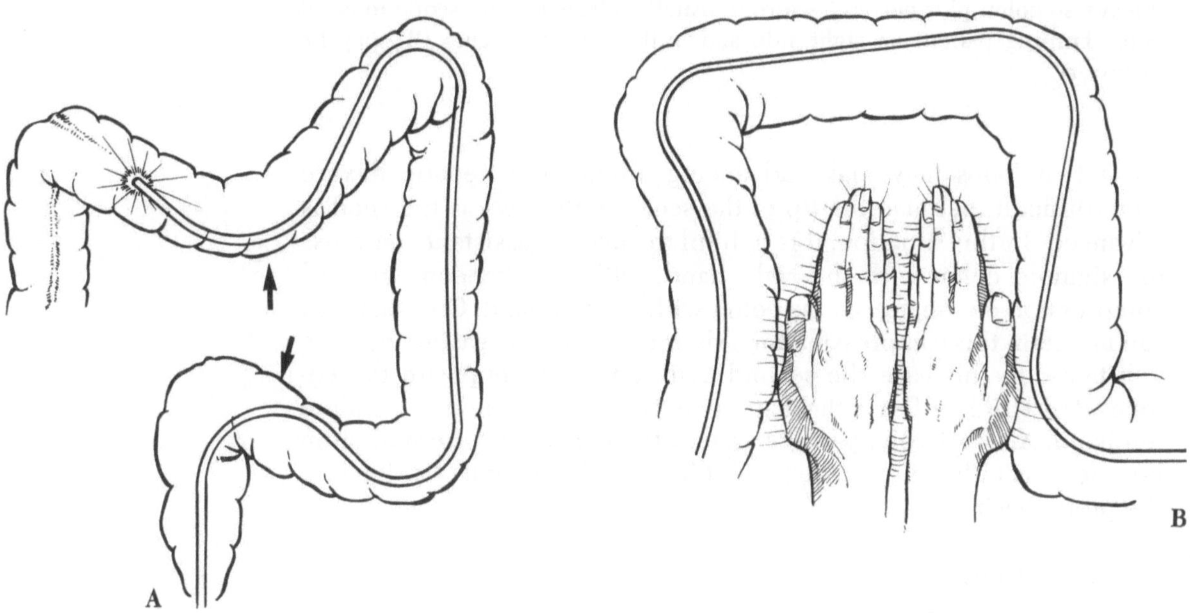

Fig. 4.36. A. With tip in proximal transverse colon, maintaining slight clockwise torque may prevent loops forming, but often both sigmoid and transverse colon loops tend to form as scope is advanced (*arrows*), so that tip may retreat as instrument is advanced. **B.** Double compression (applied once loops have been straightened) usually enables tip to be advanced around hepatic flexure.

Hepatic Flexure

Passage around the hepatic flexure does not usually present many problems, but when a sigmoid loop is present and tending to reform, and when a sagging transverse colon is present, the combination of

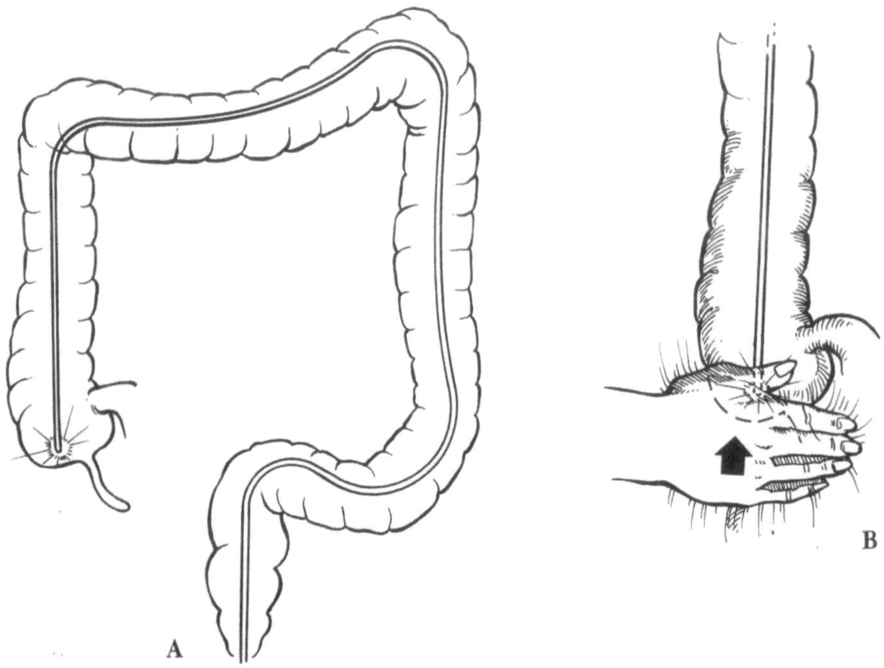

Fig. 4.37. A. When tip is arrested in midascending colon, compression of transverse colon plus clockwise torque usually advances endoscope to cecal pole. Turning patient on right side and pulling up on cecum (**B**) may be necessary.

these two loops may make advancing around the hepatic flexure more difficult, because the tip of the scope withdraws as the shaft is advanced. In this situation, it is helpful to have the assistant compress the sigmoid colon with the right hand, with simultaneous upward compression on the transverse colon with the left hand. One assistant can maintain this compression for a short time, but it is easier with two assistants; in this case the second assistant stands opposite the colonoscopist and performs the transverse colon life maneuver with the left hand. Alternatively, passage around the hepatic flexure will often be made easier by turning the patient from the left lateral position into the prone position.

Ascending Colon to Cecum

Once in the ascending colon, compression maneuvers may be helpful to prevent the sigmoid from looping or the transverse colon from sagging down into the pelvis. The method to try first, which usually is sufficient, is the application of transverse colon compression as previously described, with the assistant putting pressure in the midline and just above the umbilicus (Fig. 4.37). Should this not work, then the addition of compression of the sigmoid colon will often help to facilitate passage from the midascending colon, down to the pole of the cecum. Both these maneuvers may be helpful in obtaining the optimal position for intubation of the ileocecal valve.

The orifice of the ileocecal valve is located on the undersurface of the valve. The scope is passed to the appendix and then withdrawn slightly until the valve orifice just comes into view at the edge of the field. The tip of the scope is then very slowly angled toward the orifice, and will usually slip into the ileum once the correct angle has been established.

Passage of the endoscope to the cecum should always be attempted, even if the primary purpose of the colonoscopy is to remove a sigmoid polyp seen at barium enema, because there is often a second lesion that was overlooked on the radiographs. Ileal intubation is usually easiest with the patient supine, and should also be attempted routinely so that the skill to achieve this is available when required. Most experienced endoscopists will reach the cecum in 90%–95% of patients and intubate the ileum in 90% of those in whom the cecum has been reached [35].

A description of the techniques of polypectomy and other therapeutic aspects of colonoscopy is beyond the scope of this manual.

Defecography (Evacuating Proctography)

Indications

1. Constipation
2. Obstructed defecation
3. Incontinence
4. Rectal and perineal pain
5. Suspected intussusception, rectocele, enterocele, and prolapse
6. Postoperative assessment.

Contraindications and Precautions

The only contraindication to defecography is suspected perforation. As a precaution in patients who have had recent pouch surgery, and in whom the examination is being performed to look for leakage, water-soluble contrast should be used. In patients who have recovered from pouch surgery, liquid barium should be used rather than the barium sulfate paste [36].

Materials (Fig. 4.38)

1. Barium sulfate, 150 ml
2. Water, 400 ml
3. Electric heater
4. Potato starch, 100 g
5. 300-ml wide-tipped syringe
6. Injection pistol
7. Short wide anal catheter
8. Hollow receptacle or defecography chair (see page 96) [37]

First, 150 ml of barium sulfate is diluted in 400 ml of water. The suspension is heated, and 100 g of potato starch is gradually mixed in. Care is taken to prevent lumps. The mixture is now poured into a 300-ml syringe and cooled.

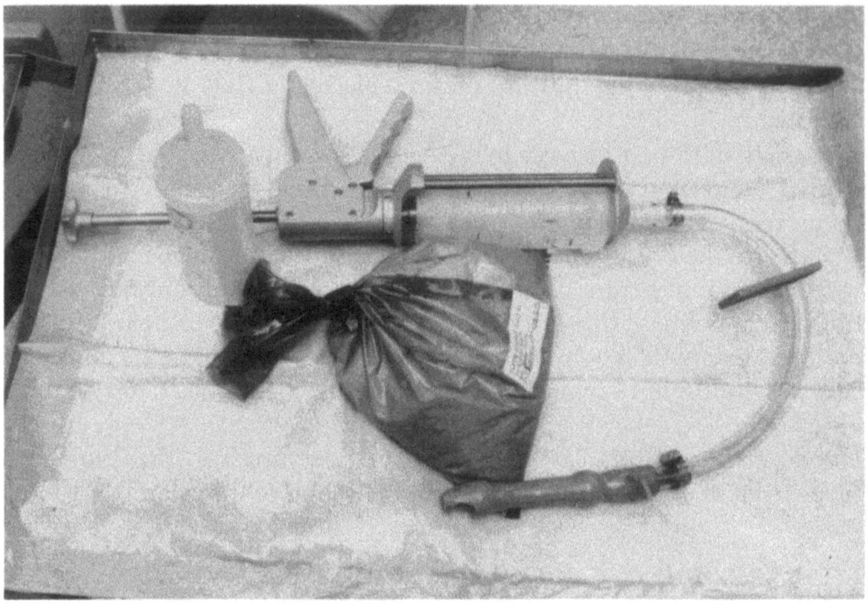

Fig. 4.38. Orthopedic cement gun with plastic syringe adapted for defecography. Barium paste is in plastic bag [38].

Preparation

No patient preparation is required. Fluid from an enema may dilute the barium and cause poor coating. A tampon soaked in water-soluble contrast is placed in the vagina in female patients.

☐ *Procedure*

Step 1. With the patient in the left lateral decubitus position, the rectal tube is inserted.
Step 2. With the injection pistol, the barium paste is introduced until the rectum is filled comfortably. Without stopping the injection the rectal catheter is withdrawn. This allows for opacification of the anal canal. The skin immediately posterior to the anal canal is marked with a smear of petroleum gel impregnated with barium.
Step 3. The patient is now seated on a hollow receptacle/defecography chair in such a way that lateral views of the rectum can be obtained.
Step 4. The examination is videotaped and spot films are taken with the patient relaxed at rest, squeezing and lifting, straining, evacuating, and at postevacuation (Fig. 4.39). Thus, five films are obtained. During videofluoroscopy the patient is asked to lift and squeeze and then relax, to strain and then relax, to cough, and finally to empty the rectum.
Step 5. Occasionally an AP film may be obtained (Fig. 4.40).
Step 6. From the films the following information is obtained: anorectal angle (Fig. 4.41) at rest, lifting, straining and evacuating; whether the anal canal is closed or open at rest, squeezing and straining, and whether any incontinence is observed; whether the puborectalis sling appears normal or is reduced; whether the sling becomes more appar-

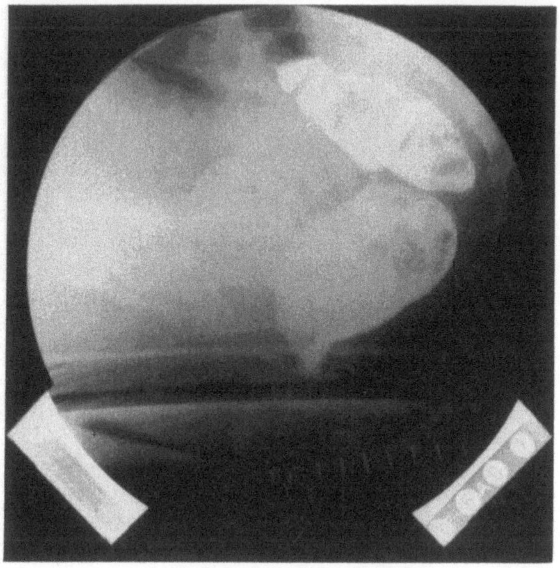

A

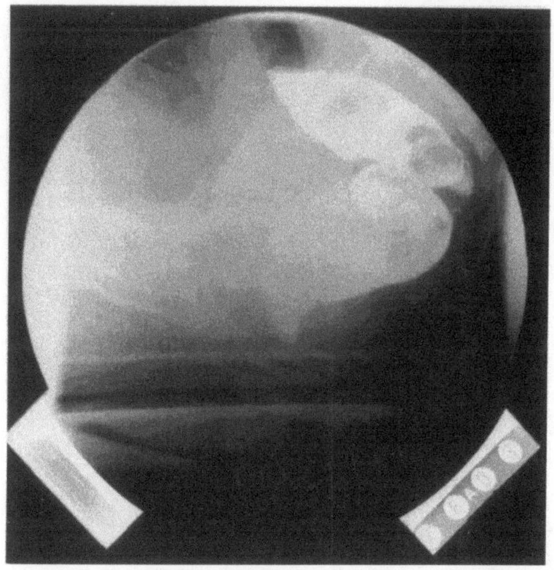

B

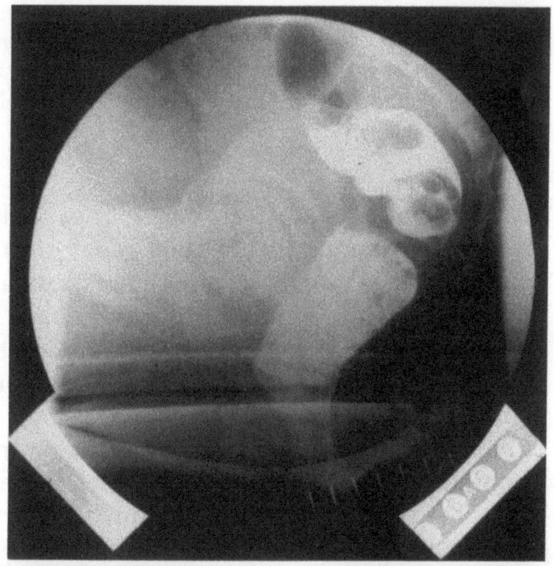

C

Fig. 4.39. Three films from evacuating proctography, at rest (**A**), during squeeze or lift (**B**), and during early evacuation (**C**). Note change in height of pelvic floor, anorectal angle, and opening of anal canal.

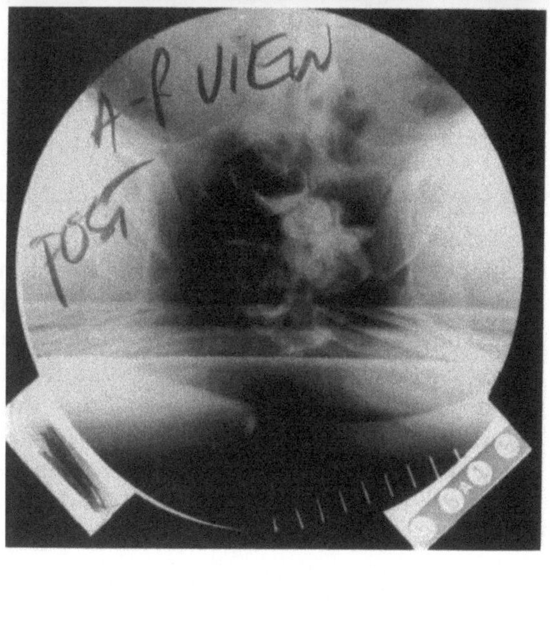

Fig. 4.40. Defecogram, AP film.

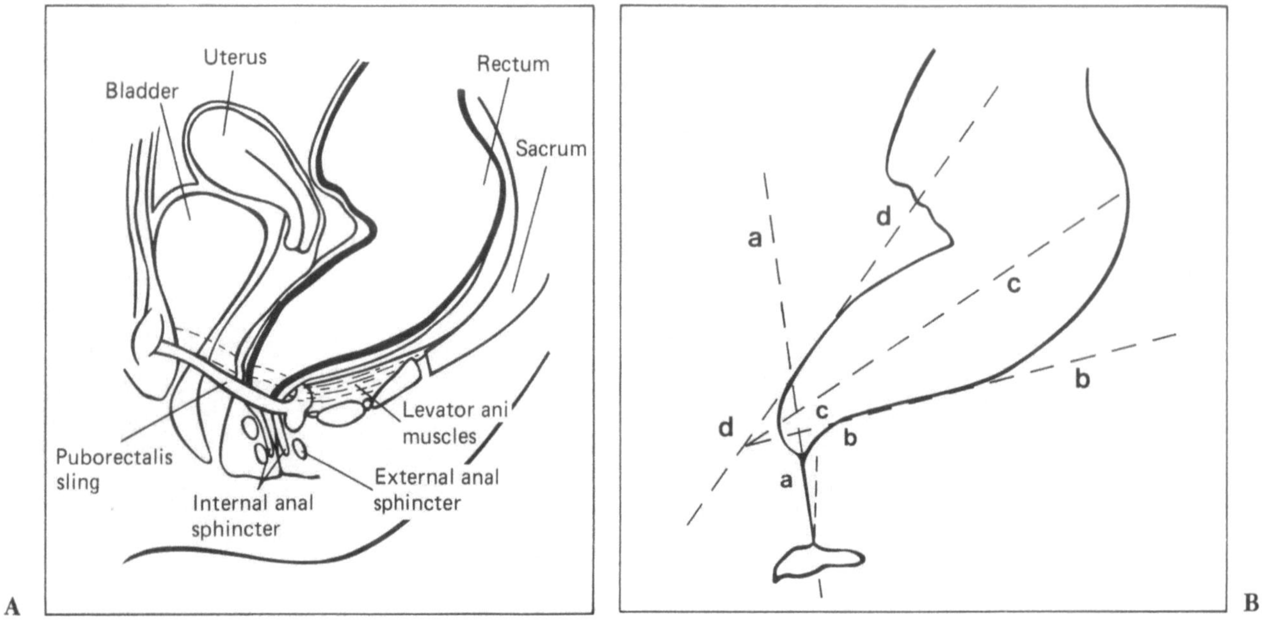

Fig. 4.41. A. Normal functional anatomy of anorectal junction. B. Problems with measuring anorectal angle. Most authors use angle of anal canal and posterior rectal wall (aa to bb), but the angle itself is of limited use. (Courtesy P.J. Shorvon).

ent during lifting and disappears during straining as it should; whether satisfactory opening of the anal canal occurs during evacuation and whether evacuation is complete. Abnormalities that are looked for include intussusception of rectal mucosa, the development of rectocele, and failure of relaxation of puborectalis sling. The amount of elevation and depression of the pelvic floor is also noted with these maneuvers.

The value of defecography is still under investigation. It is a simple examination to perform and one which patients do not find difficult. It seems to give a considerable amount of information and may be particularly useful in patients with incomplete evacuation and those with incontinence [38–40].

Defecography Throne (Fig. 4.42)

The requirements are for a comfortable commode that allows lateral fluoroscopy, produces even radiographic density from the widest part of the pelvis down to and below the line of the buttocks, and allows the anal canal to be seen without distracting glare on the screen. This necessitates a filtration device to absorb the unwanted radiation from below the seat and buttocks. Designs incorporating tubular metal in and around the seat cause a distracting number of lines on both the fluoroscopic screen and the "spot" 105-mm films that at times will block out information valuable in the interpretation of the results of the procedure. In addition, the metal used in construction will, at times,

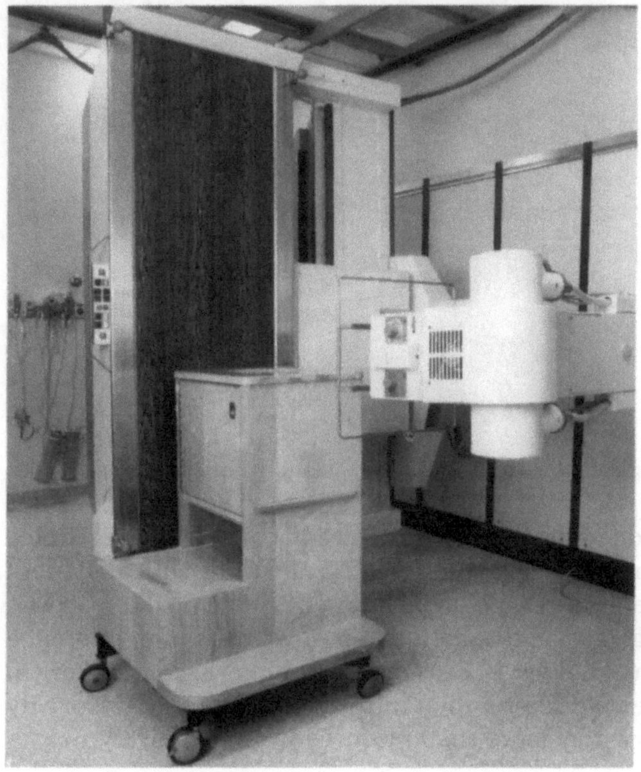

Fig. 4.42. Defecography throne.

interfere with the Automatic Brightness Control (ABC) and Automatic Exposure Control (AEC) of the fluoroscopic and spot film device.

For these reasons, we chose wood for the construction of our throne. The current seat is made of solid pine but is not ideal, as it would be better to have the wood grain perpendicular rather than parallel to the x-ray beam. Plywood should be avoided as it produces multiple distracting lines on the image. An additional toilet seat above the wooden platform to make it appear more like an ordinary toilet seat simply adds artefactual lines to the image and is therefore not recommended. The hole in the seat is circular, which makes it easier for the patient to turn sideways for AP fluoroscopy. This maneuver adds useful information when the lateral fluoroscopic views are confusing.

Radiation Filtration

Various designs have been experimented with for the radiation filtration device, and in general these may consist of either water in containers below the seat, or metal filtration plates attached to the side of the commode. When water is used, a width of about 38 cm is needed, either as a rubber or plastic doughnut beneath and in contact with the seat to avoid an air gap, or as two large plastic bottles filled with water (two 4-liter Golytely bottles are suitable). An alternative is to use 4 to 5 mm of copper filtration attached to the side of the throne and comprised of two parts, each being 2 to 2.5 mm thick. The first part lies in

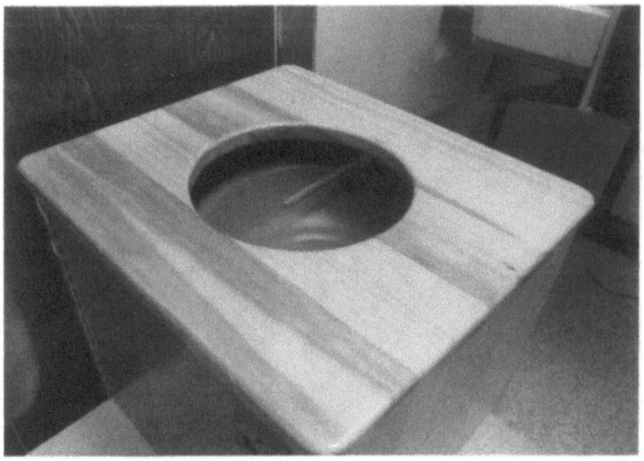

Fig. 4.43. Proctography chair shows midline plastic ruler with 1-cm marks.

contact with the side of the throne; it is 15 × 40 cm × 2–2.5 mm thick. Over it lies a second piece of copper, 2 to 2.5 mm thick with a segment cut out that represents the shape of the buttocks sitting on the seat. The crescent-shape edged is gently tapered to remove the sharp difference between the two thicknesses. Because patients being examined vary in size, we made a second filter with a different curvature that is easily exchanged for one with a more shallow curve when necessary.

Midline Measurements

A radioopaque ruler is included in the commode. This consists of a piece of plastic with 1-cm lead markers attached to the back of the seat by a spring. This allows direct measurement from the films of distances in the sagittal plane of the patient, such as anal canal length, pelvic floor movement, and separation of the rectum from the sacrum (Fig. 4.43). The ruler rests beneath the plastic bag which is used for stool collection. It indents the bag and because it is on a spring is not obtrusive to the patient.

Mobility

The addition of wheels to the commode has made it much easier for technologists to set up the room quickly, and has also facilitated centering. Small clamps on the sides of the throne are attached to the table top so that lateral table movement from the remote console permits rapid alterations in centering during the procedure. The use of wheels also allows repositioning for AP fluoroscopy for those patients who find it difficult to adjust their own position on the throne.

Height of Commode

This is dictated by how low the tube and intensifier will come when the table is upright. Since this is at least 105 cm for many tables, a system of steps is needed for patients to climb up to the appropriate height, and be seated. In addition, retractable footrests are incorporated for patients to place their feet on while sitting, both for the lateral and AP projections.

Stool Collection

A plastic bag is placed on the commode, over the midline ruler. If water is being used as the radiographic filter, the bag is placed in the centre of the water ring. If copper plates are used, it is more convenient to put the plastic bag in a bowl on the shelf and to tuck the ruler under the plastic. The bag is then changed by removing the bowl at the end of each examination.

Postoperative Colon

Early Postoperative

Indications

The two most common indications for examination in the early postoperative period are abdominal distension, pain, and fever. Patients with abdominal distension should be investigated for ileus or obstruction, and patients with pain and fever for leakage and abscess formation.

1. Ileus or obstruction?
The abdominal film often does not allow the distinction to be made as low colonic obstruction with an incompetent valve will produce dilatation of both large and small bowel, and ileus can sometimes affect predominantly either the large or small bowel. A contrast enema should be performed if doubt persists for more than 24 to 48 hours. Water-soluble contrast should be used, and some recommend that it should be diluted 25% to reduce its hypertonicity [41]. A balloon catheter is often necessary but excessive colon distension should not be allowed to occur, and relaxants (such as glucagon) should be used freely if there is spasm. Contrast medium should be run in until the clinical questions has been answered. Thus, if the plain film has shown a dilated colon down to the sigmoid, and the sigmoid obstruction was questioned, it will be sufficient to run the barium to the transverse colon. When distension is principally ileal, it will be useful to run the contrast some distance up the small bowel. Increasing colon distension during the study may prevent this from being achieved safely, and the examination should be halted rather than allowing the colon to be overdistended in an attempt to get through the ileocecal valve.
2. Suspected anastomotic leak
Water-soluable contrast medium should be used, and Gastrografin, diluted 25%, is satisfactory. The contrast should be run in slowly and the advancing edge carefully watched as it goes through the area of the anastomosis. The patient should be turned so that views at right angles can be obtained, to avoid missing small leaks or fistulae. Contrast is run well beyond the anastomosis so that a reasonable opportunity is provided for leakage to occur. A postevacuation or postdrainage film is essential as it may occasionally show a leak or a small abscess missed during the fluoroscopic part of the examination. If the patient is sick or immobile, a second technician or nurse should be present during the study to help you in the necessary turning of the patient.

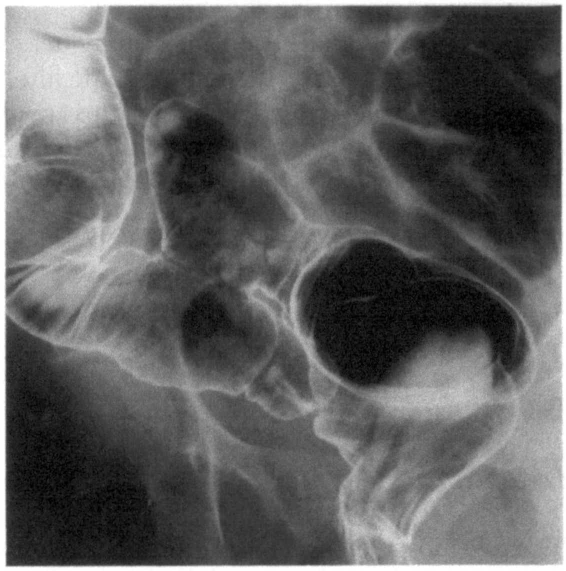

Fig. 4.44. Double-contrast demonstration of unusual side-to-side colonic anastomosis.

Late Postoperative

General Principles and Indications

Most late postoperative examinations of the colon are performed for neoplasia or inflammatory bowel disease, to look for recurrent or additional polyps and carcinomas, or to detect inflammatory bowel disease and its complications such as dysplasia, polyps, and fistulae.

A double-contrast examination will almost invariably be required, and will follow the principles discussed earlier (page 63) [42]. The caliber of anastomoses is often a concern. Every effort has to be made to obtain a true tangential view of the anastomosis, and tube angulation is helpful on remote control tables. if an anastomosis appears narrow, it is worthwhile using glucagon or Buscopan to differentiate spasm from stricture. Specific technical points are discussed next.

Although most anastomoses are made end to end, other possibilities include end to side, side to side (Fig. 4.44), and side to end. Dilatation of the blind ends associated with these side anastomoses can occur and may be associated with ulceration and bleeding, or with bacterial overgrowth. The exact nature of anastomoses should therefore be elucidated and reported. Consultation with the referring surgeon before the study is important for establishing the exact postoperative anatomy.

1. Right hemicolectomy. Reflux into the small bowel is a concern in patients with a previous right hemicolectomy for two reasons. If washouts are used as part of the preparation the ileum may be full of fluid that will impair coating of the mucosa, and barium may flood into the small bowel obscuring the sigmoid. More care than usual should therefore be taken initially to complete the examination of the left colon before barium is allowed to enter the transverse colon. For this pur-

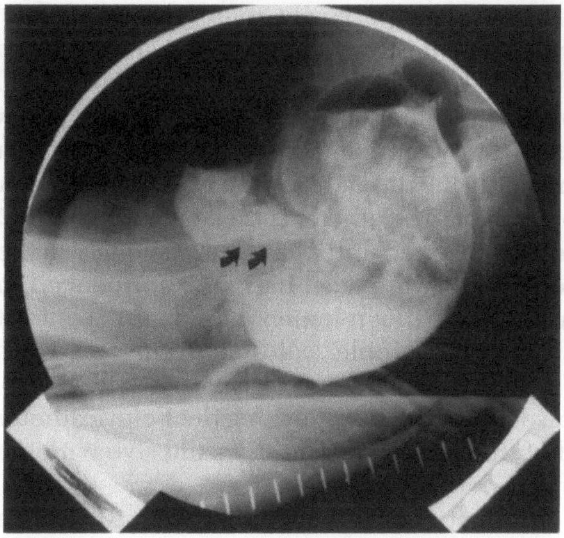

Fig. 4.45. Evacuating proctogram with liquid barium in patient with ileal pelvic pouch after total colectomy. Notice efferent limb (*arrows*) connecting pouch to anal canal. Length of this limb and its continence are important factors to assess during this examination.

pose the newer, rapidly flowing bariums are less useful (Polibar plus or Flocoat), and the slower, good-coating bariums (Polibar and HD85) are more controllable.

Once the left colon has been filmed, ample amounts of barium should be maneuvered into the ileum to mix with any residual fluid. If coating is inadequate it is worth draining the colon by putting the bag on the floor, and then running the barium in again. Spot films of the ileocolic anastomosis with intravenous relaxants are best done at the end of the examination when coating is optimal.

2. Left hemicolectomy. These examinations are often easier than standard enemas because there is less sigmoid. Occasionally adhesions make it impossible to get a tangential view of the anastomosis clear of other loops. Views of the anastomosis at right angles are helpful for detection of mucosal irregularity.

3. Ileal pelvic pouch [43]. These patients are usually difficult to examine. Indications are either incontinence or a difficulty in emptying the pouch, which may be related to difficulty in voluntary active emptying or difficulty in intubation. The problem is usually in the efferent limb connecting the pouch to the anal canal, and the radiological examination is directed to assessing this limb (Fig. 4.45). Unlike the acute problems in which water-soluble contrast is used, these delayed problems are best examined with barium, ideally double contrast.

4. Colostomy enema [44]

i. Distal. It is usually easier to examine the distal limb of a colostomy from below by inserting a catheter into the rectum and introducing barium. Having the patient apply pressure with a pad over the colostomy site with the bag in place will often allow a double-contrast examination to be performed, although a relaxant should be given as spasm is often seen. It is possible to pass a catheter into the distal limb of a colostomy, and this route is preferable when there is anal or rectal pain or tenderness, such as in severe perianal Crohn's disease.

There are several devices for colostomy enemas. The simplist is to use a Foley catheter, but leakage of barium is a major problem. Blowing up a balloon within an ostomy is not without risk and is not recommended [45]. A satisfactory method is to enlarge the hole in a teat from a baby's feeding bottle and thread it over a Foley catheter for about 6 in. The rubber balloon on the catheter is then cut with a pair of scissors. The Foley catheter is inserted until the teat sits snuggly in the colostomy, and the patient holds it in place. Barium is introduced in the main lumen, and air into the balloon lumen for a double contrast enema. Commercial air-contrast nipple colostomy tips are also available.

Adequate results can also be obtained by pushing the Foley catheter through a hole in a band of stomadhesive. The stomadhesive with the catheter is then applied to the colostomy site.

ii. Proximal. After the introduction of the catheter, barium should be introduced slowly, and the rapidly flowing varieties are best (Polibar plus or Flocoat). Most colostomies are of the descending or transverse colon, and barium will flow best if the patient is turned half on the right side, and if descending colon, also slightly head down. Air should not be started until barium is in the ascending colon, as otherwise the air often overtakes the barium, and these patients have limited mobility as they are holding the catheter in place (Fig. 4.46). An intravenous bowel relaxant should be used, and high-quality double-contrast examinations can usually be achieved.

5. Internal diversions. Ileocolic and colocolic anastomoses are sometimes made for inflammatory bowel disease or unresectable neoplasia. When the radiologist is informed about the details of previous surgery there is usually no problem in performance of the examination; however, this is not always the case. In Crohn's disease, there is an increased incidence of carcinoma in bypassed segments of both small and large bowel. Barium may flow preferentially into one or other limbs with a bypass, and it is seldom possible to demonstrate the whole segment satisfactorily.

6. Appendectomy. A leak after appendectomy is very rare, but could be shown by single-contrast enema. More often a short appendix stump may fill, or a small polyp may be found from the invaginated stump. The cecal films should be adequate to demonstrate that the nodule is at the tip of the cecum in the expected position of the appendix.

Cancer and Polyp Follow-Up: Barium Enema or Colonoscopy

After resection of carcinoma or adenoma, there is an increased incidence of further neoplasms. After cancer resection, this rises to 12% for further cancers and 83% for further adenomas after 25 years. In addition, 10% of patients who have had an adenomatous polyp resected will have another one a year later, probably overlooked at the initial colonoscopy. Furthermore, a minority, perhaps 15%, of patients with cancer who get a recurrence have their recurrence at the anastomosis, although distant metastasis is much commoner. For these reasons colonoscopy is to be preferred as the first follow-up examination, and should be carried out 1 to 2 years after colonoscopic polyp resection,

Fig. 4.46

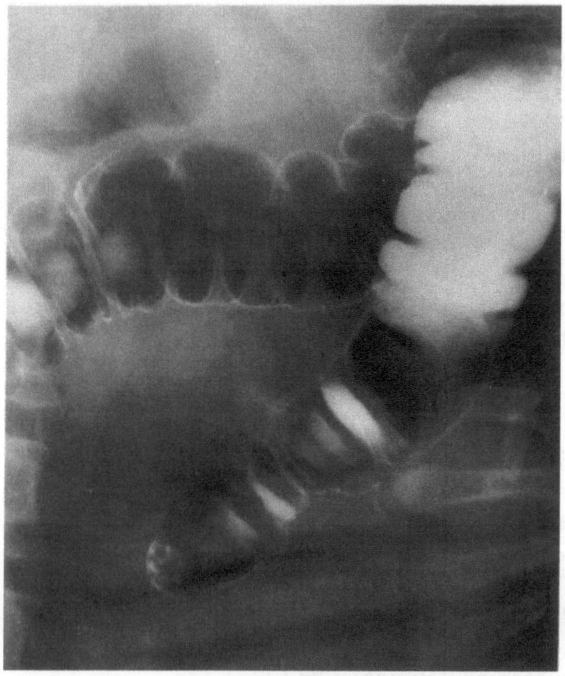

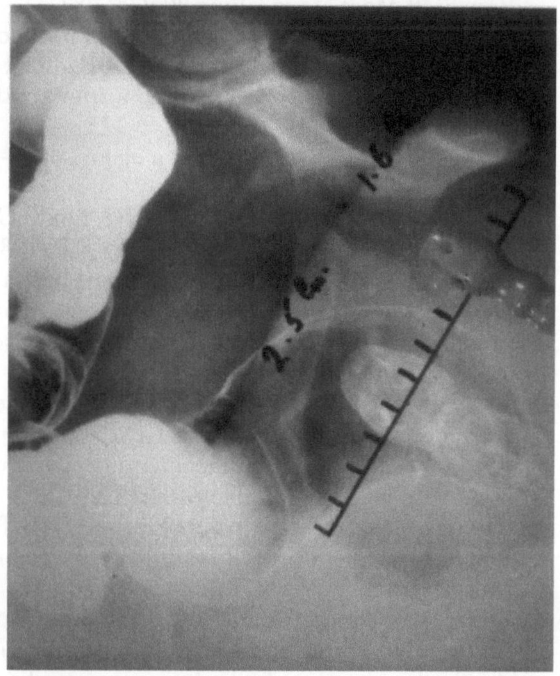

Fig. 4.47

Fig. 4.46. Double-contrast study performed through colostomy. Patient helps prevent leakage of barium by compressing over colostomy. Reproduced with permission from Stevenson GW. Technique of examination, in Margulis, Burhenne. Alimentary Tract Radiology, 3rd ed. 1983, p. 1716, Fig. 68-12.

Fig. 4.47. Polyp size can be overestimated because of magnification. Magnification factor can be established by comparing actual size of enema tube tip to size obtained on lateral rectal spot film.

and a few months after successful resection of a carcinoma. These times will be shortened if the diagnostic examinations at the time of the initial treatment were suboptimal.

Colonoscopy does miss perhaps 10% of substantial polyps, and therefore a case can be made for alternating double-contrast barium enema and colonoscopy for the follow-up of colorectal neoplasia. Although barium enema in the best hands misses 15% of substantial polyps, the combination of barium enema and colonoscopy detects almost 100% because the two techniques tend to miss lesions in different locations. An important technical point to remember when reporting polyp size from barium radiographs is that the size may be overestimated because of magnification. The magnification factor can be estimated by comparing the actual size of the barium enema tip to the size measured on the radiographs (Fig. 4.47).

References

1. Ott DJ, Chen YM, Gelfand DW, Wu WC, Munitz HA (1986). Single-contrast vs double-contrast barium enema in the detection of colonic polyps. AJR 146:993–996.

2. Pratt JH, Jackman RJ (1945). Perforations of the rectal wall by enema tips. Proc Staff Meet Mayo Clinic 20:277–283.
3. Nelson JA, Davies AU, Dodds WJ (1979). Rectal balloons: complications, causes and recommendations. Invest Radiol 14:48–59.
4. Seaman WB, Wells J (1965). Complications of the barium enema. Gastroenterology 48:728–737.
5. Barnes MR (1968). How to get a clean colon—with less effort. Radiology 91:948–949.
6. Present AJ, Jansson B, Burhenne HJ, Dodd GD, Goldberg HI, Goldstein HM, Miller RE, Nelson JA, Stewart ET (1982). Evacuation of 12 colon-cleansing regimens with single contrast barium enema. AJR 139:855–860.
7. Davis GR, Smith HJ (1983). Double-contrast examination of the colon after preparation with Golytely (a balanced lavage solution). Gastrointest Radiol 8:173–176.
8. Ernstoff JJ, Howard DA, Marshall JB, Jumshyd A, McCullough AJ (1983). A randomized blinded clinical trial of a rapid colonic lavage solution (Golytely) compared with standard preparation for colonoscopy and barium enema. Gastroenterology 84:1512–1516.
9. Girard CM, Rugh KS, Dipalma JA, Brady CE, Pierson WP (1984). Comparison of Golytely lavage with standard diet/cathertic preparation for double-contrast barium enema. AJR 142:1147–1149.
10. Chan CH, Diner WC, Fontenot E, Davidson BD (1985). Randomized single-blind clinical trial of a rapid colonic lavage solution (Golytely) vs. standard preparation for barium enema and colonoscopy. Gastrointest Radiol 10:378–382.
11. Fitzsimons P, Shorvon P, Frost RA, Stevenson GW (1987). A comparison of Golytely and standard preparation for barium enema. J Can Assoc Radiol 38:109–112.
12. Harned RK, Wolf GL, Williams SM (1980). Preliminary abdominal films for gastrointestinal examinations: how efficacious? Gastrointest Radiol 5:343–347.
13. Eisenberg RL, Hedgcock MW (1981). Preliminary radiograph for barium enema examination: is it necessary? AJR 136:115–116.
14. Laufer I (1976). The double-contrast enema: myths and misconceptions. Gastrointest Radiol 1:19–31.
15. Kelvin FM, Gardiner R, Vas W, Stevenson GW (1986). Colorectal carcinoma missed on double contrast barium enema study: a problem in perception. AJR 137:307–313.
16. Eisenberg RL, Meyers PC, May ST (1983). Optimum overhead views in double-contrast barium-enema examinations. AJR 140:505–506.
17. Johnson JO, Amberg JR (1988). Air-contrast colon examination and sigmoid hernia: avoiding perforation. AJR 150:948.
18. Maglinte DDT, Miller RE (1984). Salvaging the failed pneumocolon: a simple maneuver. AJR 142:719–720.
19. Thoeni RF, Vandeman F, Wall SD (1984). Effect of glucagon on the diagnostic accuracy of double-contrast barium enema examinations. AJR 142:111–114.
20. Harned RK, Stelling CB, Williams S, Wolf GL (1976). Glucagon and barium enema examinations: a controlled clinical trial. AJR 126:981–984.
21. Coblentz CL, Frost RA, Molinaro V, Stevenson GW (1985). Pain after barium enema: effect of CO_2 and air on double-contrast study. Radiology 157:35–36.
22. Bernier P, Coblentz C (1986). CO_2 delivery system for double-contrast barium enema examinations. Radiology 159:264.
23. Rajagopalan AJ, Mason JH, Kennedy M, Pawlikowski J (1977). The value of the barium meal in the diagnosis of acute appendicitis. Arch Surg 112: 531–533.

24. Rice RP, Thompson WM, Fedyshin PJ, Merten DF, Kelvin FM, Williford ME (1984). The barium enema in appendicitis: spectrum of appearances and pitfalls. RadioGraphics 4:393–409.
25. Scholz FJ (1989). Manual compression device for fluoroscopy. Radiology 170: 564–565.
26. Young AC (1963). The 'instant' barium enema in proctocolitis. Proc R Soc Med 56:491–494.
27. Thomas BM (1979). The instant enema in inflammatory disease of the colon. Clin Radiol 30: 165–173.
28. Bartram CI, Preston DM, Lennard-Jones JE (1983). The "air enema" in acute colitis. Gastrointest Radiol 8:61–65.
29. Farrands PA, Vellacott KD, Amar SS, Balfour TW, Hardcastle JD (1983). Flexible fiberoptic sigmoidoscopy and double-contrast barium-enema examination in the identification of adenomas and carcinoma of the colon. Dis Colon Rectum 26:725–727.
30. Harned RK, Consigny PM, Cooper N, Williams SM, Woltjen AJ (1982). Should barium enemas be performed following biopsy of the rectum or colon? Gastrointest Radiol 7:95 (abstr).
31. Maglinte DDT, Strong RL, Strate RW, Caudill LD, Dyer PA, Chernish SM, Graffis RF (1982). Barium enema after colorectal biopsies: experimental data. AJR 139:693–697.
32. Merrill CR, Steiner GM (1986). Barium enema after biopsy: current practice and opinion. Clin Radiol 37:89–92.
33. Gilbert DA, Hallstrom AP, Shaneyfelt SL, Mahler AK, Silverstein FE (1984). The National ASGE Colonoscopy Survey—Complications of colonoscopy. Gastrointest Endosc 30:156.
34. Obrecht WF, WU WC, Gelfand DW, Ott DJ (1984). The extent of successful colonoscopy: a second assessment using modern equipment. Gastrointest Radiol 9:161–162.
35. Coremans G, Rutgeerts P, Geboes K, Van den Oord J, Ponette E, Vantrappen G (1984). The value of ileoscopy with biopsy in the diagnosis of intestinal Crohn's disease. Gastrointest Endosc 30:167–172.
36. Kremers PW, Scholz FJ, Schoetz DJ, Veidenheimer MC, Coller JA (1985). Radiology of the ileoanal reservoir. AJR 145:559–567.
37. Bernier P, Stevenson GW, Shorvon P (1988). Defectography commode. Radiology 166:891–892.
38. Mahieu P, Pringot J, Bodart P (1984). Defecography: I. Description of a new procedure and results in normal patients. Gastrointest Radiol 9: 247–251.
39. Henry MM, Swash M (1985). Coloproctology and the Pelvic Floor. Pathophysiology and Management. London: Butterworth.
40. Ekberg O, Nylander G, Fork F-T (1985). Defecography. Radiology 155: 45–48.
41. Eisenberg RL, Hedgcock MW, Shanser JD, Brenner RJ, Gedgaudas K, Marks WM (1979). Iodine absorption from the gastrointestinal tract during hypaque-enema examination. Radiology 133:597–599.
42. Goldstein HM, Miller MH (1976). Air contrast colon examination in patients with colostomies. AJR 127:607–610.
43. Hillard AE, Mann FA, Becker JM, Nelson JA (1985). The ileoanal J pouch: radiographic evaluation. Radiology 155:591–594.
44. Burhenne HJ (1970). Technique of colostomy examination. Radiology 97:183–185.
45. Gelfand DW (1980). Complications of gastrointestinal radiologic procedures: 1. Complications of routine fluoroscopic studies. Gastrointest Radiol 5:293–315.

CHAPTER 5

Pediatric Gastrointestinal Examinations

Introduction

Children are not small adults. The signs, symptoms, and disease in pediatric patients often differ considerably from those in adults. A history gathered from parents suggesting a gastrointestinal cause for symptoms may be misleading. The clinician has to evaluate the entire patient and take a complete history to ensure that unnecessary examinations are not performed. It behooves the radiologist to be aware of these problems in diagnosis, and to develop a close rapport with the clinicians to ensure that the patient receives no unnecessary radiation or discomfort in solving a diagnostic dilemma.

Further, the techniques of radiologic study are different from those in adults. Morbidity and mortality are more common in children (especially infants), and procedures are more time consuming because of the time necessary to reassure the child. Most children will cooperate in favorable surroundings with confident and considerate management, especially if reassurance is constant and friendly. A frightened child becomes an uncooperative child, often leading to an unsatisfactory examination. This is most commonly the fault of the examiner. Sedation is resorted to in our hospital only for young children undergoing interventional procedures, computed tomography (CT), or magnetic resonance imaging (MR). Sedation for sonography or contrast studies is not required and may even be dangerous under certain circumstances.

Interventional techniques, endoscopy, CT, and contrast studies of the biliary or pancreatic tree are discussed under the appropriate adult sections. The other important pediatric radiological techniques are discussed in this chapter.

Sonography

In the investigation of any child, consideration should first be given to sonography because this is a radiation-free procedure, requiring little or no preparation, and is, as far as is known, a completely safe method of investigation. In children in general, the lack of fat planes and the

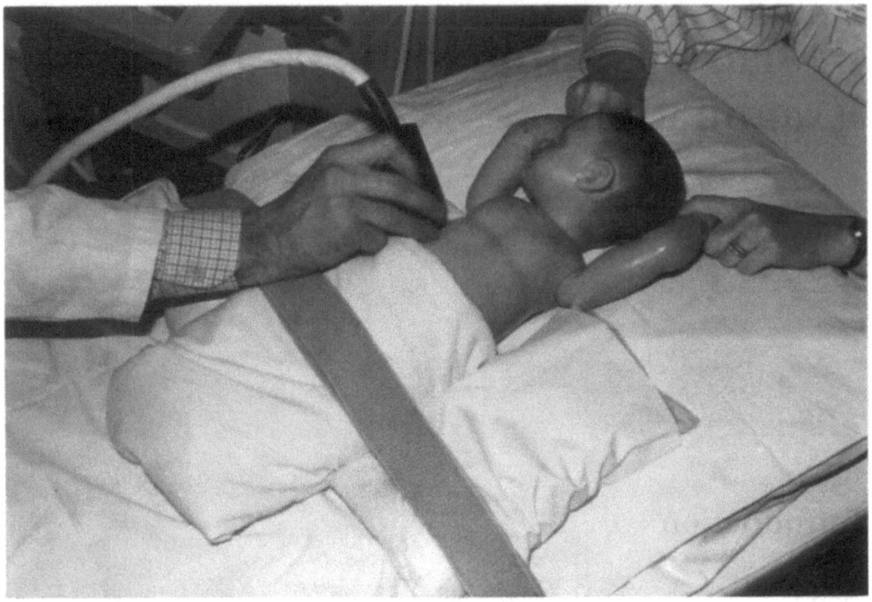

Fig. 5.1. Infant restraint. Infants can be readily restrained by binding legs in blanket and with assistant holding the arms.

smaller size of the patient make sonography easier to perform and a more reliable investigation than in adults [1].

Feeding an infant before or during the study often settles the baby enough for an adequate examination. In addition, infants can be gently restrained by binding the legs in a blanket and having an assistant hold the hands (Fig. 5.1). Explanation and reassurance is sufficient for older and many young children; sedation is unnecessary.

Indications for Examination

Mass Lesions

Sonography is the initial imaging method of choice for the investigation of abdominal mass lesions. The finding of a cystic lesion in the appropriate clinical context is often the only investigation required preoperatively. Solid lesions usually require more investigation and may require other cross-sectional imaging modalities [2]. The combination of sonography and CT as complementary techniques can give a high degree of accuracy [3].

Hypertrophic Pyloric Stenosis

Hypertrophic pyloric stenosis (HPS) in young infants is primarily a clinical diagnosis. The presence of a palpable mass, the size and shape of an olive, on the right side of the upper abdomen in a young vomiting infant is sufficient evidence to operate. Many pediatric surgeons feel that it is a matter of honor to make the diagnosis infallibly on clinical criteria, but others, including general surgeons and physicians, generally require a radiologic test to differentiate HPS from gastroesophageal reflux (GER).

Sonography, in experienced hands, is an effective modality for diagnosing HPS and can show GER [4]. The technique entails filling the stomach with dextrose saline and scanning with a 5-mHz transducer in the right hypochondrium with the baby in a right lateral decubitus position. In this way, the antrum is filled with fluid and peristalsis can be watched along with the transit of fluid from antrum to duodenum (Fig. 5.2). The presence of a pyloric muscle mass that does not open up over 15 minutes of viewing, is the major diagnostic feature of HPS, in the authors' opinion. Many measurements of the pyloric tumor have been made, and we feel that the length is the most specific [5]. The measurement taken as being abnormal varies from report to report as ranging between 14 and 16 mm [5,6]. The pylorus is accepted as being normal if it is less than 12 mm. Between 12 and 16 mm is a grey zone including some normal and abnormal patients. In addition, we have had one very premature tiny infant who developed HPS with a pyloric muscle length less than 12 mm, so these measurements should be used with caution with the overall size of the baby in mind.

Other criteria include showing continuity between stomach and duodenum through the mass [5], the presence of an antral beak and shoulders, a curved echogenic mucosal line through the center of the mass, prominent gastric peristalsis, and lack of gastric drainage (Fig. 5.3). In addition, gastroesophageal reflux is often present.

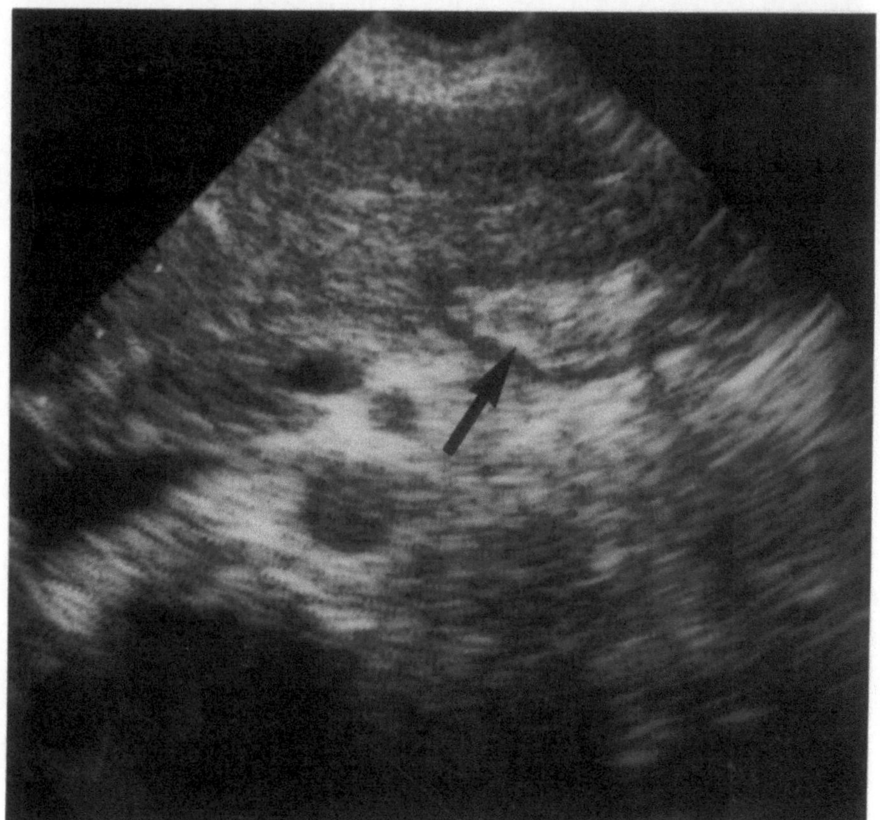

A

Fig. 5.2. Normal gastric antrum, pylorus, and duodenal cap. **A.** Transverse sonography shows gastric antrum (*arrow*) full of food, giving very echogenic center. In this patient, exact gastric wall thickness cannot be assessed and the duodenum does not fill (*continued.*)

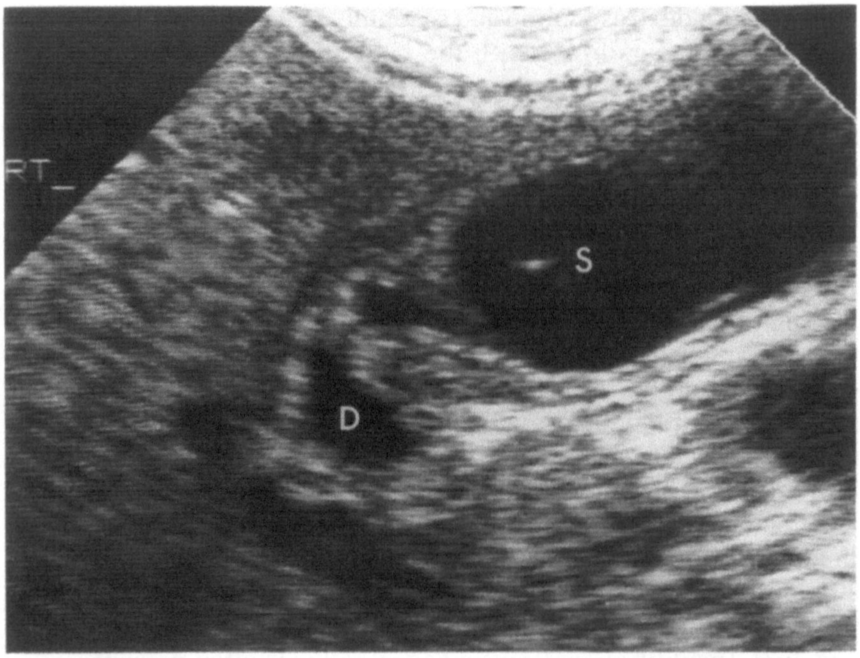

B

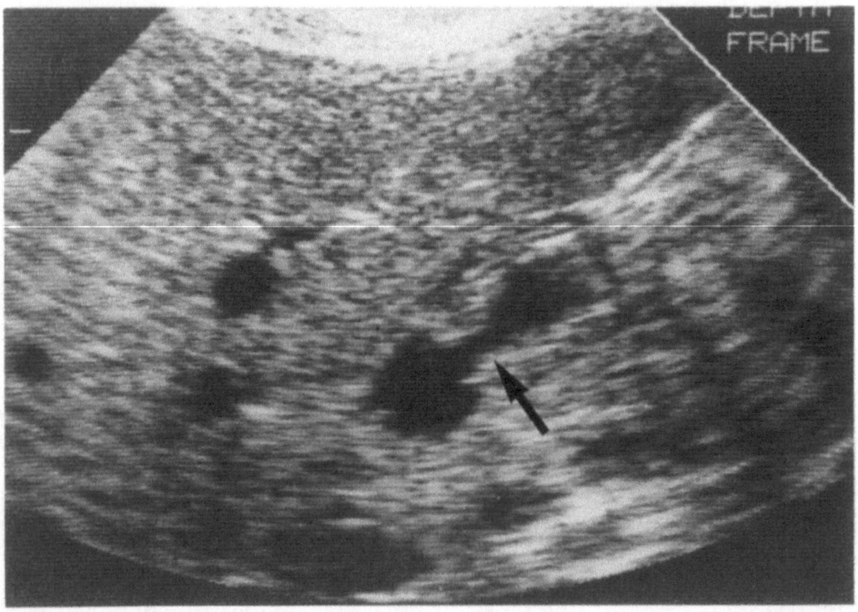

C

Fig. 5.2.B. Oblique sonography in child given clear fluids shows fluid in stomach (S) and duodenal cap (**D**). Real-time imaging of region (**C**) shows variety of appearance including normal short pyloric canal (*arrow*). In same patient, as fluid empties from gastric antrum, appearance changes (**D**) and may superficially mimic hypertrophic pyloric stenosis with apparent muscular thickening (*arrows*); however, the muscle periodically opens and fluid drains freely into duodenum.

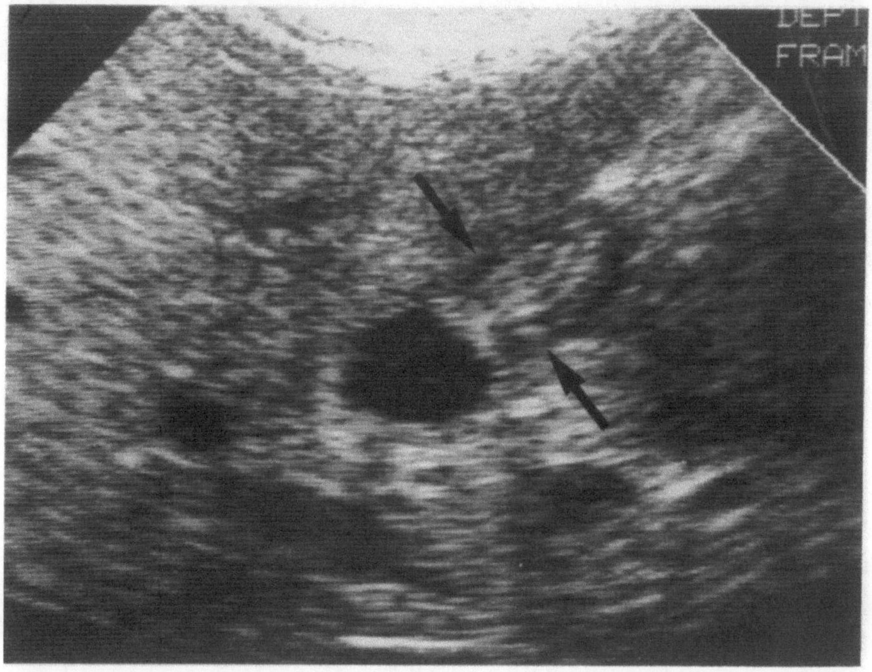

Fig. 5.2 D

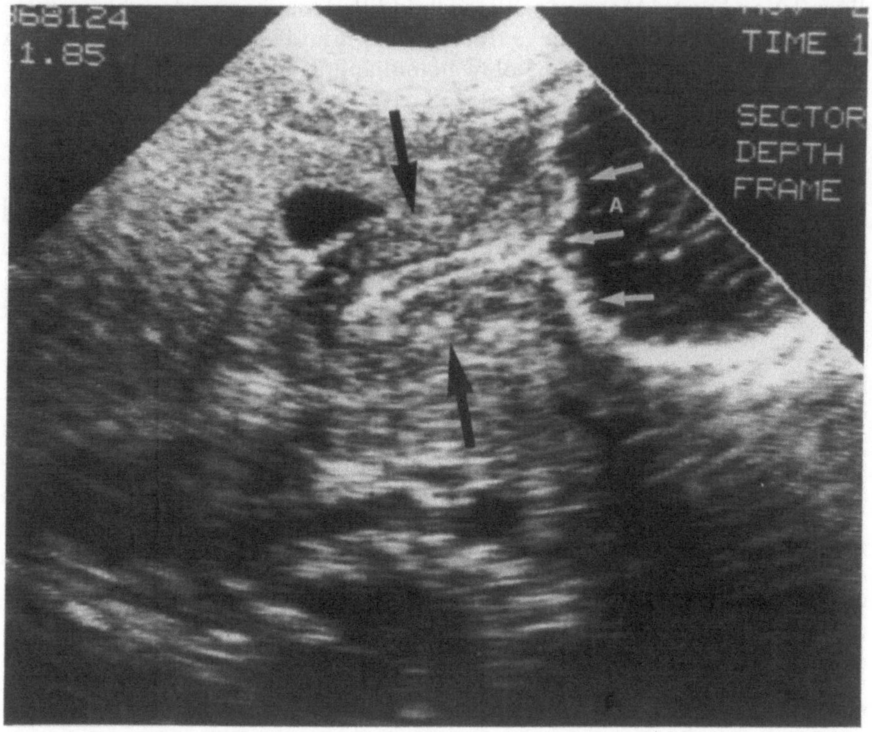

Fig. 5.3. Hypertrophic pyloric stenosis. Oblique sonography demonstrates fluid in the gastric antrum (A), a constant elongated thickened pyloric muscle (*black arrows*) and a curved echogenic mucosal line through the center of the mass. Real-time imaging demonstrates an antral beak and shoulders (*white arrows*) and prominent gastric peristalsis with lack of gastric drainage.

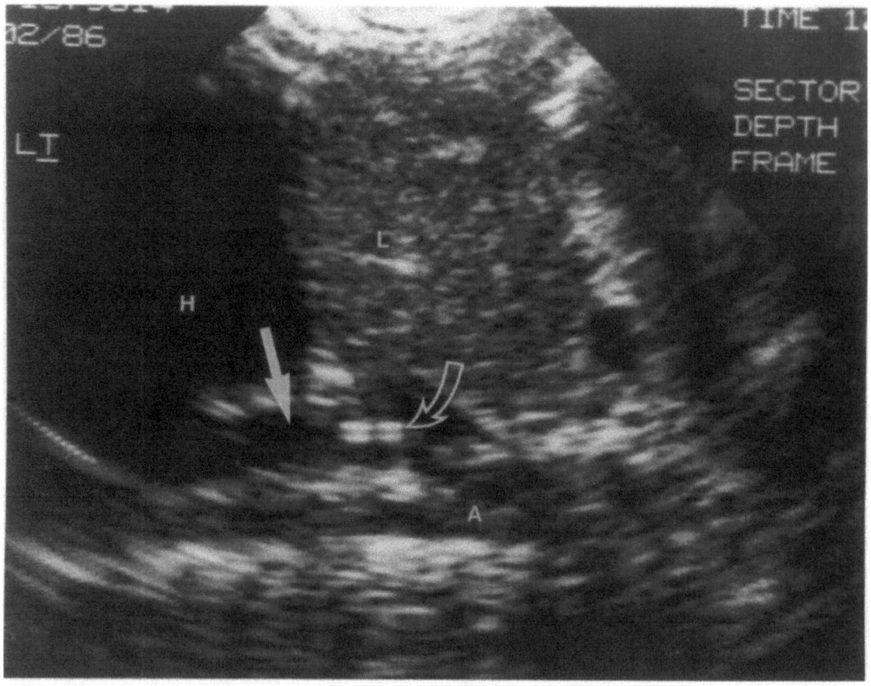

Fig. 5.4. Gastroesophageal reflux. Longitudinal sonography through heart (H), liver (L), and aorta (A) shows a dilated fluid-filled esophagus (straight arrow) in which lies a nasogastric tube (*curved arrow*). Fluid was seen to freely reflux back into the esophagus from below hemidiaphragm.

Gastroesophageal Reflux (GER)

GER can be assessed by sonography by filling the stomach with fluid and evaluating the mediastinum anterior to the descending aorta at and above the crus of the diaphragm [7,8] with the patient supine (Fig. 5.4). The sensitivity of this technique, however, is still unknown.

Gastric Wall Thickening

The gastric wall measures 2 to 3 mm in a normal child, independent of age, and consists of a hypoechoic (muscular) and hyperechoic (mucosal) layer when the stomach is full of fluid [9]. This can be used to assess many abnormalities such as inflammatory bowel disease, peptic ulcer disease, gastritis, Henoch–Schonlein purpura, and chronic granulomatous disease [9].

Small or Large Bowel

The bowel can often be evaluated in children if there is pathology. Tumors, intussusception, bowel wall thickening, acute appendicitis, and abscesses can all be diagnosed. The technique of graded compression sonography is particularly helpful in this regard. This entails gentle but gradual compression of the right iliac fossa, using the transducer, enabling visualization of the deep structures [10].

The length of large bowel atresia can also be distinguished in babies with anorectal atresia by placing the transducer on the abdomen with a moving object such as a finger adjacent to the anus or by placing the transducer on the anal dimple. The length from anal dimple to meconium-filled distal large bowel can then be ascertained, but the reliability of this technique has not yet been assessed.

Biliary Disease

As in adults, sonography is the initial imaging modality of choice for diagnosing biliary diseases or anomalies [11]. Cholelithiasis is seen more frequently than was previously thought because of sonographic demonstration of clinically unsuspected gallstones [12]. In infancy, these are often concretions of sludge and are rarely important clinically (Fig. 5.5).

Dilatation of the biliary tree, as is found in obstruction or choledochal cysts, is well demonstrated by sonography. Contrast studies of the biliary tree are now rarely, if ever, indicated in children, and so are discussed under the appropriate adult sections.

Fetal Anomalies

A raised alphafetoprotein is usually related to neural tube anomalies, but may also be found with some gastrointestinal anomalies, such as exomphalos, and esophageal or duodenal atrésia [13]. Furthermore, polyhydramnios may alert the sonographer to an anomaly [14]. Meconium ileus and peritonitis, omphalocele, gastroschisis, and diaphragmatic hernias can all be diagnosed by antenatal sonography, but discussion of these lies beyond the scope of this book [15–22].

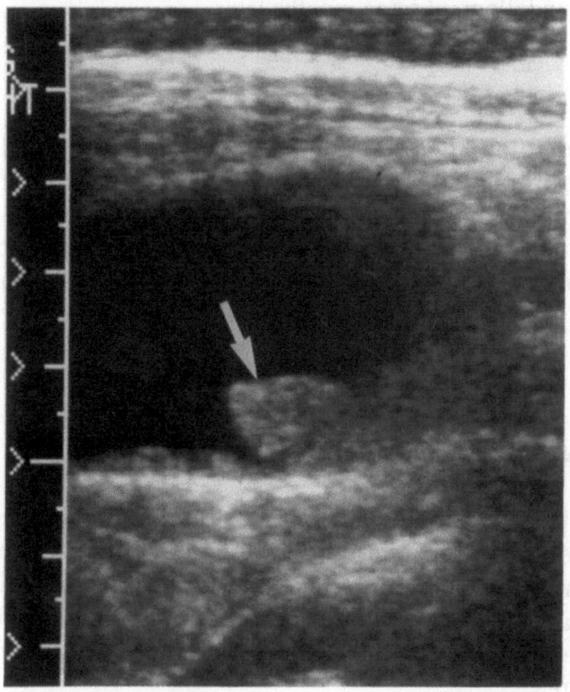

A

Fig. 5.5. Gallbladder in infancy. **A.** Concretion of sludge (*arrow*) is seen in the gallbladder (*continued.*)

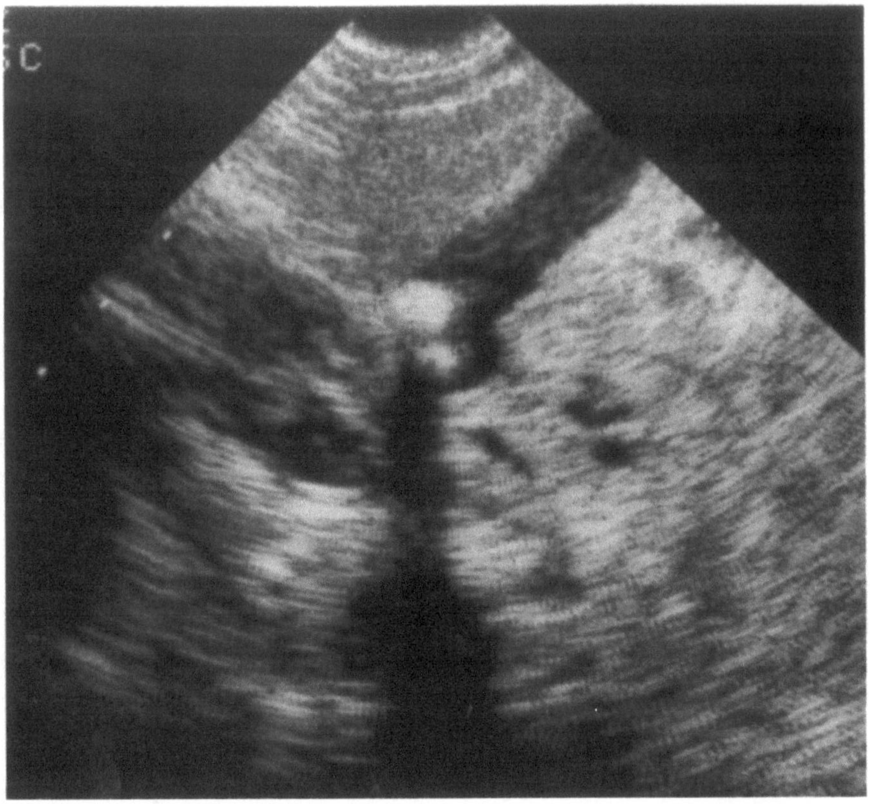

B

Fig. 5.5. B. Sludge in the gallbladder and two dense opacities, causing acoustic shadowing, are compatible with gallstones. Both these infants were asymptomatic, on total parenteral nutrition, and required no specific therapy; their gallbladders were normal on follow-up some months later.

Doppler Sonography

Duplex range-gated and colour Doppler sonography are being used increasingly to evaluate intraabdominal pathology (Fig. 5.6). It is of most value in the gastrointestinal tract in evaluating portal hypertension and hepatic blood flow in pre- or postoperative liver transplant patients [23]. In addition, major vascular thrombosis in neonates, often secondary to umbilical arterial and venous catheters, can be readily diagnosed.

Preparation for Sonographic Examinations

The biliary tree needs to be evaluated during most abdominal sonograms, and fasting is required for adequate gallbladder/biliary tree evaluation. The duration of the fast will depend on the age and clinical status of the child but average times would be 4 hours for infants, 6 hours for young children between 1 and 2 years old, and 8 hours for those over 2 years of age.

Pelvic examinations rely on the presence of a full bladder and hence young and older children are encouraged to drink plenty of fluids in the 2 hours before the examination. The normal bowel may become

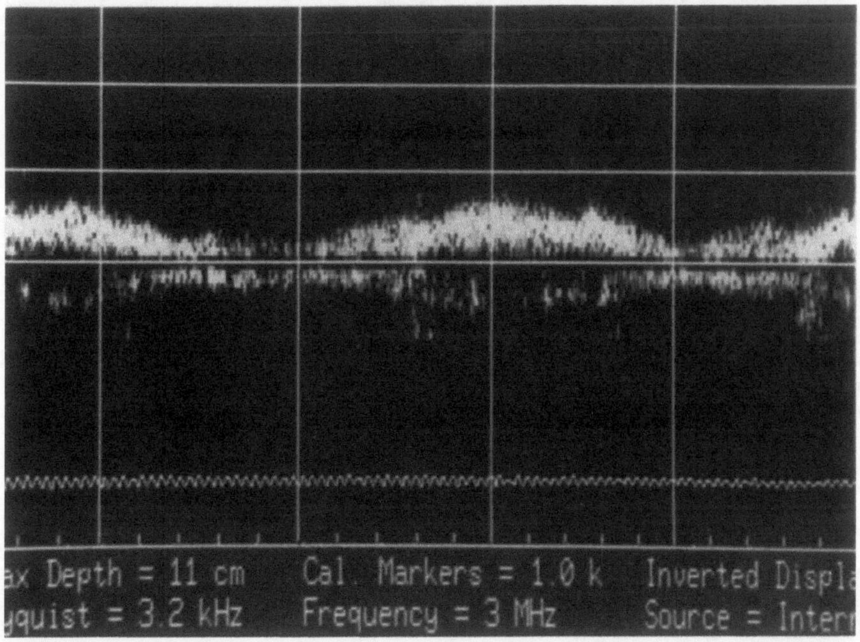

Fig. 5.6. Normal portal vein and hepatic artery blood flow. Duplex range-gated Doppler sonography demonstrates normal flow in the portal vein.

distended with fluid after a feed of dextrose saline (Fig. 5.7), and this should not be confused with an abnormality. The evaluation of infants with the utilization of a full bladder is to a large extent dependent on luck and good timing.

Upper GI Contrast Examinations in Children

Feeding Study

Indications

To evaluate an older infant or child who can be fed only with great difficulty. These children often have a degree of cerebral palsy. The study concentrates on mouth and tongue movements in relation to bolus formation of a variety of foodstuffs.

Contraindications and Precautions

There is always a risk of aspiration in these unfortunate children, especially because many have severe neurological problems. The swallowing (posterior oropharyngeal and esophageal) mechanism can also be assessed as well as the feeding (anterior oropharyngeal) function.

Materials

Barium sulfate is mixed with the everyday food that the particular child has difficulty ingesting, such as Pablum, milk, or solid food. A variety of

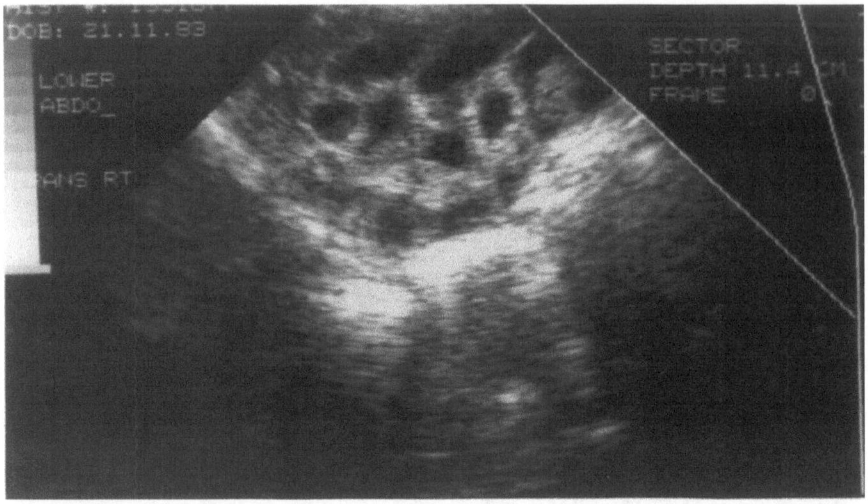

Fig. 5.7. Normal small bowel. Following a feed of dextrosaline, many small bowel loops are filled with fluid, and active peristalsis can be seen on real-time examination. This finding should not be confused with an abnormality.

prosthetic devices, spoons, syringes, and types of food can be tried for each patient.

Patient Preparation

The child is prepared as for a usual meal. The child *must* have had a prior assessment by an occupational therapist, who should be present at the radiologic examination.

□ *Procedure*

The procedure is aimed at recreating the circumstances in which the child is usually fed. This is usually upright, often supported by a tailored chair. The person who feeds the child should be the usual person involved in that child's care, whether nurse, parent, foster parent, or occupational therapist. The occupational therapist who knows the patient must be present and liaise with the radiologist during the procedure. Between them a variety of feeding devices and types of food preparation can be assessed.

We have found that the commonest abnormality of feeding is lack of coherent tongue movement. Placing the food over the dorsum of the tongus is often helpful in these patients, and can be achieved by a variety of feeding devices or maneuvers commonly used by occupational therapists.

The oropharynx is viewed in the lateral position and the examination is recorded on a dedicated videotape. Films are usually unnecessary except to document obvious aspiration or nasal escape (Fig. 5.8).

Aftercare

As per normal feed.

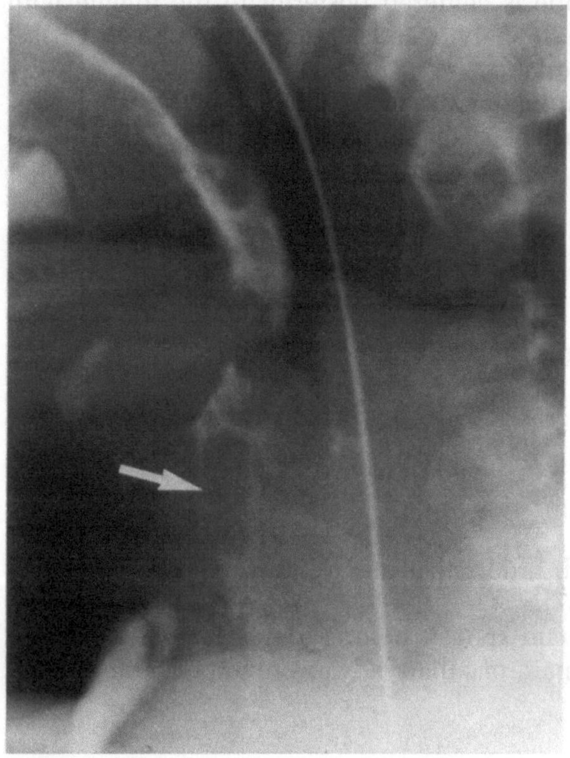

Fig. 5.8. Lung aspiration. Barium preferentially entered the trachea (*arrow*) rather than the esophagus. Position of the esophagus is indicated by a nasogastric tube. The marked aspiration seen in this child precludes oral feeding.

Swallowing Study

Indications

To assess swallowing abnormalities or difficulties affecting the posterior oropharynx including nasal escape or possible aspiration.

Contraindications and Precautions

Because of the risk of aspiration, only small amounts of contrast medium should be given initially. If there is no aspiration, larger quantities can then be given.

Materials and Preparation

As per standard esophagus, stomach, and duodenum study.

□ *Procedure*

The child is fed lying down on the right side and a video fluoroscopic recording of the posterior oropharyngeal swallowing mechanism is obtained. The fluoroscope is centered posterior to the tongue with coning to include the nasopharynx and larynx. Aspiration and nasal escape are carefully observed.

This study can be combined with a full evaluation of the esophagus, stomach, and duodenum. The examination is recorded on a dedicated video cassette and films are taken only to document any aspiration or nasal escape (Fig. 5.8).

Aftercare

As per standard esophagus, stomach, and duodenum study.

Speech Study

Indications

1. To evaluate speech disorders that may require pharyngoplasty or speech therapy [24–27].
2. Occasionally to evaluate speech before adenoidectomy, Le Fort operation, fracture repair, maxillary advancement, or other craniofacial surgery.

Contraindications and Precautions

The child needs to be cooperative and hence is usually over 5 years of age. Some cooperative 4-year olds can also be assessed.

Materials

One to 2 ml of barium sulfate 55% w/w and 100% w/v is instilled into each nostril with a syringe. We use Polibar at our institution.

Preparation

Prior speech assessment and discussion of procedure. The speech pathologist must be present during the radiographic assessment so that the findings can be fully discussed [25].

□ *Procedure*

For the examination, 1 to 2 ml of high-density barium (Polibar 56% w/w) are instilled into each nostril and sniffed back into the nasopharynx with the patient supine. The patient is sitting for the lateral, frontal, and Waters views, lying supine for the Towne view, and lying prone for the basal view. A series of phrases is repeated by the patient in each projection to assess velopharyngeal closure in a variety of speech tasks, and the entire examination is recorded on videotape with sound recording. Each patient repeats the sentences,

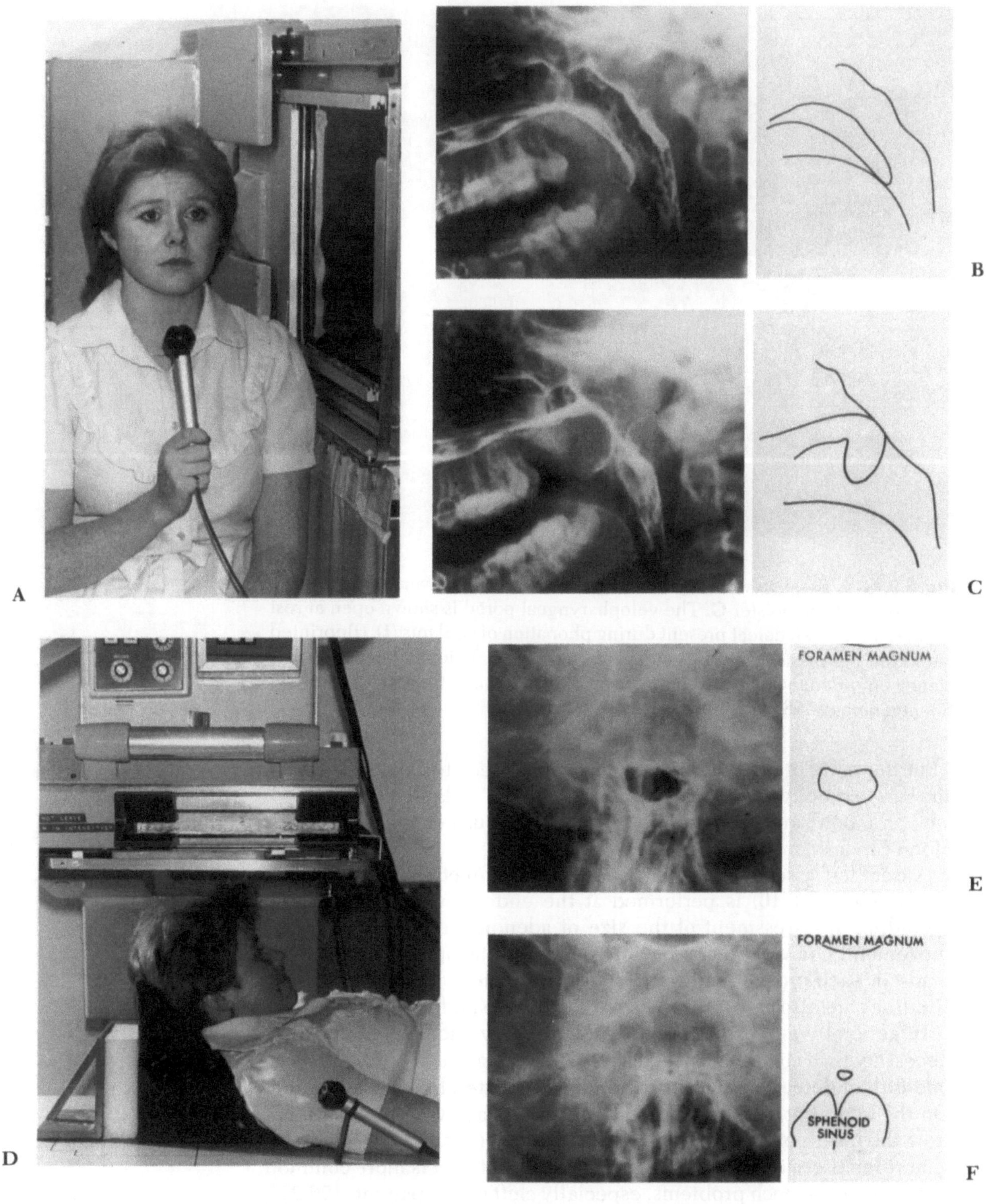

Fig. 5.9. Velopharyngeal portal evaluation. **A–C.** Lateral view. The patient sits on a footstool (**A**). The velopharyngeal portal is shown open at rest (**B**) and closed during phonation of sibilants (**C**). **D–F.** Towne view. The patient lies supine with neck extended on foam bolster (**D**). The velopharyngeal portal is shown open at rest (**E**) and with a small defect during phonation of sibilants(**F**) (*continued.*)

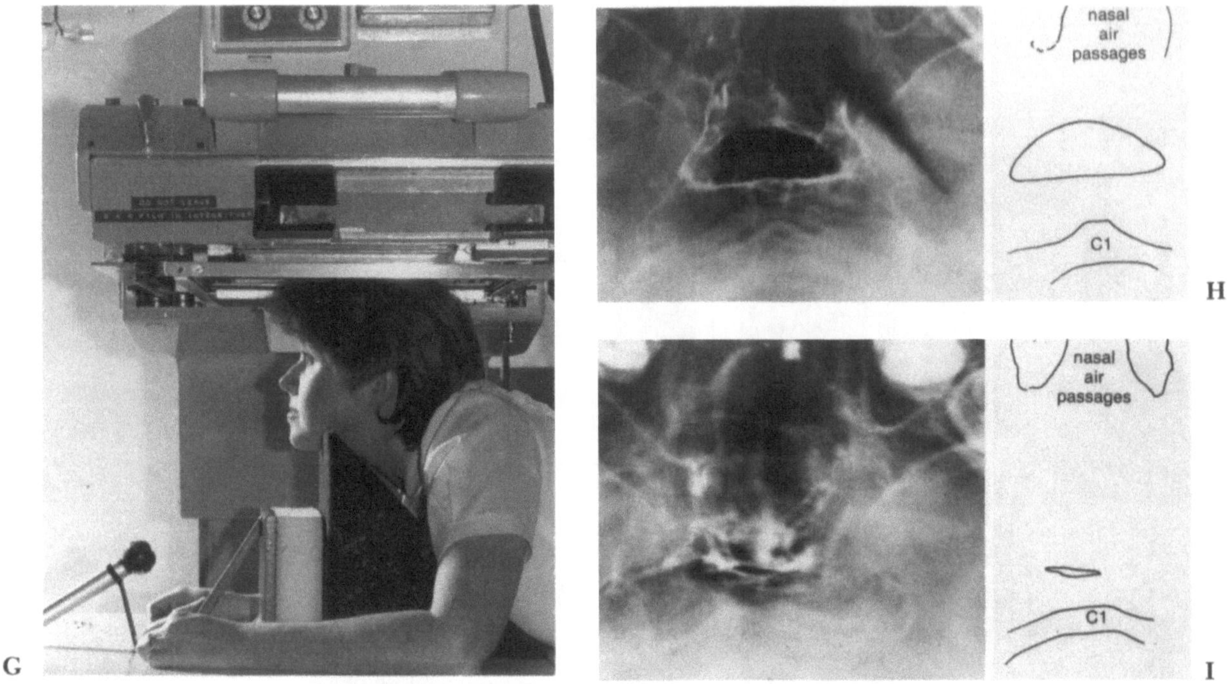

Fig. 5.9. G–I. Basal view. The patient lies prone with head vertical by resting on arms and foam bolster **G**. The velopharyngeal portal is shown open at rest (**H**) and has a small defect present during phonation of sibilants (**I**). (Reprinted with kind permission from Stringer DA, Witzel MA, Velopharyngeal insufficiency on videofluoroscopy, comparison of projections, American Journal of Roentgenology 1986;146:15–19.)

"Put the baby in the buggy; give Gary the chocolate cake; Susie sees the sun in the sky; my name is ____", as well as making the sounds 's', 'sh', and 'ooh', and counting from 1 to 10. The use of isolated sounds alone can fail to reveal all defects.

A detailed assessment of the anatomy and function on each view (Figs. 5.9 and 5.10) is performed at the end of every examination, including an assessment of the size of adenoids and consistency of movement. Drawings of the velopharyngeal portal open and closed are made in each projection. the results of the projections are compared. Findings are also assessed in terms of presence and size of adenoids.

In general we find that only the lateral view and Towne view are necessary for a complete speech assessment (Fig. 5.9A–F). As many as one-fifth of defects may be missed if only the lateral view is obtained. On the lateral projection, a prominent ridge (Passavant ridge) arising from the posterior pharyngeal wall may be seen (Fig. 5.11). This Passavant ridge is occasionally seen in normal patients but is more common in those with speech problems, especially cleft palate patients [26,27]. If lateral pharyngeal wall movement is important, the Waters view is preferable to the AP view and is performed with the patient erect [26,27].

Aftercare

Follow-up by speech pathologist.

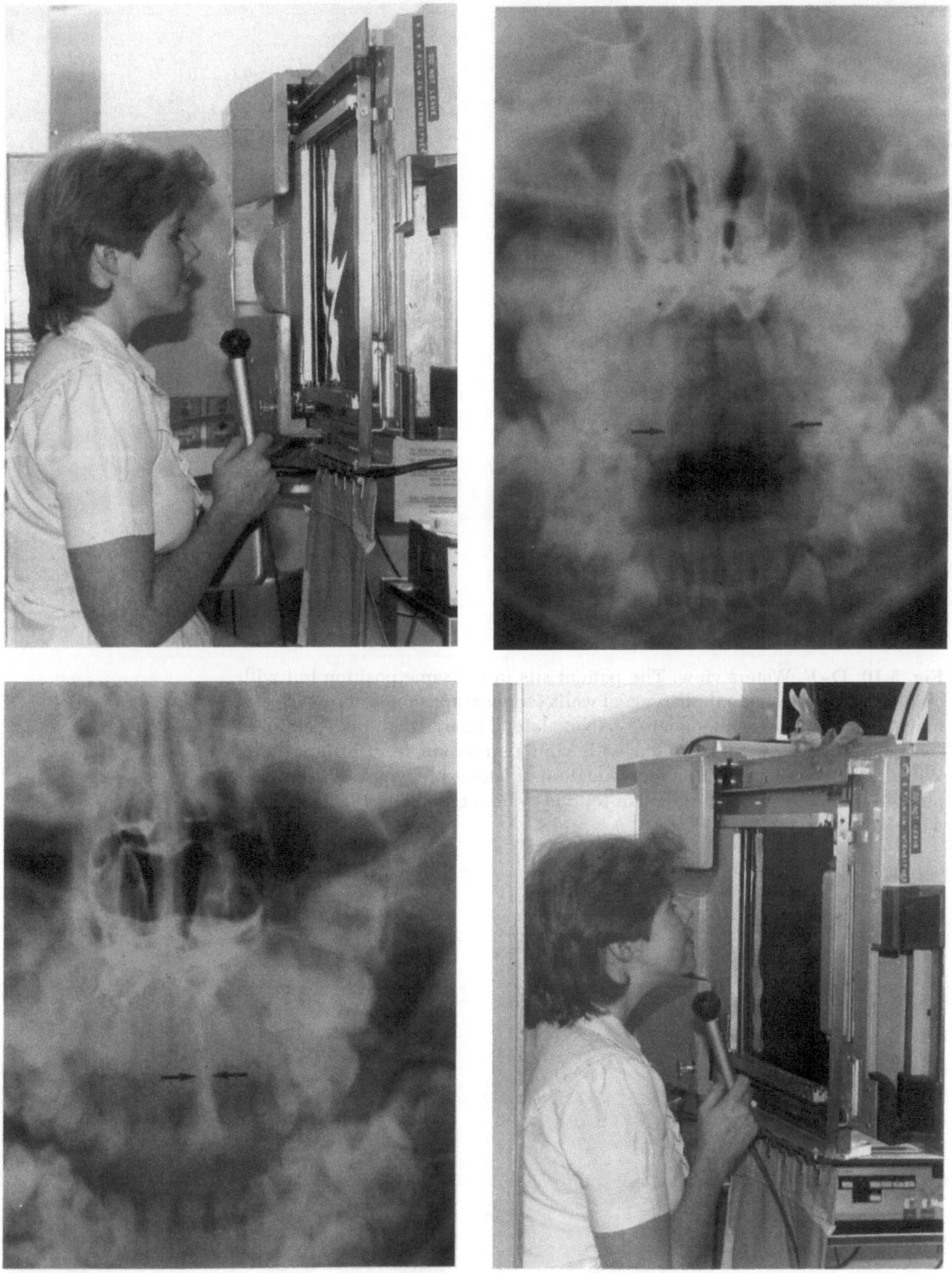

A B C D

Fig. 5.10. Velopharyngeal portal evaluation. **A–C.** Frontal view. The patient sits on a footstool (**A**). Lateral pharyngeal walls (*arrows*) are shown at rest (**B**) and during phonation (**C**) (*continued.*)

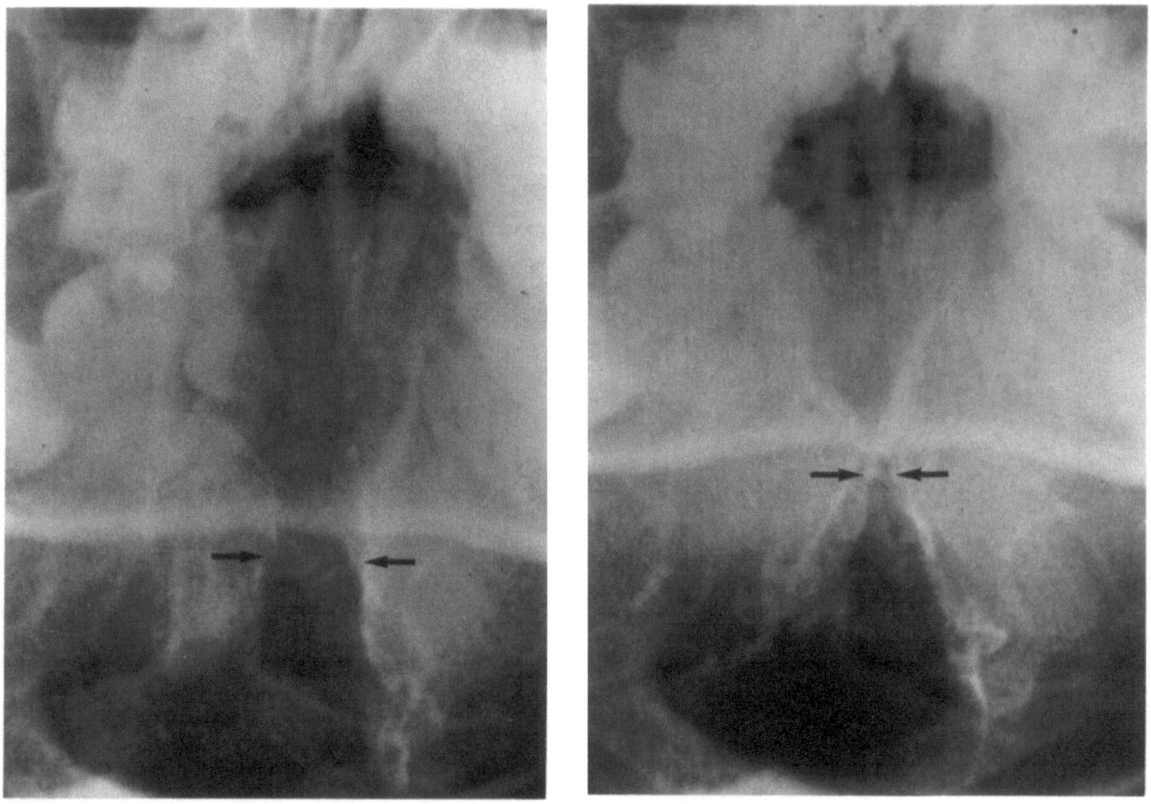

E F

Fig. 5.10. D–F. Waters view. The patient sits in the same position but with chin elevated (**D.**) Lateral pharyngeal walls (*arrows*) are shown at rest (**E**) and move medially during phonation (**F**). (Note lateral pharyngeal wall is easier to see on Waters view.) (Reprinted with kind permission from Stringer DA, Witzel MA, Waters projection for evaluation of lateral pharyngeal wall movement in speech disorders, American Journal of Roentgenology 1985;145:409–410.)

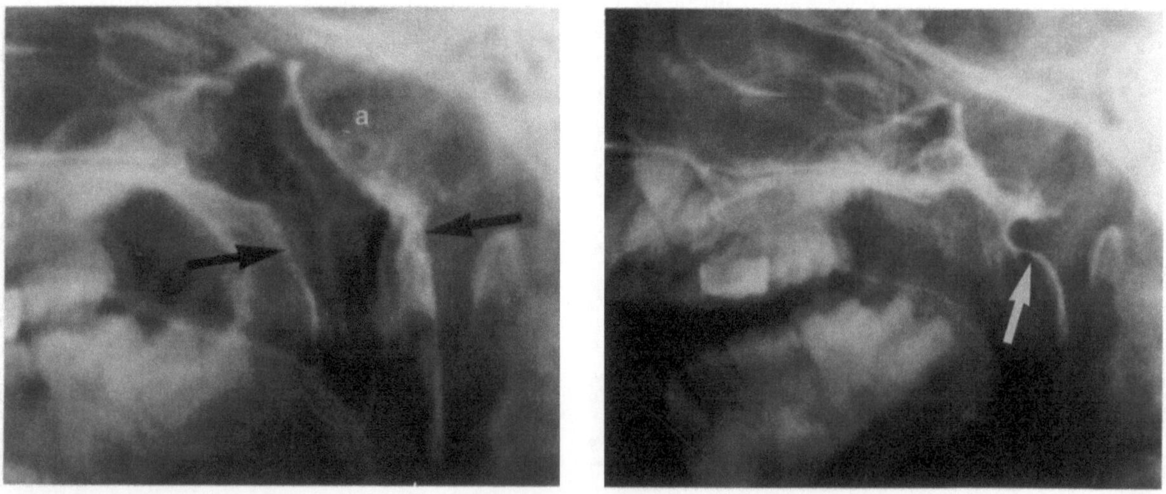

A B

Fig. 5.11. Passavant ridge. **A.** At rest, velopharyngeal portal is outlined with barium (*arrows*). Small adenoids are present (a). (**B**). On phonation, prominent bulge (*arrow*) of posterior pharyngeal wall (Passavant ridge) appears below adenoids and affects velopharyngeal portal closure.

Standard Single-Contrast Barium Meal

Indications

1. To show anatomy of the esophagus, stomach and duodenum with particular emphasis on the position of the duodenojejunal flexure to exclude malrotation.
2. To assess the functions of swallowing, competence of the gastroesophageal sphincter, and emptying of stomach contents into the duodenum.
3. To look for varices.

Contraindications and Precautions

Infants, especially those with chest problems, need to be watched carefully while they are drinking to see whether they are aspirating contrast either via the larynx or through a tracheoesophageal fistula.

Materials

One part of 56% w/w, 100% w/v barium sulfate diluted with two parts of water or sugar solution. At our hospital we used Gel-Unix when it was available, and now use Unibar 100, which has replaced this preparation in Canada. Other barium preparations may be helpful but we find that Gel-Unix is particularly well tolerated by children.

Preparations

Nil by mouth for 8 hours for a patient over 2 years of age, for 6 hours for a patient between 1 and 2 years old, and for 4 hours before the examination for patients less than 1 year of age.

□ *Procedure*

Step 1. In our hospital the upper body of the child is held steady by a parent or an assistant, and the radiologist holds the upper thighs of the patient with one hand to prevent excessive patient movement and to facilitate patient positioning. The child can be restrained by binding the lower limbs with a towel (see Fig. 5.1). Radiation is screened from the radiologist and assistants by appropriate lead or lead glass screens.

Step 2. The infant or child is lying on the right side. Barium is fed from a bottle or injected from a syringe into the mouth of the infant. A catheter can be pulled through a nipple to be more acceptable to the infant [28–30], but we found that this is rarely if ever necessary. Older children can swallow barium from a cup via a straw.

Step 3. The lateral view of the esophagus is screened with particular emphasis on the region around the carina looking for fistulae and vascular anomalies. A film of the barium-filled esophagus is taken (film

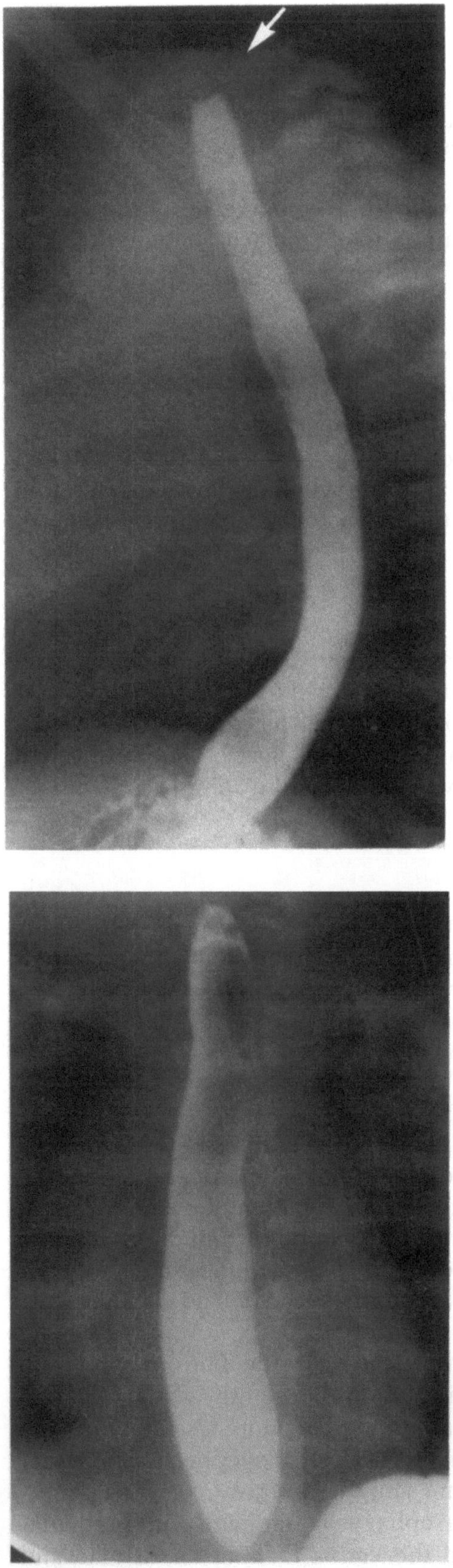

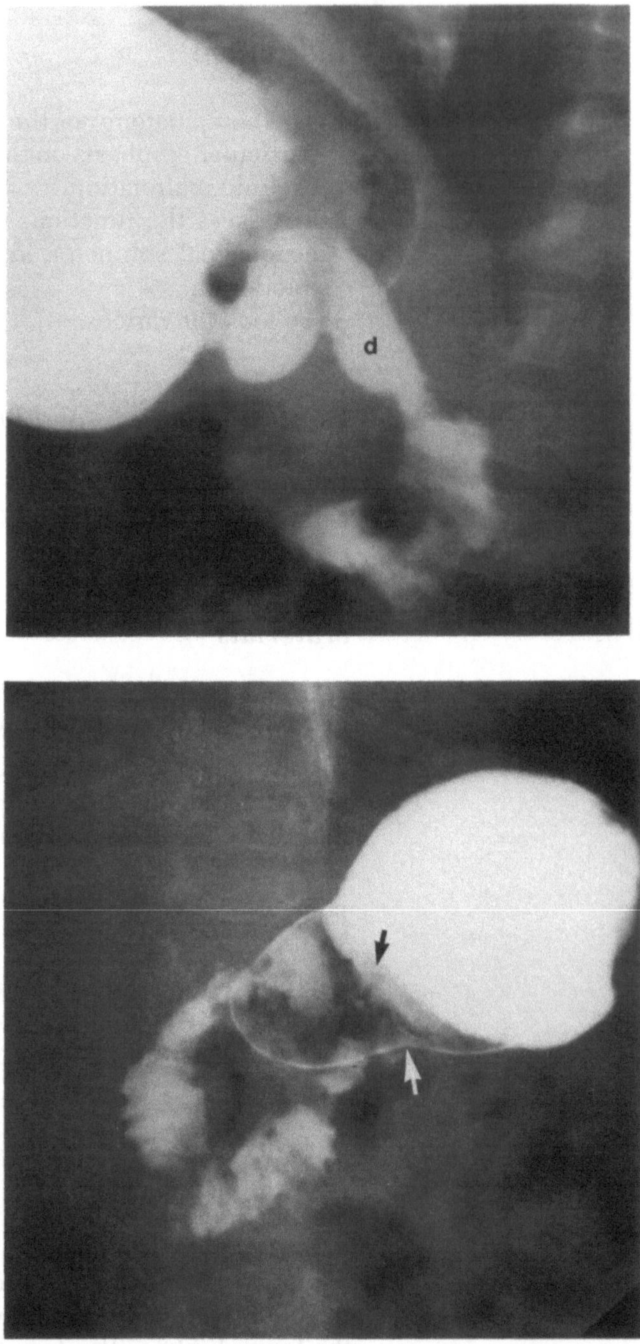

Fig. 5.12. Normal single-contrast barium meal in infant. **A.** The esophagus is filled with barium in a lateral projection. A 9-in. image intensifier is sufficient to cover esophagus from cricopharyngeus (*arrow*) to gastroesophageal junction. **B.** With the child still in a lateral position, pylorus, duodenal cap (d), and second and third parts of the duodenum are visualized. **C.** The duodenojejunal flexure (*arrow*) is seen through the air-filled gastric antrum. **D.** With the child supine, further swallows of barium outline the esophagus in AP projection.

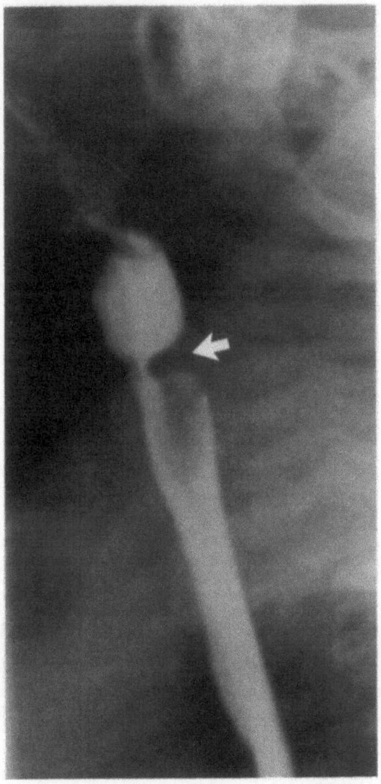

Fig. 5.13. Normal cricopharyngeus. Prominent indentation (*arrow*) of posterior aspect of the esophagus was seen to occur intermittently on fluoroscopy.

1) (Fig. 5.12A). A prominent cricopharyngeal impression is a common normal variant (Fig. 5.13).

Step 4. With the child still in the same position, if enough barium has passed into the stomach, a lateral view of the pylorus and duodenal loop can be obtained when the first bolus of barium enters the third part of the duodenum (film 2) (Fig. 5.12B).

Step 5. the child is now turned quickly supine and then onto the left-side-down position to drain the barium out of the antrum. Immediately the patient is turned supine and the duodenojejunal flexure is seen through the air-filled gastric antrum (film 3) (Fig. 5.12C). This view is the most important of the entire series as malrotation is best excluded by confirming a normal duodenojejunal flexure position to the left of the left vertebral pedicles and nearly as high as the duodenal cap. For this, the child *must* be supine. Viewing the position of the cardiac shadow is the best way to ensure that the child is truly supine at the level of the upper abdomen. The legs may have to be rotated in order to achieve a supine upper abdomen as children are often lying in a twisted fashion.

Step 6. With the child supine, further swallows of barium are taken and the esophagus is assessed in the AP projection (film 4) (Fig. 5.12D).

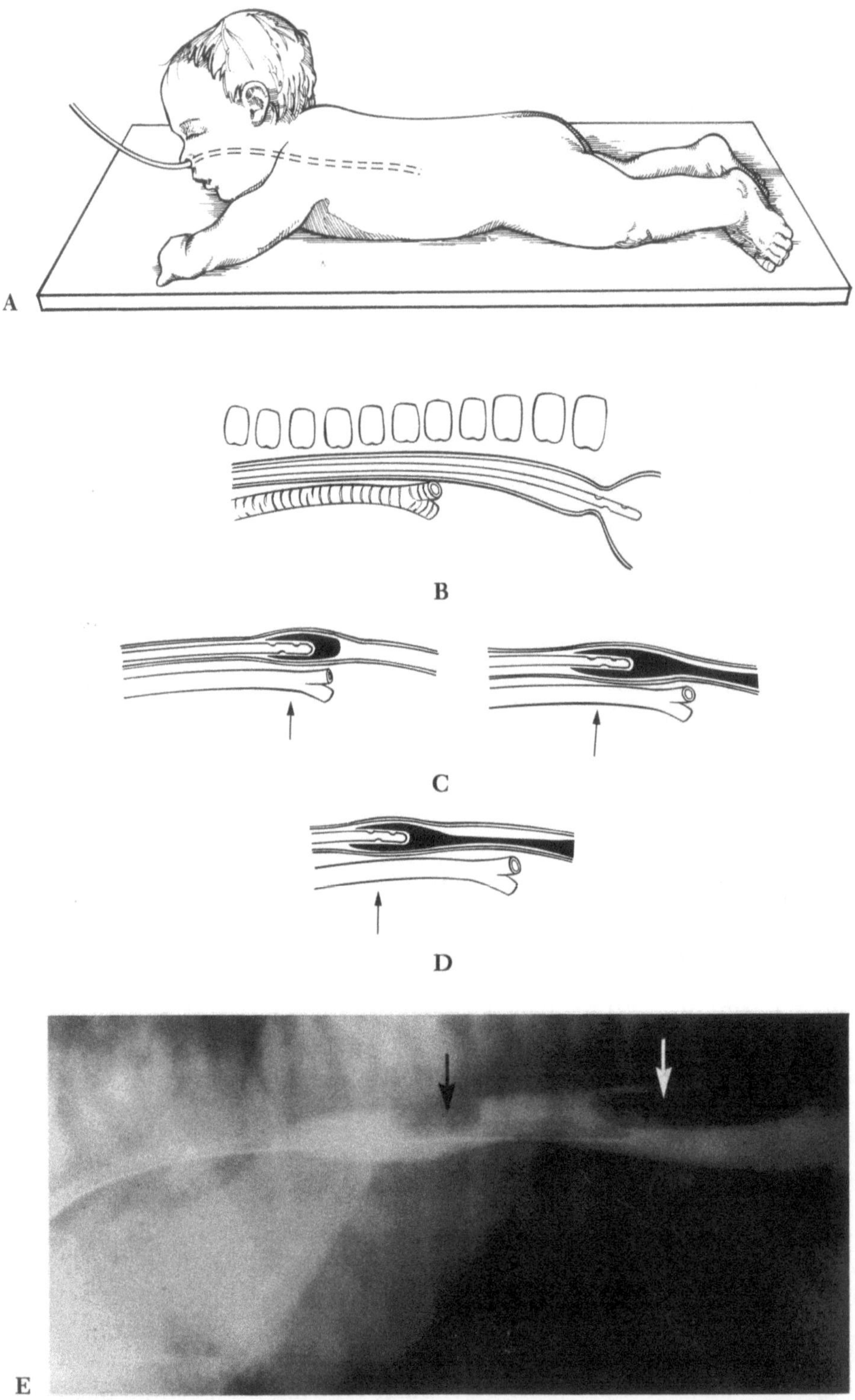

Fig. 5.14. Normal video prone esophagram. **A.** The patient is positioned prone with the tip of a feeding tube in the distal esophagus. The feeding tube is withdrawn to the level of the carina, and barium is injected relatively forcefully whilst withdrawing the catheter (**B–D**). Barium is injected into the midesophagus via a feeding tube layers preferentially on the anterior, dependent the surface of the esophagus with the patient prone (**E**). Gas bubbles (*arrows*) rise to the posterior aspect of the esophagus.

Step 7. With the stomach full of barium and after burping, reflux can be tested for with the patient in the supine position by gently rocking the child from side to side (film 5 if reflux occurs). It is our impression that the barium flowing across the gastroesophageal junction during rocking may provoke reflux. It is always necessary to burp the child as excess air has usually been swallowed. If the child is an infant, the amount of barium given should be equivalent to a normal feed of milk for that child.
NOTE: The gastroesophageal junction should be carefully screened for tenting, a finding suggestive of intermittent reflux.

In the following clinical situations the examination is extended and further views are taken.

i. 'H' Type or Recurrent Tracheoesophageal Fistula

If small, these fistulae can be extremely difficult to demonstrate and may require multiple examinations [31,32]. If this diagnosis is clinically suspected, a right lateral decubitus tube esophagram (RLDE) or video prone esophagram (VPE) should be performed [31,32] (see page 128). A video prone esophagram is technically a more cumbersome procedure to perform than a right lateral decubitus tube esophagram, but the VPE is preferable as the barium preferentially coats the anterior aspect of the esophagus (Fig. 5.14). On some equipment, larger patients may be impossible to examine using the VPE technique. If this is the case, a tube esophagram in the right lateral decubitus position can be performed. A feeding tube is inserted to the level of the suspected fistula and while fairly forcefully injecting barium with the child in the lateral projection, a video recording is made. Films are of secondary importance and should be taken only to document a fistula if easily seen. The more subtle fistulae can be seen only as small wisps of barium are forced through the tiny aperture.

ii. Hypertrophic Pyloric Stenosis

Hypertrophic pyloric stenosis (HPS) is a clinical diagnosis in most patients. In those for whom diagnostic uncertainty is present, sonography is the examination of choice [19]. If this is equivocal or unavailable, then a barium meal examination can be performed. This barium examination will also demonstrate any gastroesophageal reflux (GER), a common associated finding with any gastric outlet obstruction [7,8]. Occasionally the barium meal may exclude HPS but demonstrate that GER is the cause of the symptoms.

The initial part of the examination is identical to that already stated but when Step number 3 on page 123 is reached with the patient in the lateral position, delayed passage of barium will be seen. The pyloric canal will also be long. A degree of pylorospasm can mimic this appearance exactly and can be differentiated only by delayed fluoroscopy, which shows the constant nature of the outlet obstruction and the classical appearance of the pyloric canal in HPS. In pylorospasm, the pylorus will eventually open up with transit of barium through a normal-sized and -shaped pylorus. To be certain of the diagnosis of HPS, barium should be seen in the pyloric cap and the constant narrowing of the pylorus should be evident. If there is marked delay in passage of barium, the barium can either be gently massaged through the pylorus, or delayed fluoroscopy at 30 to 60 minutes can be performed. At the end of the examination, if GER or hypertrophic pyloric stenosis is present, a nasogastric tube should be inserted and the barium aspirated to prevent aspiration into the lungs.

iii. Peptic Ulcer or Inflammation

If ulcers are suspected, a double-contrast examination should be performed because single-contrast studies are poor at detecting mucosal disease [33].

iv. Fatigue Aspiration

Fatigue aspiration occurs toward the end of a full feed, and if clinically suspected is best demonstrated with the patient lying on the right side with fluoroscopy of the last few swallows [34]. Radiation can be kept to a minimum by coning to the hypopharynx.

v. Varices

Liquid barium is given in the prone position. Films are taken in various phases of respiration and obliquity. Small amounts of barium often demonstrate the varices best. When varices are obvious only one or two films need be taken to document this. When in doubt more films will be necessary. The Valsalva maneuver may be used on older children to increase the conspicuity of varices. Varices can also be examined with a double-contrast barium examination. If doubt still remains over the presence of varices, Buscopan can be given I.M. to relax the esophagus, although at the Hospital for Sick Children we find that this is unnecessary.

Aftercare

Stomach contents should be drained and/or the infant should be nursed erect following the procedure in all cases in which either delayed gastric emptying or significant GE reflux occurs, depending on the clinical circumstances. This is to prevent spontaneous lung aspiration.

All postprocedure orders should be written in the patient's chart.

Video Prone Esophagram

Indications

Clinical suspicion of an H-type or recurrent tracheoesophageal fistula [31,32].

Contraindications and Precautions

Care is taken to prevent or minimize aspiration, especially in infants with preexisting chest problems.

Materials

1. 10 French gauge NG tube with side holes. An 8 French gauge NG tube should be reserved for small infants if the nostril is too small.
2. One part 56% w/w and 100% w/v barium sulfate (Unibar 100) diluted with two parts water as per standard single-contrast barium meal.

Preparation

Nil by mouth for 8 hours for a patient over 2 years of age, for 6 hours for a patient between 1 and 2 years old, and for 4 hours before the examination for patients less than 1 year of age.

□ *Procedure*

1. The infant is placed prone on a cushion resting on the footstep of the fluoroscopic table with the table erect (at a chest-high position and prevented from falling by a parent or assistant) [31]. If the table top to tube or image intensifier distances are sufficient, larger children can be placed prone on a stretcher [31].
2. A nasogastric tube is positioned in the midesophagus and barium is injected forcefully. For the inexperienced, a trial practice with the syringe and NG tube to get the feel of the equipment and the barium resistance is strongly advised.

Step 3. Next the position of the tube is altered so that each part of the esophagus can be distended in turn, with barium filling each part at least twice during the examination. The whole procedure is covered by video tape fluoroscopy to allow playback. Films are less important but can be taken to document a normal or abnormal examination (see Fig. 5.14).

NOTE: To prevent aspiration following the procedure, barium should be emptied from the esophagus either via the tube or by nursing the infant erect to allow barium to drain to the stomach. Care should be taken to ensure that the nasogastric tube is in fact situated in the esophagus and not in the bronchial tree. This can be done by advancing the tube initially into the stomach, aspirating the gastric contents, and then withdrawing the tube to the appropriate position. In addition, careful fluoroscopy before injection of barium can confirm the position of the nasoesophageal tube posterior to the trachea.

Double-Contrast Examination of the Esophagus, Stomach, and Duodenum

Indications

The indications are more restricted than in adults as cancer is exceptional and ulcers are uncommon. Endoscopy is more sensitive than radiology at detecting pediatric gastric mucosal lesions, but is more invasive, and in children may require a general anesthetic [33,35–38].

1. Investigation of epigastric pain, hematemesis, or melena, if ulcers or

inflammatory bowel disease of esophagus, stomach, or duodenum are suspected and endoscopy is not indicated [33].
2. In patients with obscure diagnostic problems and possible upper GI tract disease.
3. If polyps or other mass lesions are suspected.

Contraindications and Precautions

Care is taken to prevent or minimize aspiration.

Materials

1. 85% w/w 250% w/v barium sulfate. We use E-Z-HD at our hospital.
2. Gas-producing pills (Unik Zoru). We find the pills are better tolerated than the granules.

Preparations

Nil by mouth for 8 hours for a patient over 2 years of age, for 6 hours for a patient between 1 and 2 years old, and for 4 hours before the examination for patients less than 1 year of age. Discussion of procedure with the patient (and parents).

□ *Procedure*

Step 1. The examination is started with the patient standing slightly oblique left side closer to the table. The gas tablets are swallowed with 10 to 15 ml of water. Better cooperation is obtained by giving water than barium with the gas tablets. Gas granules in children cause problems because they quickly produce frothing bubbles in the mouth. If a double-contrast study is required in young children, infants, or very sick children, the air and barium can be given through a nasogastric tube as these patients are not cooperative.
Step 2. With the patient taking swallows of barium through a straw, the esophagus is examined. With careful timing a good double-contrast view (film 1) can often be obtained (Fig. 5.15).
Step 3. The table is now put into the horizontal position with the patient prone.
Step 4. The patient is now turned first into left-side-down then supine position. If the coating is poor, the patient rolls around completely twice. The duodenojejunal flexure is localized before the cap is examined in order to exclude malrotation (see single-contrast study, p. 123) (film 2) (Fig. 5.16).
Step 5. Only a few films (occasionally one) (film 3) of the duodenal cap are obtained in the left-side-down prone position so that at least one air-filled distended cap is obtained (film 3) (Fig. 5.17). More films are obtained if there is strong clinical concern or the diagnosis is uncertain.
Step 6. A view of the gastric antrum or body of the stomach is obtained with the patient in the supine, left-, or right-side-down position if this

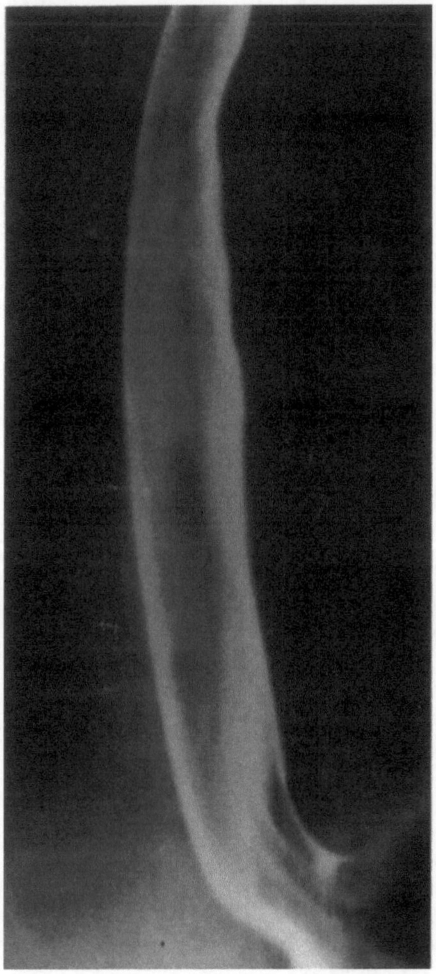

Fig. 5.15. Normal double-contrast esophagus. The esophagus distended with air and outlined by barium is well shown in a slightly oblique projection.

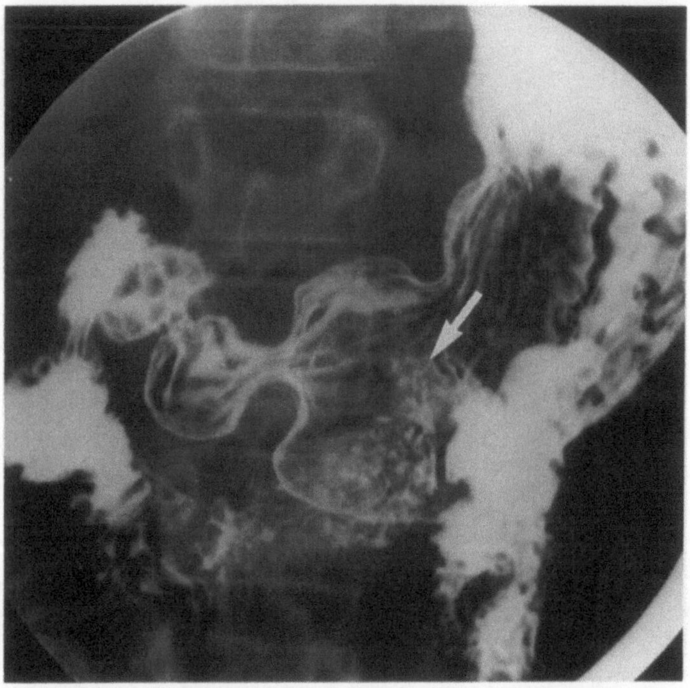

Fig. 5.16

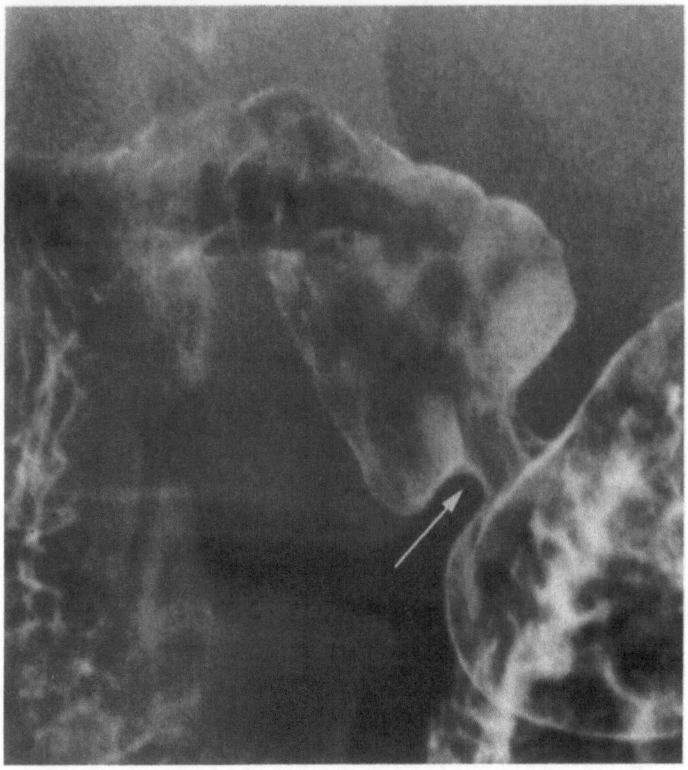

Fig. 5.17

Fig. 5.16. Normal duodenojejunal flexure. The duodenojejunal flexure (*arrow*) is seen through an air-filled gastric antrum with the patient supine. Poor gaseous distention of the stomach is a common problem in children because they cannot retain gas.

Fig. 5.17. Normal double-contrast duodenal cap. The duodenal cap is distended with air and outlined by barium. A normal short pyloric canal (*arrow*) is well seen.

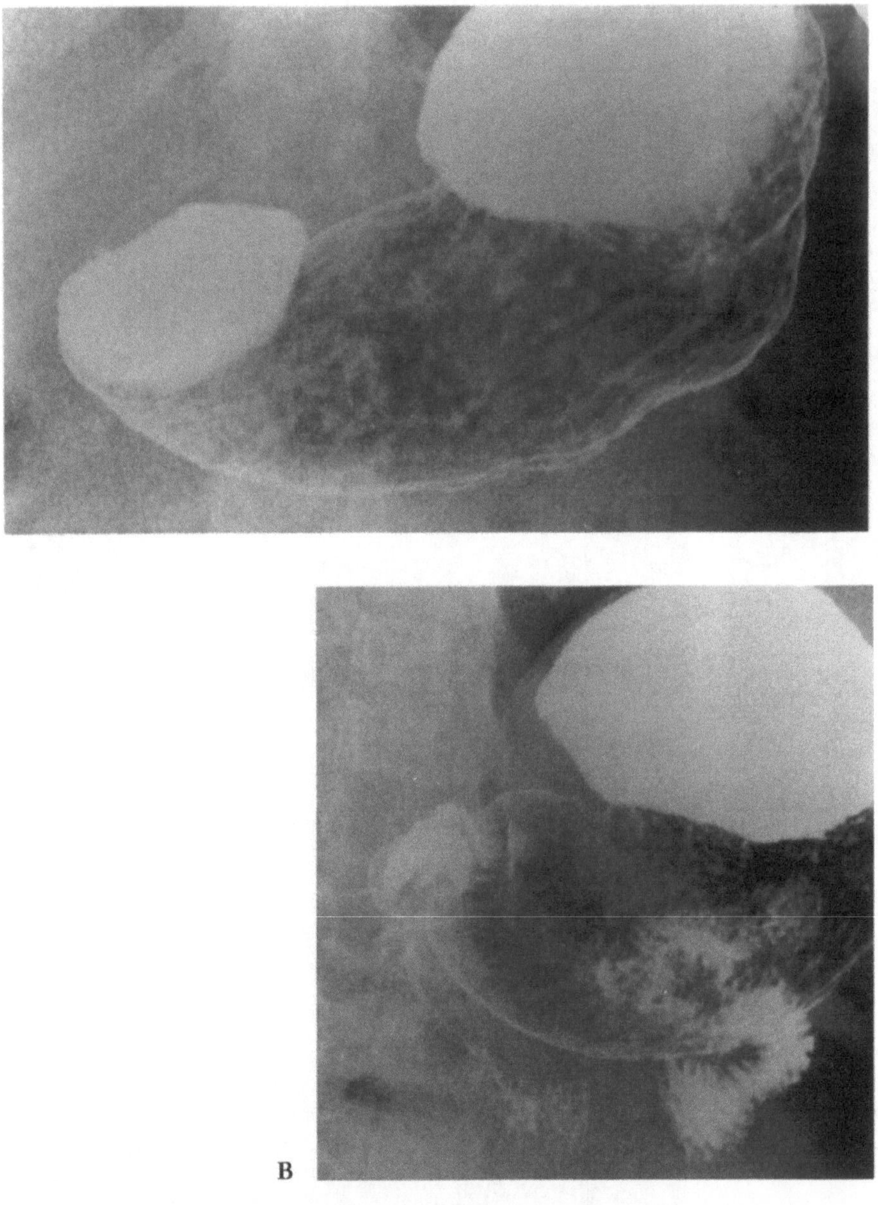

A

B

Fig. 5.18. Normal double-contrast gastric antrum and body. Views taken in the supine (**A**), left (**B**), or right (**C**) obliques can visualize different portions of the gastric antrum and body. Usually only one view is taken depending on exact anatomy of the patient.

area has not been well properly visualized on previous views (additional film 1) (Fig. 5.18).

Step 7. A view of the barium-filled cap is taken with the patient lying on their right side if there is still concern over possible duodenal cap deformity (film 4) (Fig. 5.19).

Step 8. The patient can now be brought up into the prone or the vertical position for a view of the air-filled fundus (optional film 5). The vertical position is best as it also enables a good outline to the lesser

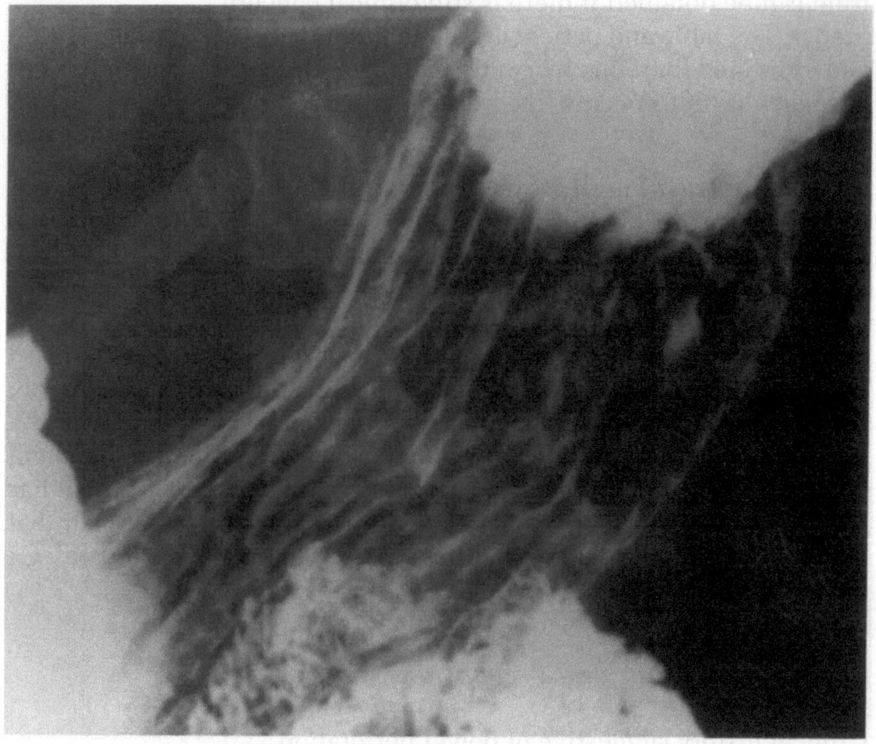

Fig. 5.18 C

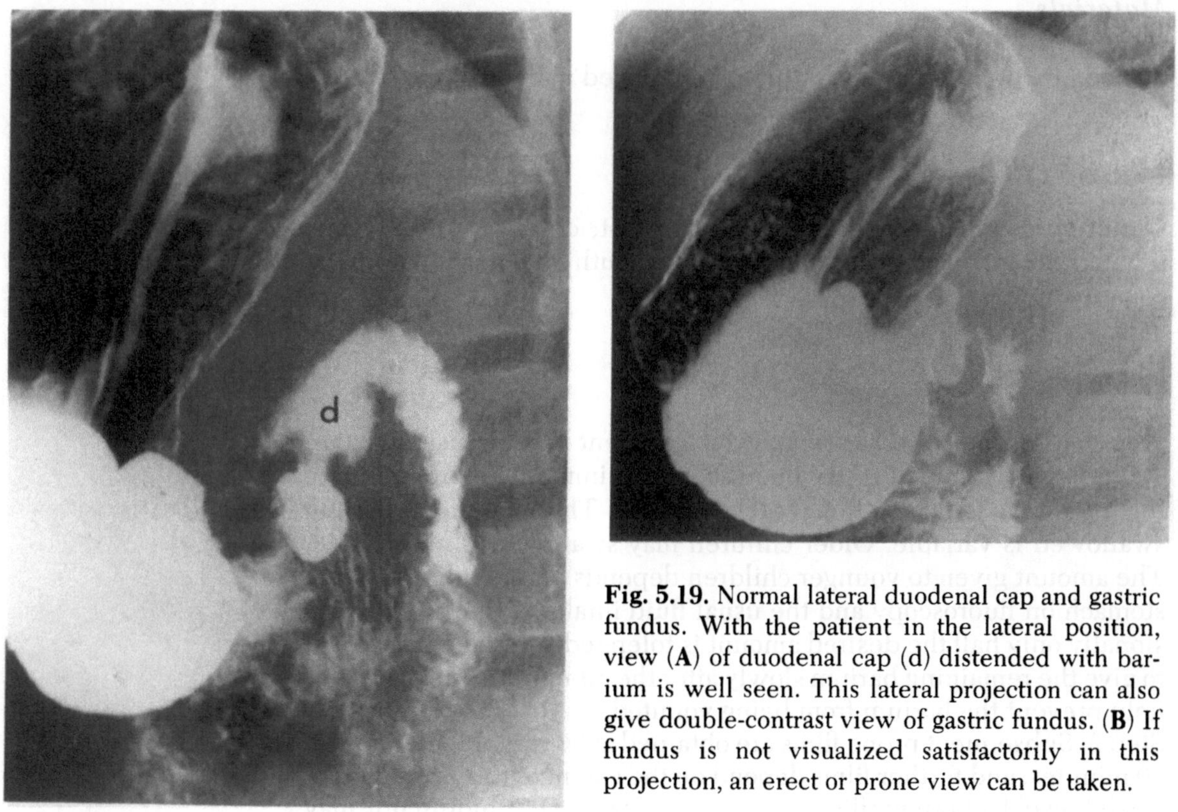

A

B

Fig. 5.19. Normal lateral duodenal cap and gastric fundus. With the patient in the lateral position, view (**A**) of duodenal cap (d) distended with barium is well seen. This lateral projection can also give double-contrast view of gastric fundus. (**B**) If fundus is not visualized satisfactorily in this projection, an erect or prone view can be taken.

and greater curvatures. Compression films of the duodenum and antrum can be obtained if there is still clinical concern.
Step 9. The table and patient are again put into the horizontal position and examined for reflux by gently rocking in the supine position. Film 6 is taken if reflux occurs (recording level of reflux).

Single-Contrast Small Bowel Meal and Follow-Through

Indications

To examine the small bowel for abnormalities of anatomy or occasionally of function. The examination is best performed after a standard single-contrast examination of the esophagus, stomach, or duodenum, but should not be combined with a double-contrast examination as the high-density barium and gas degrade the visualization of the small bowel. If no examination of the upper gastrointestinal (UGI) tract has been requested, it is wise to check with the referring physician that malrotation and other abnormalities that can be excluded on an UGI are not suspected.

Contraindications and Precautions

Clinical history suggestive of bowel perforation.

Materials

200 ml 56% w/w 100% w/v (Unibar 100) mixed with 400 ml of water.

Preparation

Children less than 1 year of age, 4-hour fast; children 1 to 2 years, 6-hour fast; and over 2 years of age, nil by mouth for 8 hours before the examination.

□ *Procedure*

Step 1. After the child has swallowed sufficient barium (usually 200–400 ml), with minimal if any fluoroscopy, an immediate prone film of the abdomen is taken (film 1) (Fig. 5.20A). The amount of barium swallowed is variable. Older children may swallow 200 ml or more. The amount given to younger children depends on the fullness of the stomach on fluoroscopy and the usual fluid intake of the child. Occasionally only half the desired amount is tolerated, and then it is wisest to give the remaining barium slowly after the 30-minute film. This will help prevent the barium from being vomited.
Step 2. Subsequent prone films are obtained at 30-minute intervals for 90 minutes, and further films depend on the extent of filling of loops of small bowel by barium (films 2, 3, 4) (Fig. 5.20B–D). Fluoroscopy may occasionally be necessary to assess progress. Rare conditions that

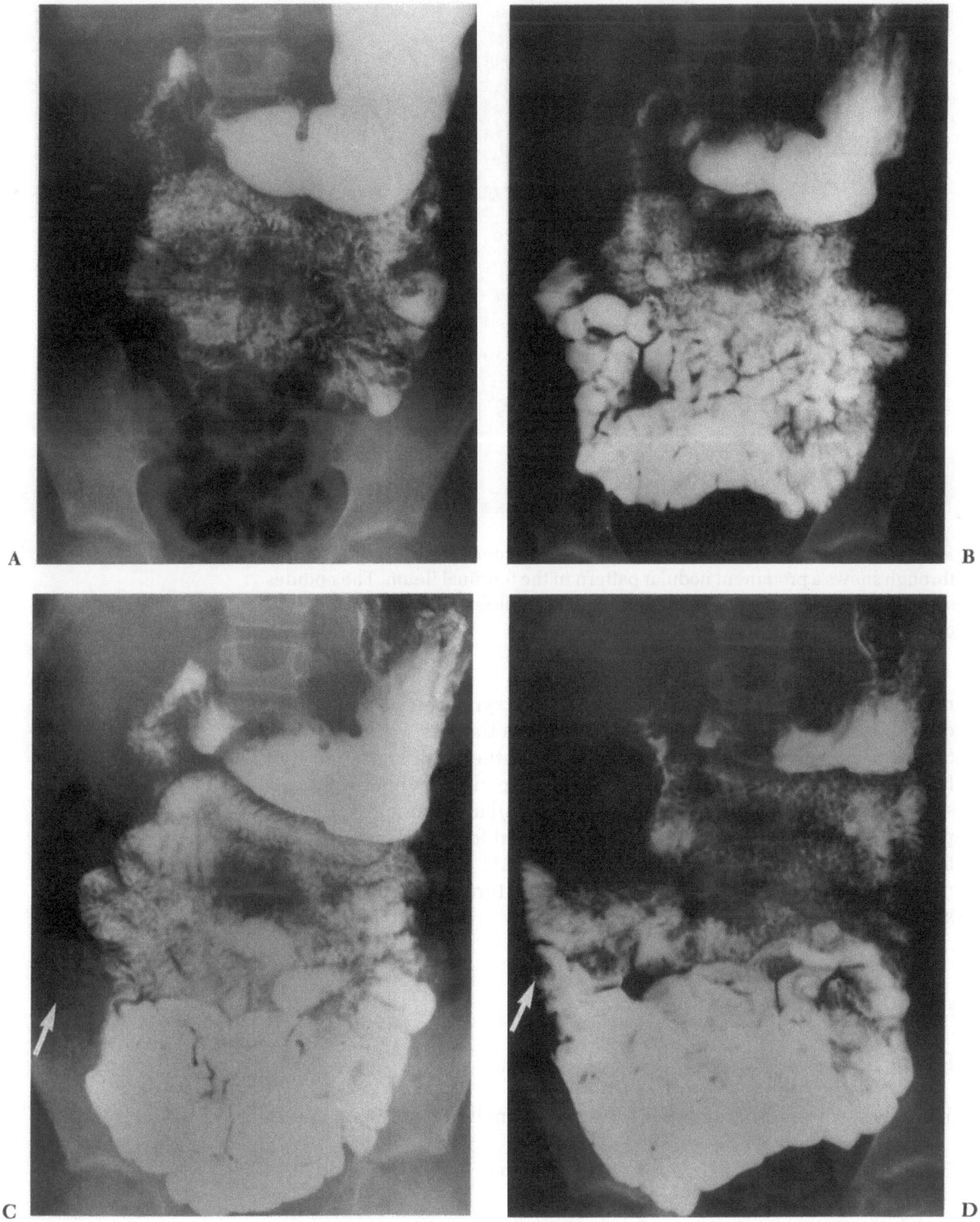

Fig. 5.20. Normal small bowel follow-through. **A.** Immediate prone film shows filling of proximal loops of small bowel. Prone films taken at 30 (**B**), 60 (**C**), and 90 (**D**) minutes show transit of barium through small bowel and into colon. The feces filled cecum seen on the 60 minute film,(**C.** *arrow*), is seen to fill with barium on the 90 minute film (**D.** *arrow*).

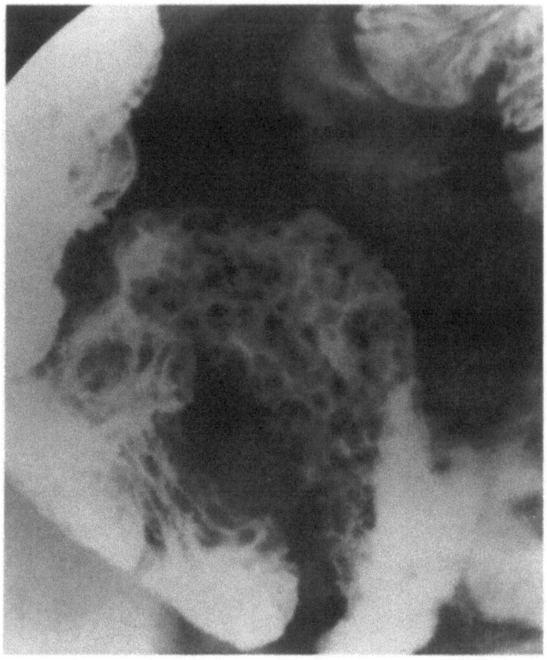

Fig. 5.21. Normal terminal ileum. A spot film from a small bowel follow-through shows a prominent nodular pattern in the terminal ileum. The nodules are very regular and of equal size because of multiple small lymphoid follicles, a normal appearance in many children.

markedly delay transit such as hypomotility syndromes may require daily films for as long as 7 to 14 days to assess transit.

Step 3. When enough barium has passed into the terminal ileum, spot films (film 5) are obtained, using an inflatable paddle or other compression device if necessary. A prominent nodular lymphoid follicular pattern may be present in children as a normal feature and should not be mistaken for abnormal pathology (Fig. 5.21). Sometimes a peroral pneumocolon examination is necessary if the terminal ileum is poorly seen [39] (see below).

Peroral Pneumocolon

Indications

1. For better visualization of the terminal ileum if not well seen on the small bowel meal [39–45] (Fig. 5.22A).
2. To aid diagnosis of fistulae if uncertain from fluoroscopy and spot films, with and without compression [39].

Materials

Disposable soft enema tips, tubing, and insufflator.

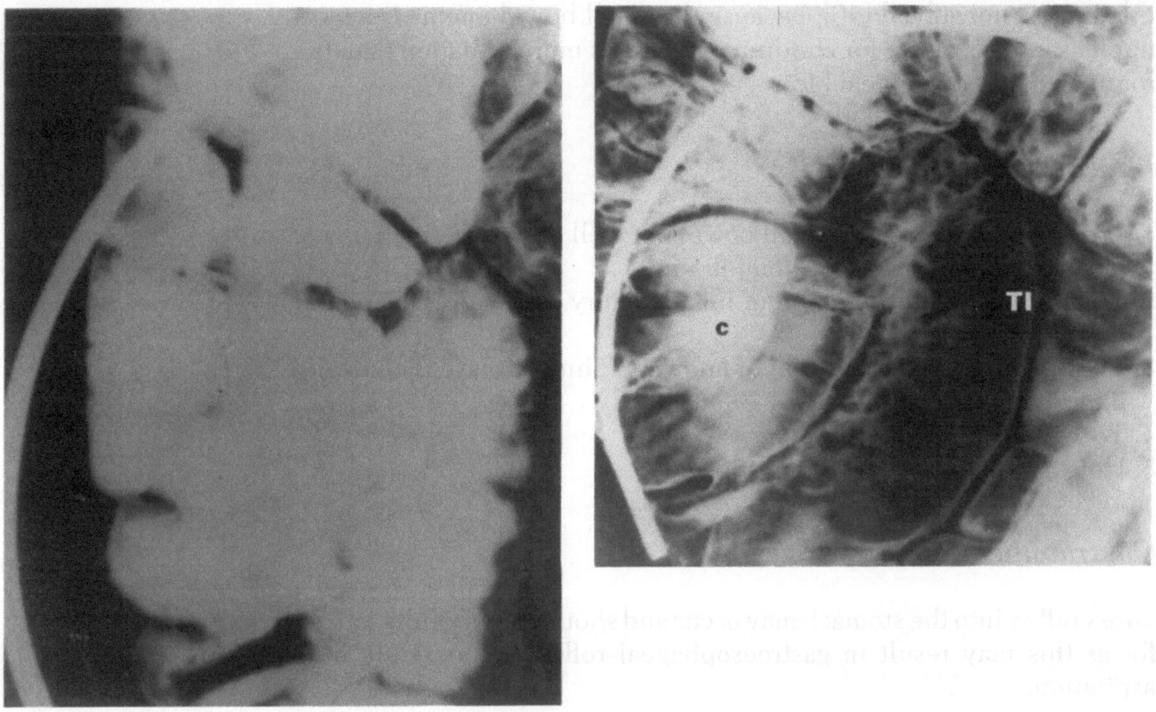

A B

Fig. 5.22. Normal terminal ileum. A. The terminal ileum was poorly visualized on a conventional small bowel follow-through despite compression. A peroral pneumocolon (B), performed immediately after film in (A), outlines cecum (c) and terminal ileum (TI). The peroral pneumocolon shows smooth mucosa on double-contrast view except for some mucosal folds and small lymphoid follicles.

☐ *Procedure*

Step 1. When a diagnostic dilemma is seen on fluoroscopy of the terminal ileum during a small bowel meal, with the patient in the lateral position left-side-down with knees and hips flexed, a soft rectal tube is inserted.
Step 2. Air is puffed into the rectum and on into the colon. Insufflation is started with the patient supine and then left-side-down.
Step 3. The patient is now turned prone to allow air to pass into the cecum and terminal ileum. The ileal cecal valve is more posterior than anterior in position so reflux of air is facilitated by the use of the prone position.
Step 4. Spot film(s) are taken when the terminal ileum is adequately visualized (Fig. 5.22B). This may be facilitated by use of compression during fluoroscopy.

Small Bowel Enema

Most diagnostic problems are solved by the small bowel meal. The small bowel enema is reserved for those very few patients for whom a dilemma is not solved [46], because the small bowel enema is a most unpleasant procedure for children and entails more radiation than the routine small bowel meal [46].

Indications

1. To demonstrate parts of small bowel not well seen on a small bowel meal or per oral pneumocolon [46–52].
2. To aid in the differentiation of inflammatory and neoplastic conditions [46].
3. To show full proximal extent of known Crohn's disease if clinically important [46,47,50].
4. To identify small nodules.
5. Unusual diagnostic problems [46].

Contraindications and Precautions

Gross reflux into the stomach may occur and should be carefully looked for as this may result in gastroesophageal reflux and possible lung aspiration.

Materials

1. Intubation tubes
   Bilbao Dotter tubes, modified (Cook's)
   a. Herlinger type, 1-135 cm 14 French, end hole
   b. Herlinger type, 2–135 cm, 12 French, end hole
   c. 10 French nasogastric tubes; only for smaller children if Bilbao-Dotter tubes are too large
2. Cook's Teflon-coated torque control guide wires for above
3. 55% w/w 100% w/v barium sulfate diluted to 15% solution. We use Polibar in our hospital; commonly mixed volumes are given below.
   Ex: 100 ml of Polibar (100% w/v 55% w/w barium sulfate) to 700 ml of water/normal saline;
   200 ml/1400 ml;
   300 ml/2100 ml.
   OR
   undiluted 55% w/w 100% w/v barium sulfate (Polibar) followed by sodium carboxymethylcellulose solution (CMC). At the Hospital for Sick Children, we prefer the dilute barium sulfate without CMC solution.
4. Two enema bags, one cold water or methylcellulose and one barium as above. (For smaller children, the water is slightly warm.)
   e. Y connector.
   f. Metal connector for different-sized tubes.

Preparation

Nil by mouth for 8 hours for a patient over 2 years of age, for 6 hours for a patient between 1 and 2 years old, and for 4 hours before the examination for patients less than 1 year of age. Discussion of procedure with the patient (and parents).

□ *Procedure*

Step 1. Some authors advocate sedation [51], but we think that this could be dangerous because of the risk of aspiration if reflux of barium occurred, and is unnecessary [46].
Step 2. The oral approach is not used because if cooperation is lost the tube can be bitten through. The tube is introduced into the nose and positioned in the stomach in the supine position. If difficulty is encountered at the level of the velopharynx or cricopharyngeus, neck flexion is often helpful, as is closing the mouth and swallowing.
Step 3. The rest of the intubation is similar to that of adults (see page 48). However, more prior discussion of the technique is necessary for the patient's cooperation to be obtained, and constant encouragement of the patient is necessary during intubation and filling of the small bowel. An assistant experienced in dealing with children is invaluable.
Step 4. 50 to 200 ml of 15% solution of barium sulfate (Polibar) is instilled under gravity. The speed of filling is varied by raising or lowering the bag of barium so that good distension of the small bowel is seen. In practice, using a 12 or 14 French Bilbao Dotter tube (the largest caliber possible for each patient), the barium column often needs to be approximately 2 meter above the patient. The exact height will depend on the length and caliber of tubes used.
Step 5. If the barium is too dense for a see-through effect, or when the proximal bowel has been examined, then cold water is instilled via the Y connector pushing the column on to more distal small bowel and causing proximal dilution. If the child is under 4 years of age, the water is tepid rather than cold to prevent hypothermia.
Step 6. Film 1 (10 × 12 or 14 × 17) or 100-mm/105-mm spot films are taken when there is good visualization of jejunum (Fig. 5.23).
Step 7. Films 2 or 3 (10 × 12 or 14 × 17) or more 100-mm/105-mm spot films are taken so that the rest of the small bowel and terminal ileum are visualized (Fig. 5.24).
Step 8. Palpation is important to visualize all loops of bowel and to adequately demonstrate the terminal ileum.

There are different ways to perform enteroclysis, and familiarity with one technique is more important than the type of technique. Compare with technique described for adults in Chapter 3.

Water-Soluble Contrast Meal

Although barium sulfate is a safe contrast media in most patients and has even been used as a bronchographic contrast agent in the past [53,54], it is sometimes safer to use a water-soluble contrast medium [55–61]. These should be the new low osmolar contrast media, namely ioxaglate, iopamidol, and iohexol, which can be used in isoosmolar concentrations with safety. Water-soluble bronchographic media may be used if these low osmolar contrast media are not available.

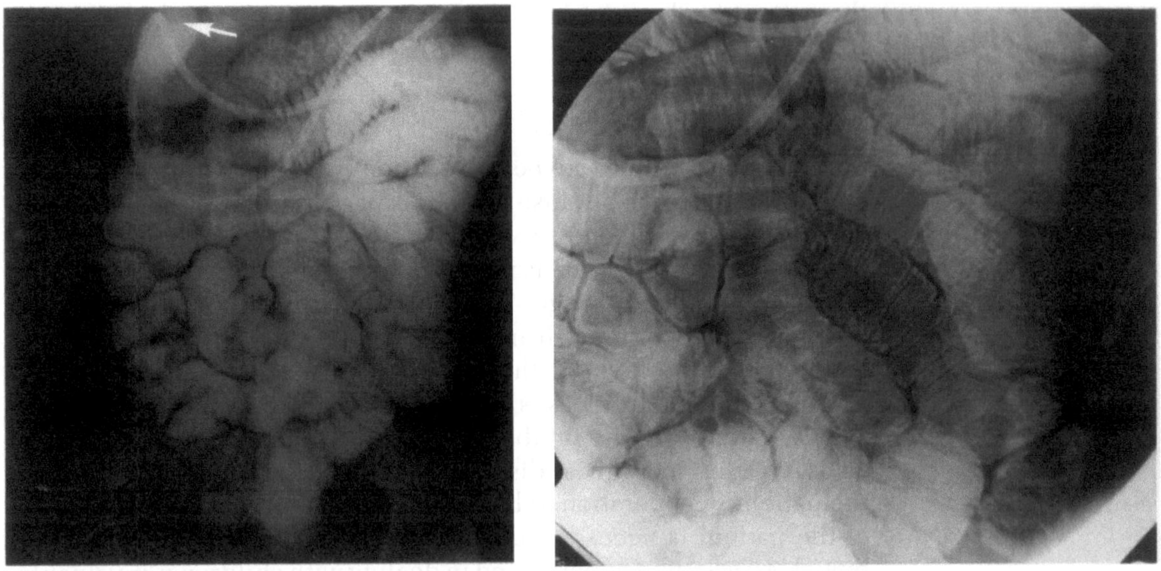

A B

Fig. 5.23. Small bowel enema. **A.** 14 × 17 in. film shows the tip of a Bilbao Dotter tube lying in the region of the duodenojejunal junction. There has been good filling of jejunum and proximal ileum and some reflux back into the stomach (*arrow*). **B.** 105-mm spot film after instillation of cold water demonstrates a good see-through effect in the jejunum. Valvulae conniventes are seen as thin linear lucencies in the lumen of the jejunum.

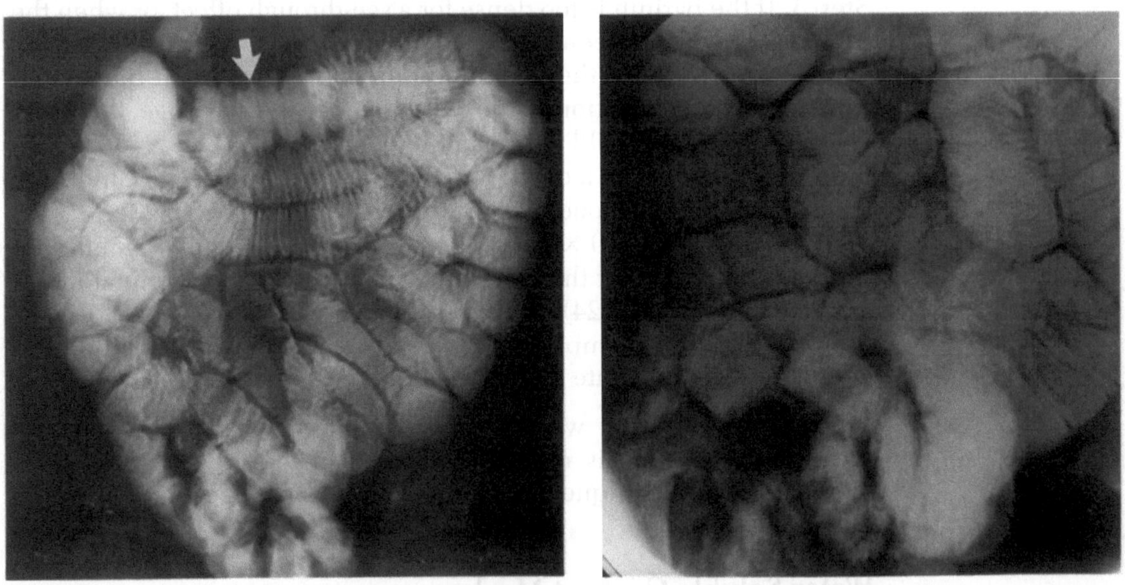

A B

Fig. 5.24. Small bowel enema. **A.** Further filling of bowel is seen with some barium present in a collapsed transverse colon (*arrow*). The cecum and ascending colon are obscured by other loops of bowel. **B.** Spot film in lower part of abdomen shows more featureless loops of ileum filled with dilute barium.

Older water-soluble contrast media should never be used because of the risk of pulmonary edema [62–64]. In particular, hyperosmolar contrast media can be very dangerous in this regard [59,60,62,63,64].

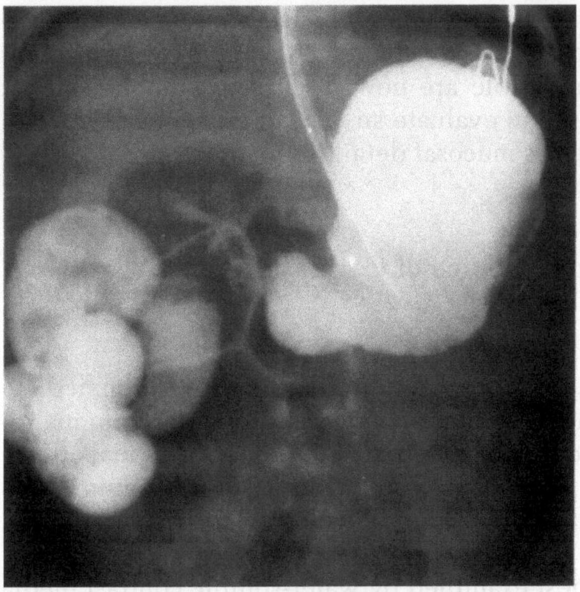

Fig. 5.25. Hexabrix meal. Stomach and nonrotated proximal small bowel are well visualized with 160-mg/ml concentration of ioxaglate in an infant after gastroschisis repair.

Indications

1. Possible perforation of the upper gastrointestinal tract.
2. Suspected lung aspiration.
3. Possible inspissation of barium in the large bowel.
4. Small bowel obstruction in neonates [56].
5. Possible neonatal necrotizing enterocolitis [56].

Materials

At our hospital, we use an 160-mg/ml concentration of ioxaglate as it is cheaper than the other contrast agents and in a prospective study gave good results with no deleterious effects on the patients. We find that this concentration gives good visualization (Fig. 5.25). Isoosmolar iopamidol or iohexol could also be used.

The examination is otherwise identical to that of a standard single-contrast barium meal. Occasionally the examination may be continued and the small bowel examined as well.

Lower GI Tract Contrast Examinations in Children

General Considerations

In children, the diagnostic problems encountered differ from those of adults. Tumors are very rare, nearly all polyps are benign juvenile polyps, and inflammatory bowel disease is very rare under 8 years of age. Hence, the majority of contrast enemas performed are single-contrast studies looking for gross anatomy and function. In addition, water-soluble contrast media are commonly used in infancy for diagnostic and therapeutic purposes, and the relative merits of the different single-contrast media available are now discussed. Double-contrast studies are primarily used to evaluate suspected inflammatory bowel disease in older children as mucosal detail is far superior [65].

Single-Contrast Enema: Choice of Contrast Media

In Neonates

Bowel obstruction is a relatively common finding in the immediate newborn period, and may be from many causes, ranging from malrotation with volvulus requiring immediate surgery or intestinal atresia requiring rapid rather than immediate surgery, to meconium ileus or functional immaturity of the large bowel, treated by enemas [60, 66–76].

These neonates are best examined by water-soluble contrast media because of the risk of enema perforation, or a distal atretic segment of ileum which on some occasions opens directly into the peritoneum [60,73,75]. However, the contrast media, such as Gastrografin or other ionic hyperosmolar contrast media, are absorbed and can cause serious side effects including changes in circulating plasma volume, colitis, and necrotizing enterocolitis, and may increase the risk of perforation [60,66–76]. Great care and continuous intravenous hydration are necessary if these contrast media are used.

Ideally, the new low osmolar contrast media such as ioxaglate, iopamidol, or iohexol are used in isoosmolar concentrations. We use a 160-mg/ml concentration of ioxaglate in our hospital, which we find gives good opacification of the neonatal colon (Fig. 5.26).

In Older Infants and Children

Barium sulfate is the usual contrast medium of choice in older infants and children unless perforation or distal intestinal obstruction syndrome are suspected. If there is a possible perforation, water-soluble contrast medium is used in a similar technique to that described for a single-contrast barium enema. Because the new isoosmolar contrast media are so expensive in the necessary quantities, at our hospital we generally use a dilute (nearly isoosmolar) water-soluble contrast media such as Cysto-Conray, 17%.

i. Distal Intestinal Obstruction Syndrome. The distal intestinal obstruction syndrome (or meconium ileus equivalent) is found in patients with cystic fibrosis and pancreatic insufficiency, which give very sticky bowel contents that can cause an ileocecal obstruction. Gastrografin or other water-soluble contrast media have been advocated in the treatment of this condition, but we have found that oral Golytely (a balanced electrolyte solution) gives better results, is better tolerated by the patient, and is cheaper [77–79].

ii. Intussusception Reduction. Barium sulfate and water-soluble contrast media have both been commonly used for intussusception

A 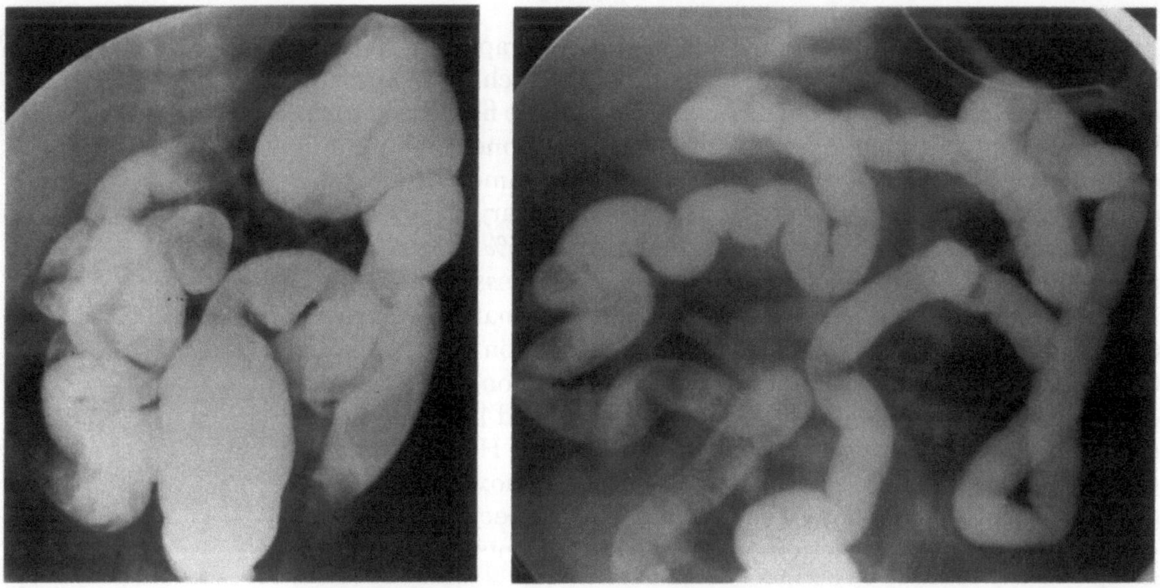 B

Fig. 5.26. Water-soluble contrast enema in infant. **A.** Isotonic ioxaglate gives good opacification throughout the large bowel and terminal ileum. In another infant (**B**), pellets of meconium in the terminal ileum and a microcolon empty of meconium confirm the diagnosis of meconium ileus in a newborn infant with distal intestinal obstruction.

reduction in North America, Europe, and Australia; however, there are risks from both of these contrast media because of the possibility of perforation. Barium in the peritoneum is to be avoided as it may lead to barium peritonitis and adhesions, and water-soluble contrast media, if not isoosmolar, may result in dramatic electrolyte and plasma volume changes that are especially dangerous in the young sick infant. In China, and in the nineteeth century in North America, air has been used to reduce intussusceptions. This has been investigated at our hospital and has now replaced the liquid contrast media as the medium of choice [80,81]. This is discussed further (see page 148).

Water-Soluble Enema in Neonates

Indications

Intestinal obstruction, e.g., clinical history of bilious vomiting and/or distended abdomen. There are many causes for this including:

1. Small bowel atresia
2. Meconium ileus
3. Malrotation with or without volvulus
4. Hirschsprung disease
5. Functional immaturity of the large bowel (which includes the hypoplastic left hemicolon syndrome and meconium plug syndrome)
6. Large bowel atresia.

Contraindications and Precautions

The study should not be performed if there is free intraperitoneal air. It is often extremely difficult to fill the colon in these children as many have a microcolon. The pressure that one has to use to fill the colon can be relatively high, and the study therefore has to be done very carefully and sometimes slowly over a prolonged period of time. Fluoroscopy during this time should be limited to what is necessary.

Concentrations of contrast media greater than 25% should not be used as the osmolarity is too high and draws in excessive fluid. This may dehydrate the baby and distend the bowel proximal to the obstruction, leading to perforation [60,66–76]. (See discussion under General Considerations.) Ideally, the new low osmolar nonionic contrast media, ioxaglate, iopamidol, or iohexol, should be used [60]. These are diluted with water to give an isotonic solution. At the Hospital for Sick Children, we use a 160-mg/ml concentration of ioxaglate as it is cheaper than the other contrast agents, and in a prospective study gave good results with no deleterious effects on the patients.

Materials

1. Size 8 or 10 French Foley catheter
2. Low osmolar contrast media such as ioxaglate, iopamidol, or iohexol mixed to an isoosmolar concentration.
3. Tape to strap the buttocks together
4. 60-ml disposable syringes.
5. 30 ml of *N*-acetylcysteine (Mucomyst) (200 mg/ml) can be added to each 30–60 ml of contrast media if meconium ileus is suspected [60].

Preparation

The test is discussed with the parents and also the clinicians, particularly because these infants are most at risk from this procedure.

□ *Procedure*

Step 1. Plain films of the abdomen in supine and erect position are obtained before the examination. Usually these have already been obtained before the test is ordered.
Step 2. The soft catheter, such as a Foley catheter, is inserted just inside the rectum and the buttocks of the child are taped together. The balloon is NOT inflated.
Step 3. With the patient prone, contrast is injected into the rectum manually through a syringe attached to the catheter. The child is fluoroscoped intermittently. Spot films of the lateral rectum (film 1), cecum (film 2), and encountered abnormalities (film 3) are obtained (Fig. 5.26) (see Chapter 6).
Step 4. If meconium is encountered, contrast medium is slowly and gently injected so that it passes around the plugs and hence facilitates the passage of this material.

Step 5. After the diagnosis has been established, a single abdominal film is obtained (film 4).
Step 6. Occasionally, if the large bowel is very convoluted, using normal saline or water after the initial injection of contrast can facilitate visualization of more proximal bowel as the contrast medium is pushed on from the distal large bowel.

Single-Contrast Barium Enema

Indications

1. To show position of cecum and hence exclude malrotation
2. To show Hirschsprung disease and investigate other causes of constipation.
3. To demonstrate gross anatomy of the colon.

Contraindications and Precautions

1. A recent deep biopsy of the rectum or colon, through a rigid or wide-bore flexible sigmoidoscope. If a deep biopsy has been taken, wait at least a week and preferably 10 days. A superficial biopsy from a narrow-bore flexible sigmoidoscope need not be a contraindication [65, 82–85].
2. The possibility of perforation is a contraindication. Use water-soluble contrast or, preferably, low osmolar nonionic media if an enema is essential.
3. Toxic megacolon is a contraindication.
4. Rectal bleeding or possible colitis requires a double-contrast examination [65].
5. In Hirschsprung disease, the colon should not be filled with barium proximal to the zone of transition as the barium may inspissate precipitating obstruction.

Materials

1. 1 part 55% w/w 100% w/v barium sulfate (Polibar) diluted with 5 parts water.
2. 5 ml (10 mg) of Dulcolax per liter of barium is usually used at the Hospital for Sick Children (unless there is a contraindication such as colitis, rectal bleeding, or the patient is generally unwell. It should be remembered that the patients with colitis and rectal bleeding need a double-contrast barium enema). Further contraindications are the investigation of possible intussusception and the examination of small or sick infants.
3. Disposable soft enema tips and enema bags.

Preparation

Discussion of procedure with the patient (and parents).

□ *Procedure*

Step 1. After the rectal tube has been inserted, the patient is put into the right lateral (left-side-down) position. As the barium is introduced, a lateral film of the rectosigmoid region is taken (film 1) (Fig. 5.27A).
Step 2. The patient is now put into the prone position and more barium is introduced until the rest of the large bowel is filled, as shown by filling of the appendix or terminal ileum. The prone position is best as the transverse colon is then dependent. If there is any delay in filling of the ascending colon, the patient can be turned lateral, right-side-down. However, as soon as the cecum fills a spot film must be obtained (film 2) (Fig. 5.27B), in the oblique or supine position, to show the relationship of the cecum to the right iliac wing to exclude malrotation.
Step 3. The barium is always introduced under fluoroscopic control but using short flashes of exposure to minimize radiation dose. Spot films are obtained if any abnormalities are identified (optional film 1).
Step 4. When the large bowel is full, a preevacuation film is taken of the entire abdomen (film 3) (Fig. 5.27C). This film should be taken without delay to prevent excessive patient discomfort and can be taken prone or supine for expediency.
Step 5. A postevacuation film (film 4) is taken after evacuation (Fig. 5.27D).

Intussusception Reduction

Indication

Clinical suspicion of intussusception.

Relative Contraindications and Precautions

The risk of perforation is mostly related to infants under 6 months of age with small bowel obstruction. The patient should be examined by a surgeon, preferably pediatric, before the procedure for two reasons. First, they are usually the most experienced at detecting peritonitis and those children at risk of perforation, and second, they should be aware of the patient before the radiologic study, because a well-recognized complication of the enema is perforation, requiring reasonably rapid surgery.

Absolute Contraindication

Clinical evidence of peritonitis or perforation.

Materials

1. One part 55% w/w, 100% w/v barium sulfate (Polibar) diluted with five parts water *OR* air reduction pump
2. Foley catheter
3. Tape to tape the buttocks together.

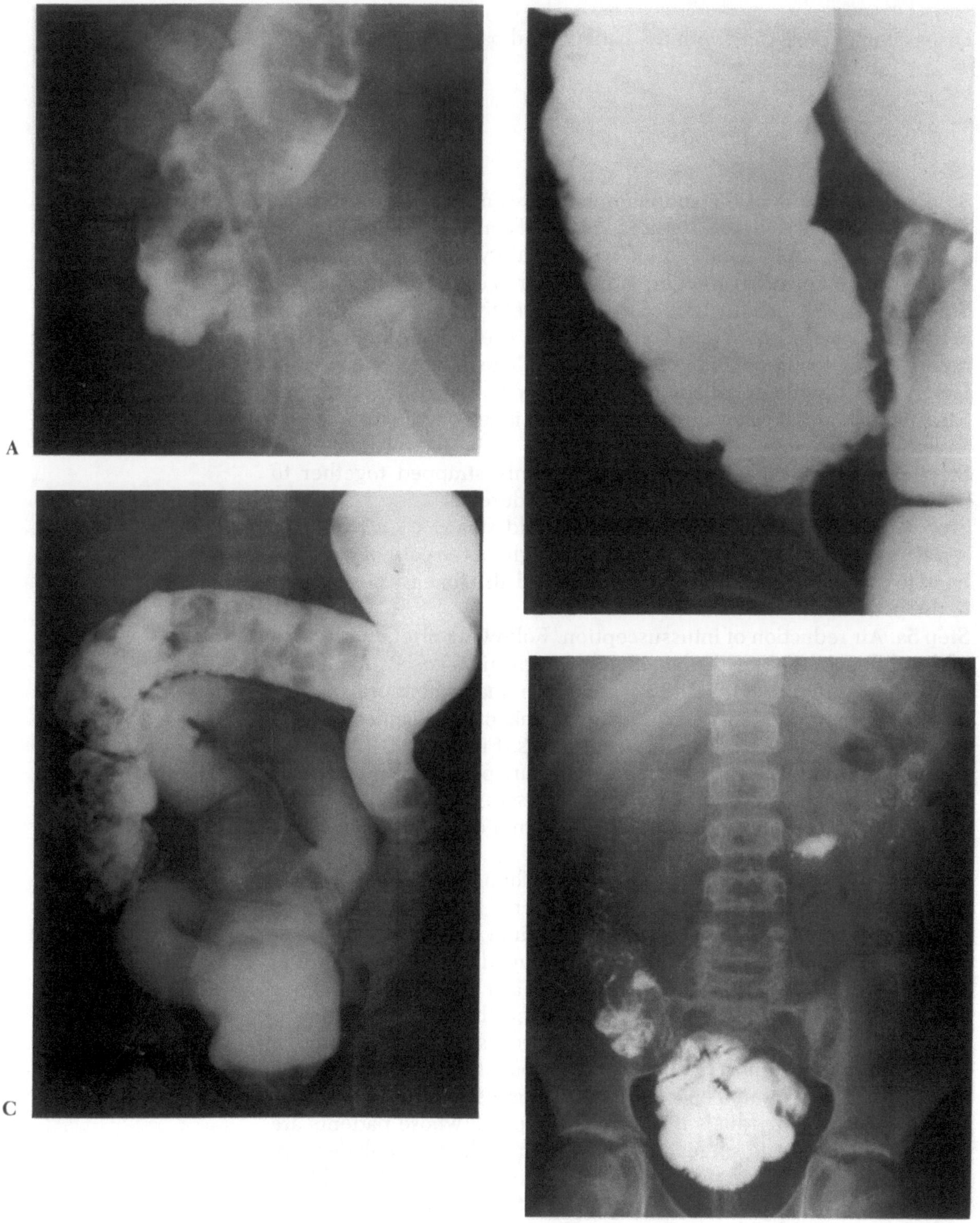

Fig. 5.27. Normal single-contrast enema. Spot films of rectum (A) and cecum (B) are taken before obtaining a pre-evacuation film (C). Ten minutes later, if Dulcolax has been used, a postevacuation film (D) is taken.

Preparation

Discussion of procedure with the patient (and parents).

□ *Procedure*

Step 1. A scout film of the abdomen is not essential except in infants and in those whose clinical status is a cause of concern. The plain films cannot exclude an intussusception with certainty, and are useful only to show small bowel obstruction in infants or to exclude perforation.
Step 2. With the patient prone, a *soft* catheter is inserted into the rectum. In our hospital, a Foley catheter is used. Some radiologists inflate the balloon to 5 ml in older children. The author obtains satisfactory results without balloon inflation. If the balloon is inflated, *only* 5 ml of air should be used and it should be inflated only just above the anus.
Step 3. The buttocks are carefully but firmly strapped together to prevent leakage of contrast during the procedure.
Step 4. The upper body of the child is held steady by a parent or assistant. The radiologist holds the upper thighs of the patient with one hand to prevent excess patient movement and also for easy positioning of the patient.
Step 5a. Air reduction of intussusception. Following brief fluoroscopy of the abdomen to show the bowel gas pattern, air is gently insufflated using a hand pump so that the air pressure remains at approximately 80 mm of mercury. This is sufficient to make the diagnosis in all patients and to reduce most intussusceptions (Fig. 5.28A). In those in whom reduction does not occur, an air pressure pump (so long as it has an adequate safety release valve) can be used. The pressure in the system and patient can be raised above 80 mm of mercury but never above 120 mm of mercury.

At the Hospital for Sick Children, we have found this technique to be simple, quick, and safe, and it gives us an overall reduction rate of over 80%, better than our reduction rate with barium sulfate.
Step 5b. If barium or water-soluble contrast media is used, it is run in at a steady rate, initially with the barium bag at a 1-meter height above the patient. Particular attention is paid when the intussusception is encountered and when reduction starts, because this is the time at which perforation is most likely to occur. A spot film is obtained (film 1) when the barium column encounters the intussusception (Fig. 5.29A).

Experienced individuals in pediatric hospitals whose patients are screened by pediatric surgeons often disregard the textbook descriptions of intussusception reduction. At the Hospital for Sick Children, Toronto, Canada, the length of clinical symptoms before and length of time for attempted reduction are not adhered to. If the surgeons are happy that the child's clinical condition is satisfactory, symptoms of many days duration (e.g., after transport over long distances) will not preclude radiologic reduction. If barium is used, the barium column is often raised above the 1-meter standard, especially if resistance at the ileocecal level is found. The ceiling is the maximum height used and in

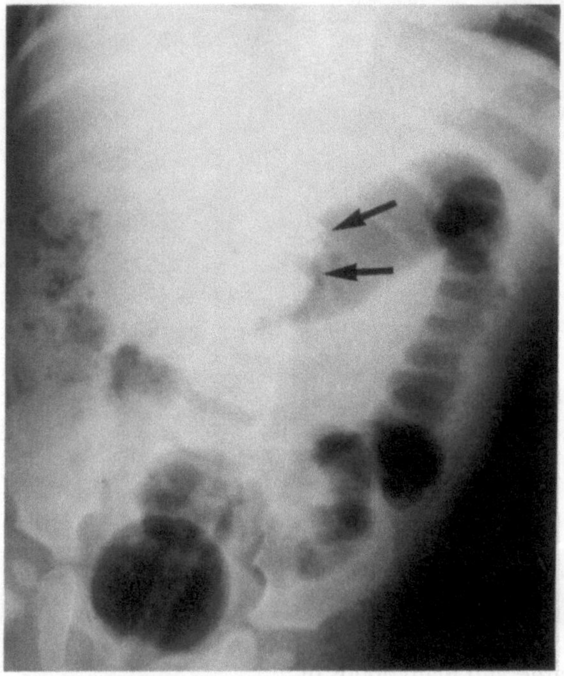

A

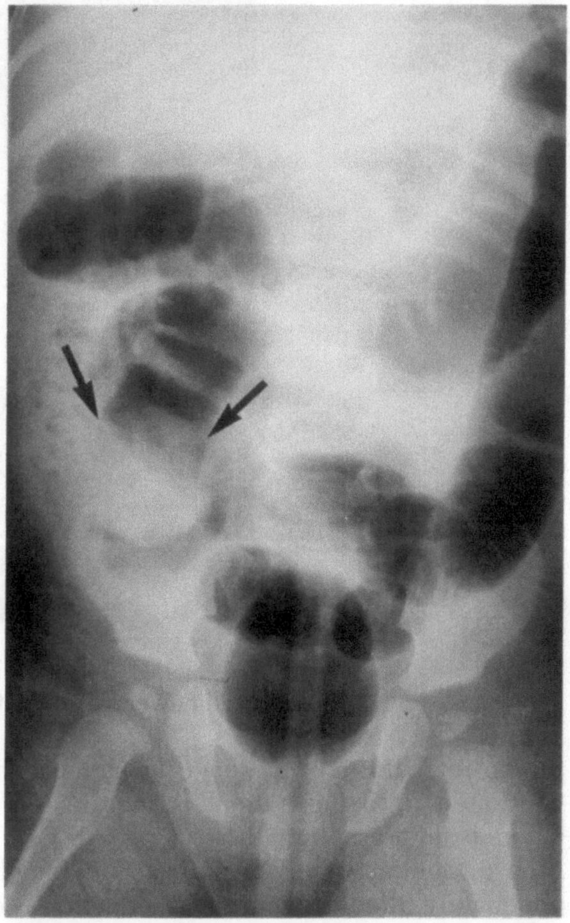

B

Fig. 5.28. Air reduction of intussusception. **A.** Air outlines filling the defect of an intussusception (*arrows*). **B.** With further air insufflation, the intussusception is reduced to the level of cecum (*arrows*). Note that the Foley balloon catheter has been overinflated in the rectum (See text).

Fig. 5.29. Colon. Barium reduction of intussusception. A. Intussusception is shown outlined by barium in ascending colon (*arrows*), and cecum (B-arrows) (*continued*)

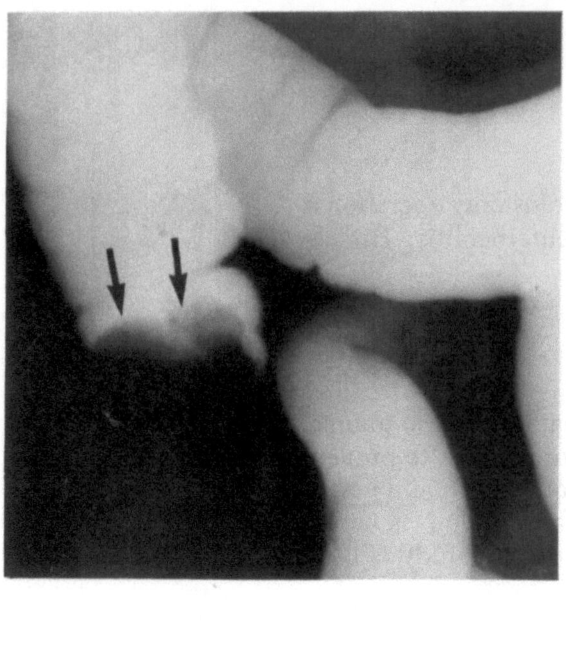

A

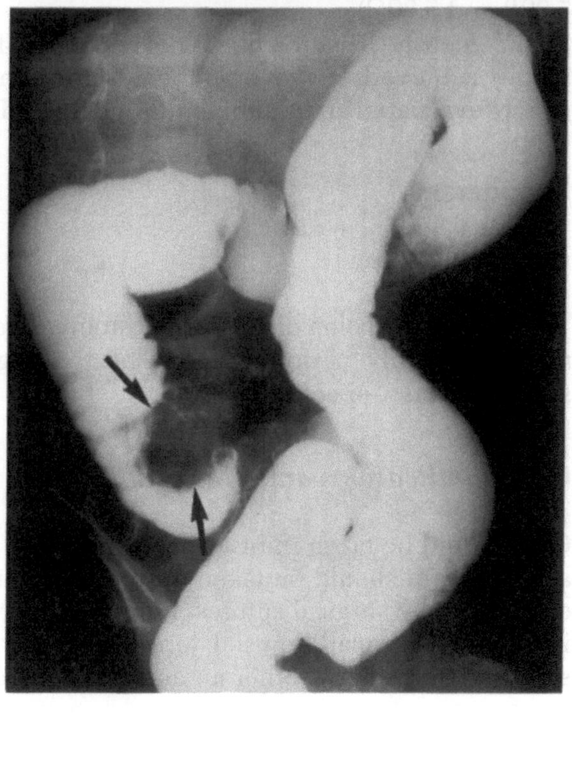

B

C 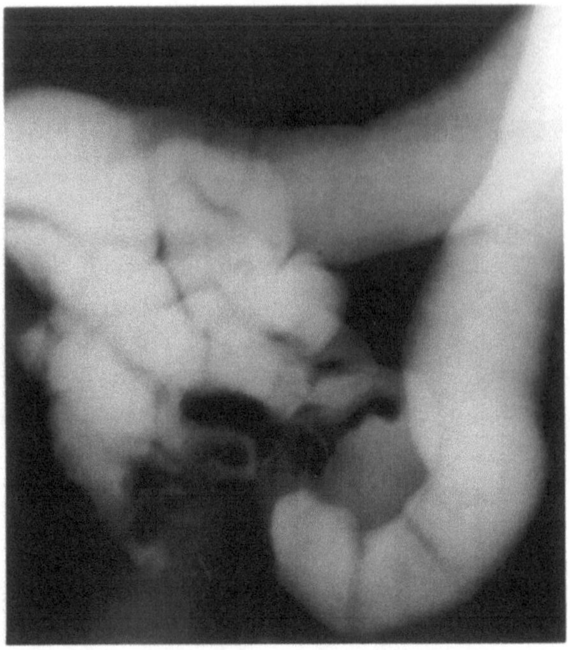

Fig. 5.29. C. Barium fills large and many loops of small bowel post reduction.

our hospital, this is 6 feet above the patient! The attempt at reduction is continued until the patient is inordinately distressed or fatigued. There is no preset time limit.

Step 6. Contrast is given until a number of small bowel loops are adequately filled to ensure that reduction is complete. A supine spot film of the abdomen is obtained before evacuation (film 2) (Figs. 5.28B, 5.29B and 5.29C)

Step 7. A postevacuation film is not necessary if full reduction has been readily achieved. However, if there is any clinical concern, the bowel is now evacuated and a supine full-length abdominal film is taken.

Loopogram

Indications

To examine the colon distal to a colostomy. The colostomy operation is most commonly performed after necrotizing enterocolitis, Hirschsprung disease, or colitis.

Contraindications and Precautions

Care should be taken in inserting catheters so that there is no trauma, and also care should be taken during injection of contrast to prevent damage to the surgical sutures. Foley catheter balloons should not be inflated in the small bowel. Close liaison with the surgeons is necessary to determine whether an antegrade or retrograde study is best.

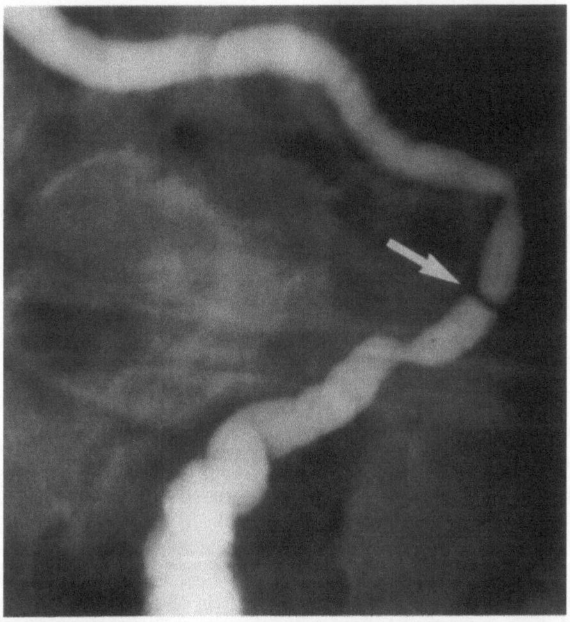

Fig. 5.30. Loopogram. Water-soluble contrast media injected through a colostomy in a follow-up examination in an infant who had necrotizing enterocolitis shows a short segment stricture (*arrow*) at junction of descending and sigmoid colon overlying the left iliac wing.

The general rule is to insert the catheters in the opening furthest away from the site of major surgery; for example, insert through colostomy if a rectal pull-through has been performed.

Materials

1. Iothalamate meglumine 17.2% (Cysto-Conray 11) is used at our hospital. Low osmolar contrast media such as iohexol or iopamidol can be used but are expensive. They should be reserved for those patients for whom complications are suspected.
2. Occasionally barium is used (5 parts barium to 1 part water) if no risk of perforation or leak is present, or after a normal water-soluble contrast examination. However, inspissation could occur.
3. Soft nasogastric tubes, Foley catheters, or disposable soft enema tips may be used, depending on whether the study is performed antegrade or retrograde.

□ *Procedure*

Contrast is run throughout the loop to demonstrate patency and exclude leaks. Spot films are taken if any abnormalities are encountered (Fig. 5.30). One spot film of the entire bowel is taken if no abnormalities are seen.

Double-Contrast Barium Enema

Indications

The indications are more restricted than in adults as cancer is almost unheard of.

1. Rectal bleeding of unknown cause
2. To show polyps or masses
3. To show fine mucosal detail, for example, extent of involvement in inflammatory bowel disease.

Colonoscopy is very effective at diagnosing the foregoing conditions [35,36,86–89], but is more invasive and more hazardous with reports of perforations, hemorrhage, and even explosions [90–92]. Colonoscopy and double-contrast barium enemas may both miss lesions [88,93–95], and in children should be considered as a complementary investigation [94].

Contraindications

a. Bowel perforation
b. Toxic megacolon
c. Recent *deep* (not narrow-bore colonoscopic) large bowel biopsy. (See Single-Contrast Colon Exam, page 145.)

Materials

1. Undiluted 55% w/w, 100% w/v barium sulfate (Polibar).
   It is essential to use a high-density barium sulfate preparation to obtain adequate coating [94]. A lymphoid follicular pattern will be seen in nearly all pediatric patients and can be used as an indication of the effectiveness of mucosal coating [96].
2. Disposable enema bags and *soft* enema tips.

Preparation

Step 1. Over 2 years of age

a. Clear fluids for 36 hours before the examination.

b. Castor oil, 1 ml/kg body weight, or magnesium citrate or other purgative the afternoon before the examination, if not clinically contraindicated.

c. Saline or Fleet enema the evening before and the morning of the examination.

Step 2. Under 2 years of age

Under 2 years of age, we find that it is safest to prepare the patient in the department.

The patient arrives unprepared. A very limited distal colonic enema with 5 ml (10 mg) per liter concentration of Dulcolax is performed with dilute contrast media instilled to the splenic flexure or midtransverse colon, depending on amount of fecal residue.

The double-contrast study is performed 30 to 60 minutes post evacuation, and is most easily performed by syringes of barium and air with spot films taken as each area of the large bowel is distended. Often the only large films then required are the decubitus views.
Step 3. The procedure is explained to the patient and parents.

□ *Procedure in Children over 2 Years of Age*

Step 1. The patient is lying on the left side with both hips and knees flexed. The enema tube is inserted and secured with tape to the buttocks. With the tube in position the patient is now turned prone.
Step 2. Under intermittent fluoroscopic control the barium is run up to the midtransverse colon under hydrostatic pressure and then stopped. Occasionally in older, more cooperative teenagers, less barium can be used and the barium flow is stopped when the column has reached the splenic flexure.
Step 3. The patient is turned on the right side and excess barium is drained from the rectum. This will also allow the barium to pass around the hepatic flexure.
Step 4. When enough barium has passed around the hepatic flexure, the patient either sits up or the head of the table is elevated. No air is insufflated until some barium has descended to the cecum. This is because the air insufflation is the uncomfortable part of the examination when the child's cooperation can rapidly disappear. Hence it is only when enough barium is present wherever it is needed and when barium has stopped draining from the rectum that air is insufflated.
Step 5. Air is insufflated very slowly. In this way the rectal distension, the most uncomfortable part of the procedure, is kept to a minimum. Carbon dioxide has been advocated in adults instead of air as it causes less discomfort [97,98], but it is not widely used in children.
Step 6. Enough air having been insufflated to give adequate distension of the bowel, the patient is rotated twice through 360° in each direction to obtain good coating of the mucosa.
Step 7. With the patient on one side a lateral rectum film is obtained. The side on which the patient lies is determined by the image seen fluoroscopically as that giving the best double-contrast view (Fig. 5.31A). Occasionally this is best obtained with the patient erect or by a cross-table lateral prone film.
Step 8. With the patient lying with the left side down and half onto the back, a film is taken of the air-filled cecum and terminal ileum (Fig. 5.31B). The left-side-down position helps fill the cecum with air.
Step 9. The following overhead films are then taken:

- a. supine abdomen (Fig. 5.31D) (Fig. 5.31C)
- b. prone abdomen (a 20° to 25° angled caudal view is sometimes useful in unfolding the sigmoid colon and does not change radiation dosage in smaller children)
- c. left lateral decubitus (Fig. 5.31E)
- d. right lateral decubitus (Fig. 5.31F)

Step 10. Further spot films are taken as necessary. No postevacuation film is taken.

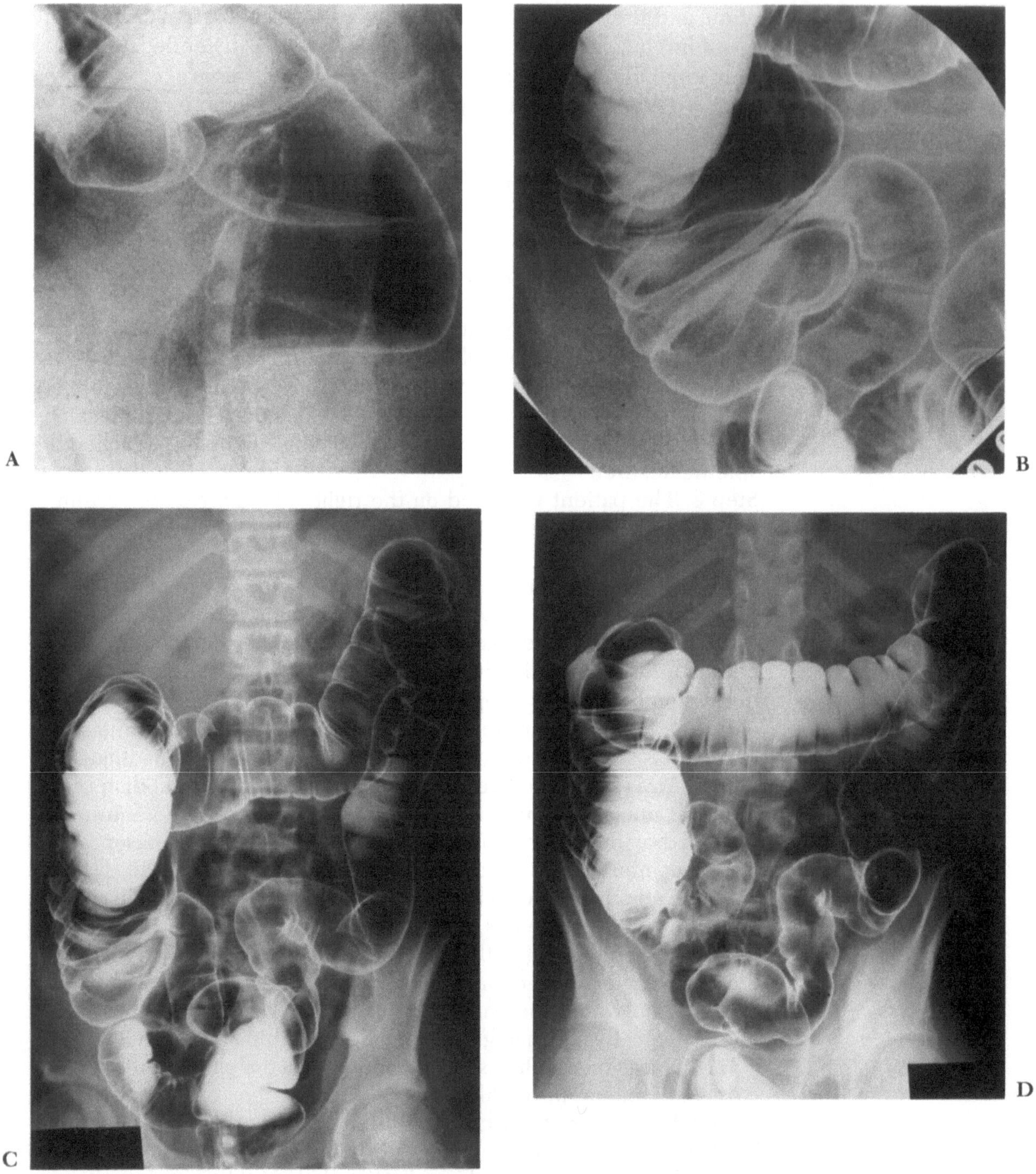

Fig. 5.31. Normal double-contrast barium enema in older children. Spot films of lateral rectum (**A**) and oblique cecum (**B**) are taken when visualized optimally. Then, full-length films of the abdomen are taken with the patient supine (**C**), and prone (**D**). Decubitus films are taken with the patient lying on left side (**E**) and right side (**F**). With these views, most diagnostic problems in children can be readily solved.

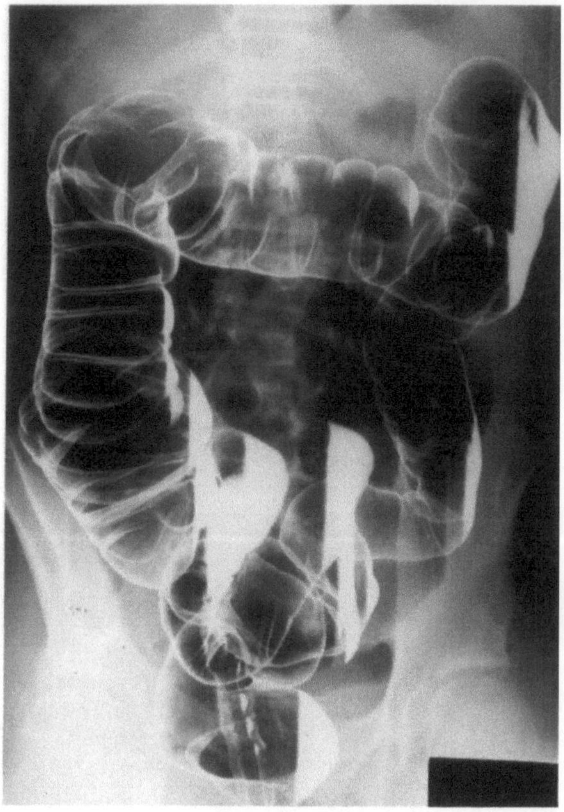
E

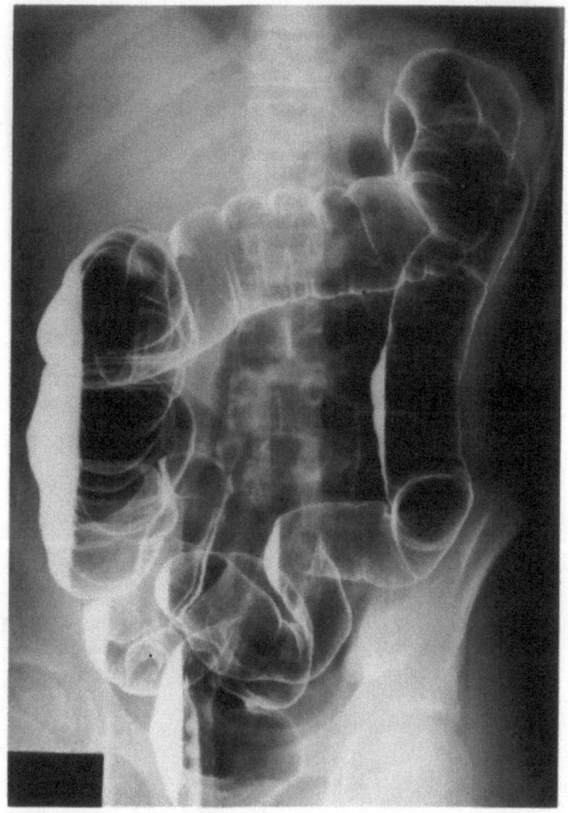
F

□ *Procedure in Children Under 2 Years of Age*

The procedure is modified in younger children. The barium is slightly diluted with water and is injected by hand using a syringe. Excess barium is aspirated and air is injected via a syringe; spot films are taken rapidly as each part of the large bowel is outlined. This enables a quick examination to be performed with films taken at optimum filling (Fig. 5.32). At the end of the procedure, other views, such as supine, prone, or decubitus projections, may be helpful (Fig. 5.33), especially if all areas have not been seen well, provided the infant is retaining the barium and air. It is sometimes helpful to insufflate a small amount of air before each large film to facilitate distension of bowel loops.

Lymphoid Follicular Pattern

A lymphoid follicular pattern of slightly raised, sometimes umbilicated nodules measuring less than 3 mm (Fig. 5.34) is almost always present in children, especially the younger ones, and is a normal finding. It is useful as it indicates good mucosal coating [96].

Defecogram

The value of defecography in children as in adults is still being evaluated [99,100]. The basic procedure is similar to that in adults [99–102] (see pages 93 and Figs. 4.39 and 4.40).

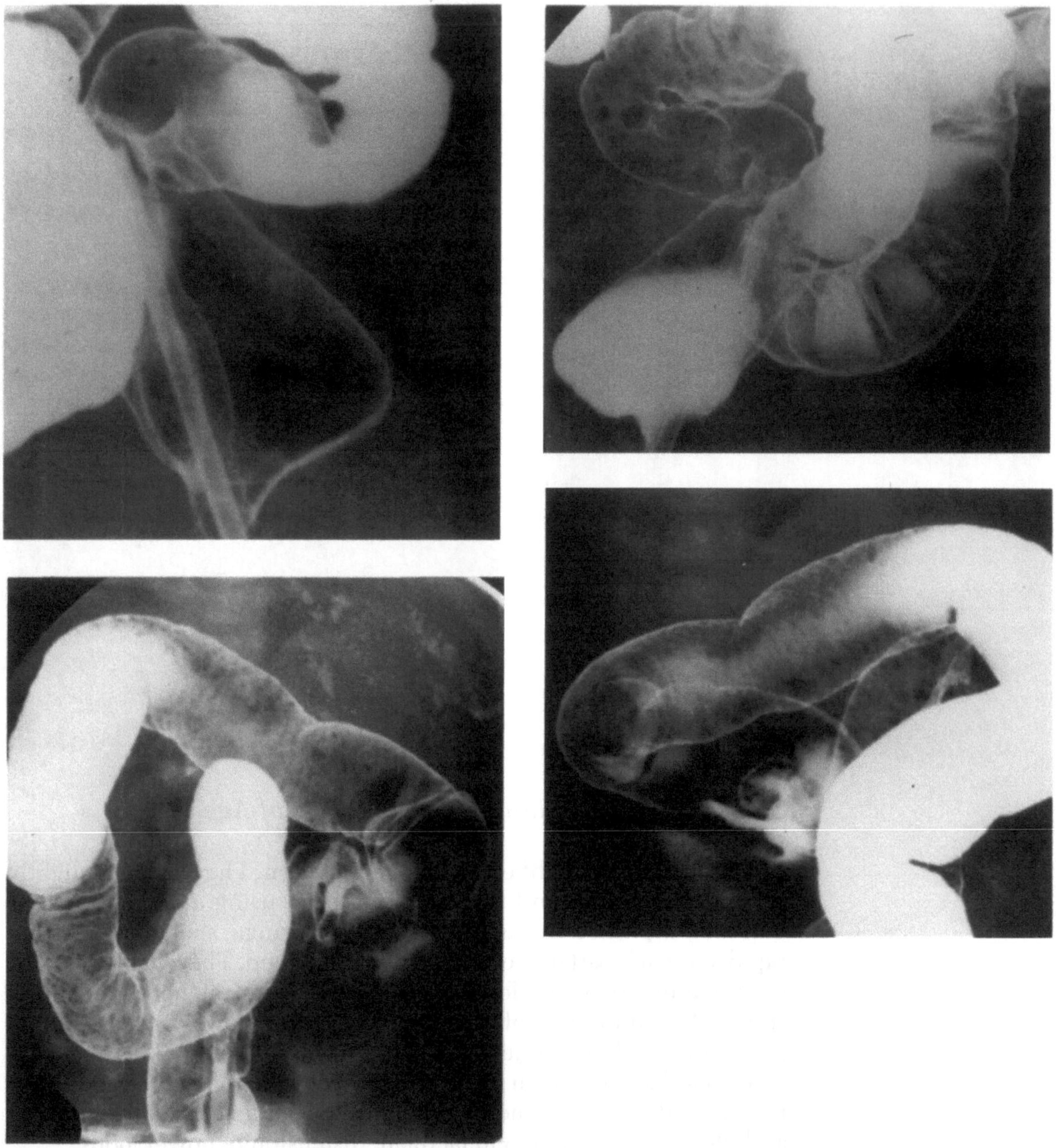

A B C D

Fig. 5.32. A–D. Double-contrast barium enema in infant. Four spot films in various projections show most portions of the large bowel.

Indications

The major indication is the investigation of rectal constipation or incontinence secondary to anorectal malformations and Hirschsprung disease, especially in the long-term postoperative phase.

Contraindications

As per adults (page 93).

A 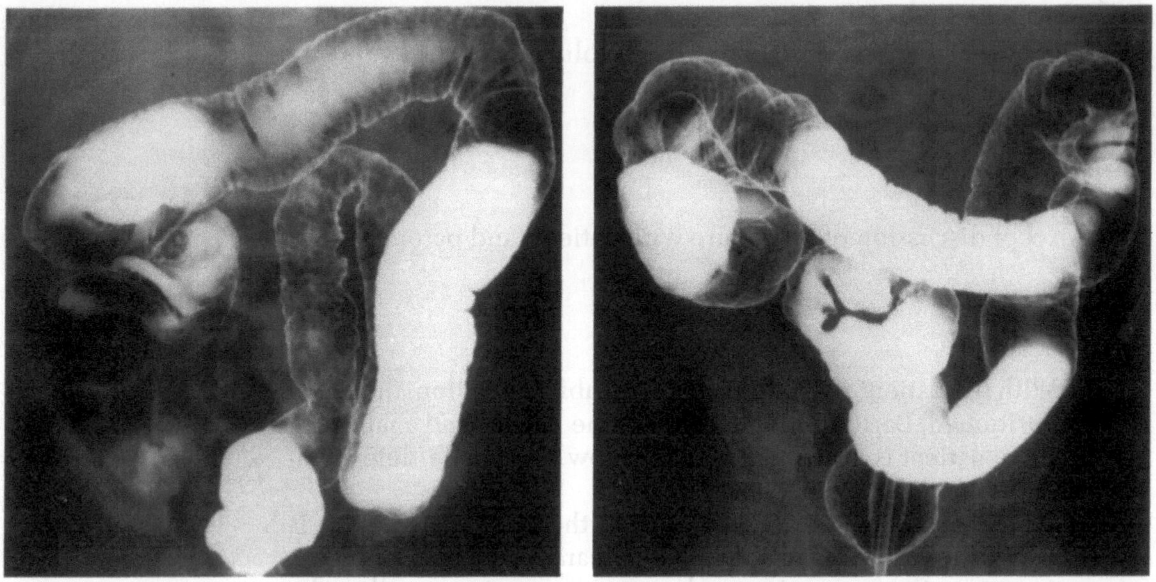 B

Fig. 5.33. Double-contrast barium enema in infant. Supine (**A**) and prone (**B**) views show most of the large bowel. The cecum is high in position and is pointing laterally. In an asymptomatic child, this probably represents a variant of mobile cecum but malrotation would have to be considered in any symptomatic child, and if there is any clinical concern a barium meal would be indicated to demonstrate the position of the duodenojejunal flescure.

A 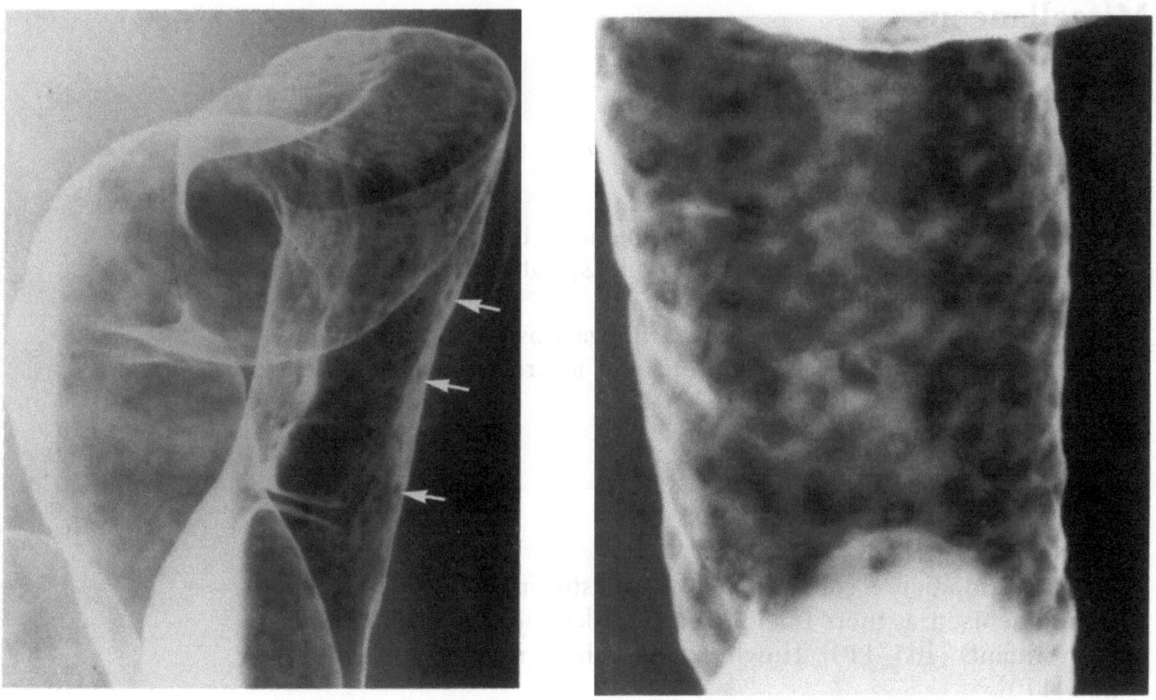 B

Fig. 5.34. Lymphoid follicular pattern. Double-contrast barium enema spot films show slightly raised nodules measuring less than 3 mm (*arrows*) in the splenic flexure (**A**) **B**. Spot film from descending colon shows a small central collection of barium in some of the nodules.

Preferred Materials

1 part 55% w/w, 100% w/v barium sulfate (Polibar).
Soft rectal catheter.

Preparation

None except discussion of procedure with patient (and parents).

□ *Procedure*

Step 1. With the patient in the left lateral decubitus position, the rectal tube is positioned. Barium is injected to fill the rectum and anal canal, and then the patient is seated erect on a hollow receptable/defecography chair (as in adults, page 93).
Step 2. The mechanism of defecation from the lateral projection is videotaped with spot films to show the appearance at rest, straining, evacuating, stopping evacuation, and evacuating again as well as the postevacuation appearance. In children, it is unusual to get sufficient cooperation to be able to see all these parts of defecation, and the procedure is modified according to the individual.
Step 3. The videotape is played back to the referring surgeon, and it is only with this close cooperation that the test can be fully evaluated.

Miscellaneous

Intestinal Tube Placement

Indications

1. Nasal or oral gastrojejunal tubes, nasojejunal tubes, small bowel biopsy capsules, and pancreatic enzyme aspiration tubes often require fluoroscopy for accurate placement.
2. A feeding tube can be positioned via the gastrostomy into the jejunum when a gastrostomy is present and gastroesophageal reflux prevents gastrostomy feeding [103,104].

Contraindications and Precautions

1. Malrotation or risk of volvulus.
2. Risk of perforation. A soft tube such as a silastic or Erythrothane tube should be used, as there is an increased risk of bowel perforation in these infants [105–113]. However, even these may cause perforation [113].
3. Time of fluoroscopy. By allowing plenty of time for tubes to pass into the small bowel without screening, fluoroscopy can be kept to an absolute minimum.

Materials

The correct tube for the purpose: feeding nasojejunal tubes, often necessary in small infants, are the most commonly positioned tubes. Familiarity with the type of tube to be inserted is essential before starting the procedure as there are many types of nasojejunal tubes, few of which permit the use of conventional guide wires. Some of the tubes contain a polymer guide wire, which can be removed but not reinserted.
Appropriate guide wires.
(Metoclopramide).

Preparation

As for a barium meal.

□ *Procedure*

Step 1. The patient is positioned supine and the tube is passed into the stomach. Slightly prebending the tube and flexing the patient's neck may facilitate passage of the tube past the velopharynx and larynx, respectively.
Step 2. When the tube is in the stomach, the patient lies on the right side so that the tube tip is carried by peristalsis and gravity to the pylorus. The tube is gently advanced with the guide wire under fluoroscopic guidance through the pylorus. A variable time can elapse before the tube can be advanced through the pylorus and care should be taken to keep fluoroscopy to a minimum.
Step 3. A guide wire is invaluable at aiding control of the tube, and this can be further aided by giving the end of the guide wire a slight kink. If metal, however, the kink should not be so marked that the guide cannot be removed at the end of the procedure and so should be tested for ease of withdrawal before insertion into the patient.
Step 4. If a gastrostomy is present, an endotracheal tube can be used as a guide to facilitate tube placement and to steer the tube to the pylorus (104).
Step 5. Intramuscular metoclopramide is used in some institutions to aid the passage of the tubes, but is not used in our hospital as we find that with care the tubes can be passed relatively easily.

Foreign Body Removal

Indications

Removal of blunt foreign bodies such as coins (114–117).

Contraindications and Precautions

1. The safety of the procedure. Although this technique has been used regularly with excellent results in some centers, the safety of the

procedure has been seriously questioned because of the possibility of aspiration [118]. Hence, great caution is advised with care being taken to protect the airway throughout the procedure, and the technique should not be attempted by the inexperienced [119].

2. Sharp foreign bodies. Generally, only uncomplicated smooth radioopaque foreign bodies with no esophageal abnormality should be removed. However, with experience, some successes with nonopaque foreign bodies or in esophageal atresia repair patients are recorded [120]. Sharp foreign bodies are not amenable to removal by this method because of the fear of esophageal perforation [114,116].

3. Route of catheter passage. The nasal route of catheter passage occasionally results in the foreign body being deposited in the nasal air passages [119], and hence the oral route is preferred.

4. Failure of removal. Failure of removal of smooth foreign bodies probably occurs because of esophageal edema, and this is found especially in infants [121]. The lateral chest radiograph may be useful in predicting chances of success with widening of the tracheoesophageal interspace being associated with failure of foreign body removal [121].

5. Other complications. In a survey of the Society of Pediatric Radiology, in 2500 esophageal foreign body removals, one child with congenital heart disease was observed to experience severe hypoxia during the procedure [119]. In two other children, a small amount of blood streaking of mucus was seen, presumably from mild esophageal mucosal injury.

Materials

1. 14 French Foley catheter
2. 5–7 ml of isoosmolar water-soluble contrast medium
3. Laryngoscope and resuscitation equipment.

Preparations

As per barium meal.

□ *Procedure*

Step 1. A 14 French Foley catheter is passed, preferably through the mouth or possibly through the nose, and beyond the foreign body.

Step 2. The inflatable balloon is filled with 5–7 ml of isoosmolar water-soluble contrast medium.

Step 3. The catheter is withdrawn under fluoroscopic control with the child slightly inverted in the prone oblique position.

Step 4. Inversion of the fluoroscopic table helps prevent aspiration of the foreign body during withdrawal. If the table cannot be inverted, then someone experienced in laryngoscopy should be present in the fluoroscopy suite in case aspiration occurs [116,117].

References

1. Cremin BJ (1985). Real time ultrasonic evaluation of the paediatric abdomen: technique and anatomical variations: a personal view. Br J Radiol 58:859–868.
2. Holm HH, Smith EH, Bartrum RJ (1977). The relationship of computed tomography and ultrasonography in diagnosis of abdominal disease. J. Clin Ultrasound 5: 230–237.
3. Brasch RC, Abols IB, Gooding CA, Filly RA (1980). Abdominal disease in children: a comparison of computed tomography and ultrasound. AJR 134:153–158.
4. Pilling DW (1983). Infantile hypertrophic pyloric stenosis: a fresh approach to diagnosis. Clin Radiol 34:51–53.
5. Stundar RJ, Le Quesne GW, Little KET (1986). The improved ultrasound diagnosis of hypertrophic pyloric stenosis. Pediatr Radiol 16:200–205.
6. Hayden CK, Swischuk LE, Lobe TE, Schwartz MZ, Boulden T (1984). Ultrasound: the definitive imaging modality in pyloric stenosis. Radiographics 4:517–530.
7. Naik DR, Bolia A, Moore DJ 91985). Comparison of barium swallow and ultrasound in diagnosis of gastroesophageal reflux in children. Br Med J 290:1943–1945.
8. Naik DR, Moore DJ (1984). Ultrasound diagnosis of gastroesophageal reflux. Arch Dis Child 59:366–379.
9. Stringer DA, Daneman A, Brunelle F, Ward K, Martin DJ (1986). Sonography of the normal and abnormal stomach (excluding hypertrophic pyloric stenosis) in children. J Ultrasound Med 5:183–188.
10. Puylaert JBCM (1986). Acute appendicitis: US evaluation using graded compression. Radiology 158:355–360.
11. McGahan JP, Phillips HE, Cox KL (1982). Sonography of the normal pediatric gall bladder and biliary tract. Radiology 144:873–875.
12. Brill PW, Winchester P, Rosen MS (1982). Neonatal cholelithiasis. Pediatr Radiol 12:285–288.
13. Farrant P, Dewbury KC, Meire HB (1981). Antenatal diagnosis of duodenal atresia. Br J Radiol 54:633–635.
14. Alexander ES, Spitz HB, Clark RA (1982). Sonography of polyhydramnios. AJR 138:343–346.
15. Benacerraf BR, Greene MF (1986). Congenital diaphragmatic hernia: US diagnosis prior to 22 weeks gestation. Radiology 158:809–810.
16. Brown B St. J (1985). The prenatal ultrasonographic features of omphalocele: a study of 10 patients. J Can Assoc Radiol 36:312–315.
17. Chinn DH, Filly RA, Callen PW, Nakayama DK, Harrison MR (1983). Congenital diaphragmatic hernia diagnosed prenatally by ultrasound. Radiology 148:119–123.
18. Denholm TA, Crow HC, Edwards WH, Simmons GM, Marin-Padilla M, Bartrum RJ (1984). Prenatal sonographic appearance of meconium ileus in twins. AJR 143:371–372.
19. Grignon A, Filiatrault D, Yasbeck S (1986). Gastroschisis and omphalocele: prenatal ultrasonographic diagnosis and postnatal evolution. Presented at the 29th Annual Meeting of the Society for Pediatric Radiology, Washington, April 9–13, 1986.
20. Lince DM, Pretorius DH, Manco-Johnson ML, Manchester D, Clewell WH (1985). The clinical significance of increased echogenicity in the fetal abdomen. AJR 145:683–686.
21. McGahan JP, Hanson F (1983). Meconium peritonitis with accompanying pseudocyst: prenatal sonographic diagnosis. Radiology 148:125–126.
22. Nelson PA, Bowie JD, Filston HC, Crane LM (1982). Sonographic diagnosis of omphalocele in utero. AJF 138:1178–1180.

23. Stringer DA, Daneman A, St. Onge O (1985). Doppler assessment of abdominal and peripheral vessels in children. Presented at the 71st Meeting of the Radiological Society of North America, Chicago, November 1985.
24. Skolnick ML (1970). Videofluoroscopic examination of the velopharyngeal portal during phonation in lateral and base projections. A new technique for studying the mechanics of closure. Cleft Palate J 7:803–816.
25. Skolnick ML (1977). A plea of an interdisciplinary approach to the radiological study of the velopharyngeal portal. Cleft Palate J 14:329–330.
26. Stringer DA, Witzel MA (1985). Waters projection for evaluation of lateral pharyngeal wall movement in speech disorders. AJR 145:409–410.
27. Stringer DA, Witzel MA (1986). Velopharyngeal insufficiency on multiview videofluoroscopy: comparison of projections. AJR 146:15–19.
28. Becker MH, Genieser NB (1972). A new device for feeding infants during fluoroscopy. J Pediatr 80:291–292.
29. Hyde I, Danby B (1980). An aid to barium meal examinations in infants. Br J Radiol 53:997–998.
30. Poznanski A (1969). A simple device for administering barium to infants. Radiology 93:1106.
31. Stringer DA, Ein SH (1984). Recurrent tracheoesophageal fistula: a protocol for investigation. Radiology 151:637–641.
32. Thomas PS, Chrispin AR (1969). Congenital tracheoesophageal fistula without esophageal atresia. Clin Radiol 20:371–374.
33. Drumm B, Rhoads M, Stringer DA, Sherman PM, Ellis LE, Durie PR (1988). Peptic ulcer disease in children: etiology, clinical findings, and clinical course. Pediatrics 82:410–414.
34. Cumming WA, Reilly BJ (1972). Fatigue aspiration. Radiology 105:387–390.
35. Burdelski M (1978). Endoscopy in pediatric gastroenterology. Eur J Pediatr 128:33–39.
36. Cadranel S, Rodesch P, Peeters JP, Cremer M (1977). Fiberendoscopy of the gastrointestinal tract in children: a series of 100 examinations. Am J Dis Child 131:41–45.
37. Gyepes MT, Smith LE, Ament ME (1977). Fiberoptic endoscopy and upper gastrointestinal series: comparative analysis in infants and children. AJR 128:53–56.
38. Hyslop JS, Mitchelmore AE, Cox RR, Wells IP (1982). Double contrast barium meal examination: a comparison of two high density barium preparations, E-Z-HD and X-Opaque. Clin Radiol 33:83–85.
39. Stringer DA, Sherman PM, Liu P, Daneman A (1986). Value of the peroral pneumocolon in pediatrics. AJR 146:763–766.
40. Heitzman ER, Berne AS (1961). Roentgen examination of the cecum and proximal ascending colon with ingested barium. Radiology 76:415–421.
41. Kellett MJ, Zboralske FF, Margulis AR (1977) Per-oral pneumocolon examination of the ileocecal region. Gastrointest Radiol 1:361–365.
42. Kelvin FM, Gedgaudas RK, Thompson WM, Rice RP (1982). The peroral pneumocolon: its role in evaluating the terminal ileum. AJR 139:115–121.
43. Kressel HY, Evers KA, Glick SN, Laufer I, Herlinger H (1982). The peroral pneumocolon examination. Radiology 144:414–416.
44. Laufer I (1979). Upper gastrointestinal tract: technical aspects. In: Laufer I (ed), Double Contrast Gastrointestinal Radiology with Endoscopic Correlation. Philadelphia: WB Saunders, pp. 59–77.
45. Pochaczevsky R (1974). Oral examination of the colon: "the colonic cocktail". AJR 121:318–325.
46. Stringer DA, Cloutier S, Daneman A, Durie PR (1986). The value of the small bowel enema in children. J Can Assoc Radiol 37:13–16.
47. Ekberg O (1977). Crohn disease of the small bowel examined by double

contrast technique: a comparison with oral technique. Gastrointest Radiol 1:355–359.
48. Eklof O, Erasmie U (1978). The small bowel enema: an improved method of examination and its indications in childhood. Ann Radiol (Paris) 21:143–148.
49. Herlinger H (1979). Small bowel. In: Laufer I (ed), Double Contrast Gastrointestional Radiology with Endoscopic Correlation. Philadelphia: WB Saunders, pp. 423–494.
50. Herlinger H (1982). The small bowel enema and the diagnosis of Crohn disease. Radiol Clin North Am 20:721–742.
51. Ratcliffe JF (1983). The small bowel enema in children: a description of a technique. Clin Radiol 34:287–289.
52. Sellink JL (1974). Radiologic examination of the small intestine by duodenal intubation. Acta Radiol [Diagn] (Stockh) 15:318–332.
53. Nelson SW, Christoforidas AJ, Pratt PC (1964). Further experience with barium sulfate as a bronchographic contrast medium. AJR 92:595–614.
54. Nice CM, Waring WW, Killelea DE, Hurwitz L (1964). Bronchography in infants and children: barium sulfate as a contrast agent. AJR 91:564–570.
55. Cohen MD, Smith JA, Slabaugh RD, Rust RJ (1982). Neonatal necrotizing enterocolitis shown by oral metrizamide (Amipaque). AJR 138:1019–1023.
56. Cohen MD, Weber T (1982). Metrizamide in neonatal and childhood small bowel obstruction. AJR 139:689–692.
57. Ginai AZ (1985). Experimental evaluation of various available contrast agents for use in the gastrointestinal tract in case of suspected leakage: effects on peritoneum. Br J Radiol 58:969–978.
58. Ginai AZ, ten Kate FJW, ten Berg RGM, Hoornstra K (1984). Experimental evaluation of various available contrast agents for use in the upper gastrointestinal tract in case of suspected leakage: effects on lungs. Br J Radiol 57:895–901.
59. Ratcliffe JF (1983). The use of loxaglate in the pediatric gastrointestinal tract: a report of 25 cases. Clin Radiol 34:579–583.
60. Ratcliffe JF (1985). Low osmolality water soluble (LOWS) contrast media and the pediatric gastrointestinal tract. Radiology Now 8:8–11.
61. Willson JKV, Rubin PS, McGee TM (1959). The effects of barium sulfate on lungs: a clinical and experimental study. AJR 82:84–94.
62. Chiu CL, Gambach RR (1974). Hypaque pulmonary edema—a case report. Radiology 111:91–92.
63. Huston J, Wallach DP, Cunningham GJ (1952). Pulmonary reaction to barium sulphate in rats. Arch Pathol 54:430–438.
64. Reich SB (1969). Production of pulmonary edema by aspiration of water soluble nonabsorbable contrast media. Radiology 92:367–370.
65. Winthrop JD, Balfe DM, Shackelford GD, McAlister WH, Rosenblum JL, Siegel MJ (1985). Ulcerative and granulomatous colitis in children: comparison of double- and single-contrast studies. Radiology 154:657–660.
66. Grantmyre EB, Butler GJ, Gillis DA (1981). Necrotizing enterocolitis after renografin-76 treatment of meconium ileus. AJR 136:990–991.
67. Harris PD, Neuhauser EBD, Gerth R (1964). The osmotic effect of water soluble contrast media on circulating plasma volume. AJR 91:694–698.
68. Leonidas JC, Burry VF, Fellows RA, Beatty EC (1976). Possible adverse effect of methylglucamine diatrizoate compounds on the bowel of newborn infants with meconium ileus. Radiology 121:693–696.
69. Lutzger LG, Factor SM (1976). Effects of some water-soluble contrast media on the colonic mucosa. Radiology 118:545–548.
70. Noblett HR (1969). Treatment of uncomplicated meconium ileus by gastrografin enema: a preliminary report. J Pediatr Surg 4:190–197.

71. Poole CA, Rowe MI (1976). Clinical evidence of intestinal absorption of gastrografin. Radiology 118:151–153
72. Poole CA, Rowe MI (1976). Distal neonatal intestinal obstruction: the choice of contrast material. J Pediatr Surg 11:1011–1022.
73. Seltzer SE, Jones B (1978). Cecal perforation associated with gastrografin enema. AJR 130:997–998.
74. Shaw A (1969). Safety of *N*-acetylcysteine in treatment of meconium obstruction of the newborn. J Pediatr Surg 4:119–125.
75. Wolfson JJ, Williams H (1970). A hazard of barium enema studies in infants with small bowel atresia. Radiology 95:341–343.
76. Wood BP, Katzberg RW, Ryan DH, Karch FE (1978). Diatrizoate enemas: facts and fallacies of colon toxicity. Radiology 126:441–444.
77. Bowring AC, Jones RFC, Kern IB (1970). The use of solvents in the intestinal manifestations of Mucoviscidosis. J Pediatr Surg 5:338–343.
78. Cleghorn GJ, Stringer DA, Forstner GG, Durie PR (1986). Treatment of distal intestinal obstruction syndrome in cystic fibrosis with a balanced intestinal lavage solution. Lancet i(8470):8–11.
79. Koletzko S, Stringer DA, Cleghorn GJ, Durie PR (1989). Lavage treatment of distal intestinal obstruction syndrome in children with cystic fibrosis. Pediatrics. 83:727–733
80. Campbell JB, Dunbar JS (1986). Contrast in Intussusception, Controversy II. Presented at the 29th Annual Meeting of the Society for Pediatric Radiology, Washington, April 9–13, 1986.
81. Gu L, Alton DJ, Daneman A, Stringer DA, Liu P, Wilmot DM, Reilly BJ (1988). Intussusception reduction in children by rectal insufflation of air. AJR 150: 1345–1348.
82. Harned RK, Consigny PM, Cooper NB, Williams SM, Woltjen AJ (1982). Barium enema examination following biopsy of the rectum or colon. Radiology 145:11–16.
83. Lappas JC, Miller RE, Lehman GA, Eskridge JM, Morton JA (1983). Post endoscopy barium enema examinations. Radiology 149:655–658.
84. Maglinte DDT, Strong RC, Strate RW, Caudill LD, Dyer PA, Chernish SM, Graffis RF (1982). Barium enema after colorectal biopsies: experimental data. AJR 139:693–697.
85. Merrill CR, Steiner GM (1986). Barium enema after biopsy: current practice and opinion. Clin Radiol 37:89–92.
86. Gans SL, Ament M, Christie DL, Liebman WM (1975). Pediatric endoscopy with flexible fiberscopes. J Pediatr Surg 10:375–380.
87. Habr-Gama A, Alves PRA, Gama-Rodrigues JJ, Teixeira MG, Barbieri D (1979). Pediatric colonoscopy. Dis Colon Rectum 22:530–535.
88. Laufer I, Mullens JE, Hamilton J (1976). Correlation of endoscopy and double contrast radiography in the early stages of ulcerative and granulomatous colitis. Radiology 118:1–5.
89. Williams CB, Laage NJ, Campbell CA, Douglas JR, Walker-Smith JA, Booth IW, Harries JT (1982). Total colonoscopy in children. Arch Dis Child 57:49–53.
90. Bigard M-A, Gaucher P, Lassalle C (1979). Fatal colonic explosion during colonoscopic polypectomy. Gastroenterology 77:1307.
91. Geenen JE, Schmitt MG, Wu WC, Hogan WJ (1975). Major complications of colonoscopy: bleeding and perforation. Am J Dig Dis 20:231–235.
92. Kozarek RA, Earnest DL, Silverstein ME, Smith RG (1980). Air pressure induced colon injury during diagnostic colonoscopy. Gastroenterology 78:7–14.
93. Laufer I, Smith NCW, Mullens JE (1976). The radiological demonstration of colorectal polyps undetected by endoscopy . Gastroenterology 70:167–170.
94. Stringer DA, Sherman PM, Jakowenko N (1986). Correlation of double-

contrast high density barium enema, colonoscopy and histology in children with special attention to disparities. Pediatr Radiol 16:298–301.
95. Thoeni RF, Menuck L (1977). Comparison of barium enema and colonoscopy in the detection of small colonic polyps. Radiology 124:631–635.
96. Miller M, Stringer DA, Chui-Mei T, Daneman A, Juodis E (1987). Lymphoid follicular pattern in the colon: an indicator of barium coating. J Can Assoc Radiol 38:256–258.
97. Coblentz CL, Frost RA, Molinaro V, Stevenson GW (1985). Pain after barium enema: effect of CO_2 and air on double-contrast study. Radiology 157:35–36.
98. Grant DS, Bartram CI, Heron CW (1986). A preliminary study of the possible benefits of using carbon dioxide insufflation during double contrst barium enema. Br J Radiol 59:190–191.
99. Nussle D, Genton N, Bozic C (1976). Functional radiological findings in Hirschsprung's disease and in other causes of dyschezia. Ann Radiol (Paris) 19:111–112.
100. Brown BSJ (1965). Defecography or anorectal studies in children including cinefluorographic observations. J Ca Assoc Radiol 16:66–76.
101. Ekberg O, Nylander G, Fork FT (1985). Defecography. Radiology 155: 45–48.
102. Mahieu P, Pringot J, Bodart P (1984). Defecography: I. Description of a new procedure and results in normal patients. Gastrointest Radiol 9:247–251.
103. McLean GK, Rombeau JL, Caldwell MD, Ring EJ, Freiman DB (1982). Transgastrostomy jejunal intubation for enteric alimentation. AJR 139:1129–1133.
104. Strife JL, Dunbar JS, Rice S (1985). Jejunal intubation via gastrostomy catheters in pediatric patients. Radiology 154:249.
105. Cheek JA, Staub GF (1973). Nasojejunal alimentation for premature and full-term newborn infants. J Pediatr 82:955–962.
106. Boros SJ, Reynolds JW (1974). Duodenal perforation: a complication of neonatal nasojejunal feeding. J Pediatr 85:107–108.
107. Chen JW, Wong PWK (1974). Intestinal complications of nasojejunal feeding in low-birth-weight infants. J Pediatr 85:109–110.
108. Sun SC, Samuels S, Lee J, Marquis JR (1975). Duodenal perforation: a rare complication of neonatal nasojejunal tube feeding. Pediatrics 55: 371–375.
109. Rhea JW, Ahmad MS, Mange MS (1975). Nasojejunal (transpyloric) feeding: a commentary. J Pediatr 86:451–452.
110. Siegle RL, Rabinowitz JG, Sarasohn C (1976). Intestinal perforation secondary to nasojejunal feeding tube. AJR 126:1229–1232.
111. Perez-Rodrigues J, Quero J, Frias EG, Omenaca F, Martinez A (1978). Duodenorenal perforation in a neonate by a tube of silicone rubber during transpyloric feeding. J Pediatr 92:113–114.
112. Merten DF, Mumford L, Filston HC, Brumley GW, Effman EL, Grossman H (1980). Radiological observations during transpyloric tube feeding in infants of low birth weight. Radiology 136:67–75.
113. McAlister WH, Siegel MJ, Shackelford GD, Perlman JM, Ternberg JL, Bower RJ (1985). Intestinal perforations by tube feedings in small infants: clinical and experimental studies. AJR 145:687–691.
114. Shackelford GD, McAlister WH, Robertson CL (1972) The use of a Foley catheter for removal of blunt esophageal foreign bodies from children. Radiology 105:455–456.
115. Carlson DH (1972). Removal of coins in the esophagus using a Foley catheter. Pediatrics 50:475–476.
116. Campbell JB, Davis WS (1973). Catheter technique for extraction of blunt esophageal foreign bodies. Radiology 108:438–440.

117. Campbell JB, Quattromani FL, Foley LC (1983). Foley catheter removal of blunt esophageal foreign bodies: experience with 100 consecutive children. Pediatr Radiol 13:116–119.
118. Berdon WE (1983). Editorial comment. Pediatr Radiol 13:119.
119. Campbell JB, Condon VR (1985). Catheter removal of blunt esophageal foreign bodies in children: survey of the Society for Pediatric Radiology. Presentation at the 28th Annual Meeting of the Society of Pediatric Radiology, Boston, 1985.
120. Nixon GW (1979). Foley catheter method of esophageal foreign body removal: extension of applications. AJR 132:441–442.
121. Lederman H, Towbin R, Ball WS, et al. (1985). Esophageal edema as a predictor of unsuccessful balloon extraction of esophageal foreign bodies. Presented at the 28th Annual Meeting of the Society for Pediatric Radiology, Boston, 1985.

CHAPTER 6

Special Procedures

Sinograms and Fistulograms

Most sinus and fistula tracts can be examined by insertion of a small catheter (such as a 5 or 8 French neonatal feeding tube) into the orifice of the tract. The tube is inserted until resistance is felt, taking care that kinking of the catheter does not occur. Water-soluble contrast is then slowly injected, and spot films outlining the course of the sinus tract are obtained. These films should be taken in at least two projections (Fig. 6.1).

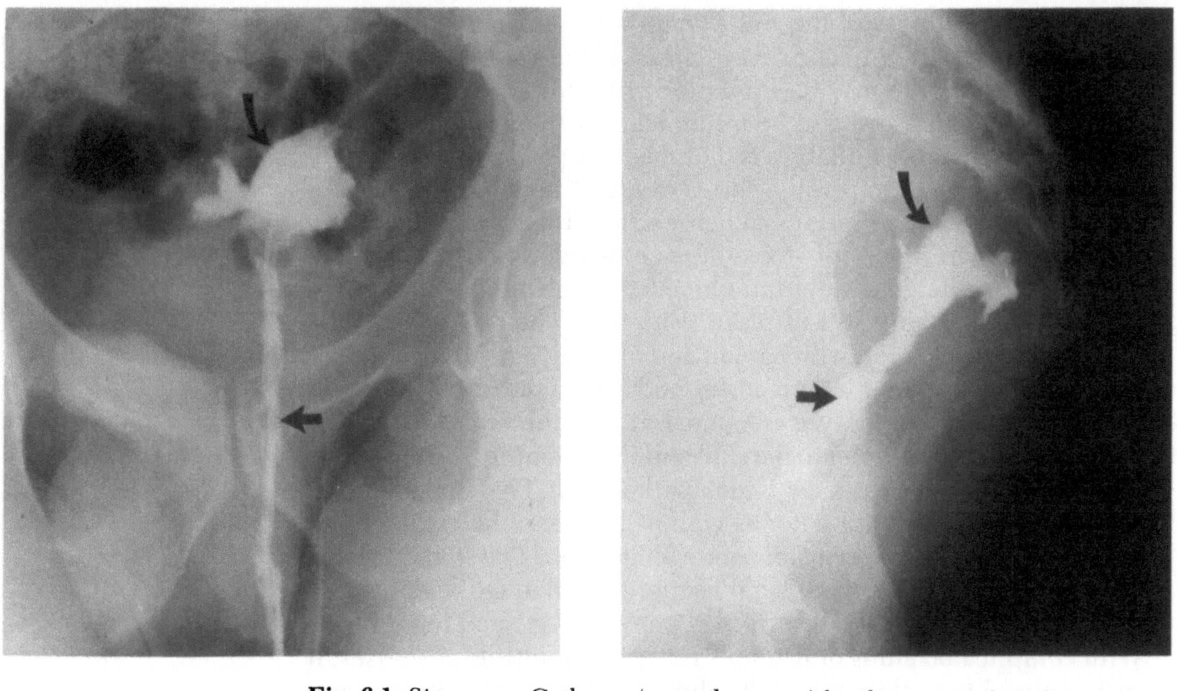

A B

Fig. 6.1. Sinogram. Catheter (*straight arrow*) has been introduced into sinus tract. Sinus cavity (*curved arrow*) has been opacified with contrast, and spot films in anteroposterior (**A**) and lateral (**B**) positions are obtained. Lateral position shows posterior, presacral location of cavity.

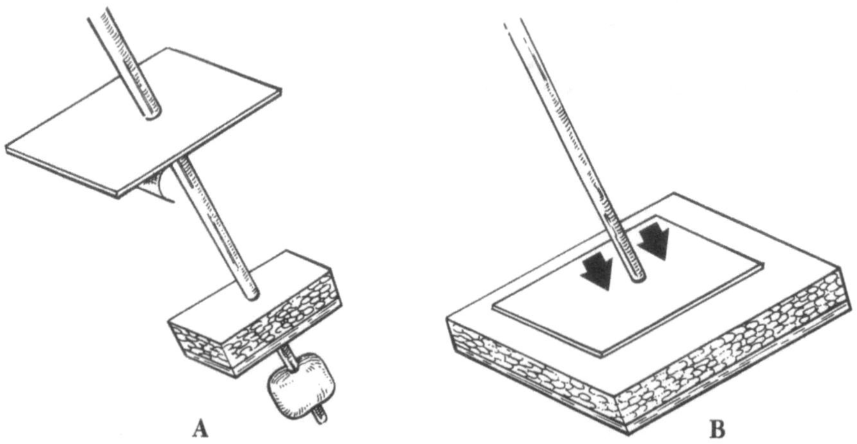

Fig. 6.2. Catheter is pushed through hole in stomadhesive and tip positioned in sinus tract (**A**). Plastic covering on undersurface of stomadhesive is removed, and stomadhesive is firmly applied to skin (**B**).

Leakage of contrast around the catheter during sinogram or fistulogram study creates a problem with performance of the procedure as well as interpretation of obtained radiographs. The leakage results from an inadequate seal between the catheter used for the study and the skin. With each injection contrast flows along the path of least resistance, frequently to the skin surface. The problem of leakage can be minimized in several ways. A Foley catheter instead of a feeding tube can be inserted into the tract and leakage prevented by insufflating the balloon. Many sinus tracts, however, are small, and do not permit insertion of even the smallest Foley catheter. A second problem arises from the softness of the Foley catheters, making it difficult to advance them within a tract. Nevertheless, if the caliber of the tract permits, the procedure may be attempted with this type of catheter.

Leakage of contrast can also be minimized by the use of stomadhesive. With this method, initially a catheter size appropriate to the study is selected. We have prepared a series of metal punches the sizes of which correspond to the various catheter sizes. Holes were previously made in 6 × 6 cm pieces of stomadhesive, which were resterilized. The selected catheter is now introduced through the stomadhesive with the paper backing still in place (Fig. 6.2). The skin around the sinus or fistula is cleaned with Savlon and alcohol, and allowed to dry completely. The catheter is then positioned within the tract. The paper backing on the stomadhesive is removed, and the stomadhesive is advanced along the catheter to the skin and then compressed against it, making sure that the catheter is not withdrawn. The stomadhesive forms a seal around the catheter as well as between the catheter and skin. The patient is now ready for contrast injection. The stomadhesive works well if the surface to which it is applied is flat. Difficulty with a proper skin seal occurs if the surface is uneven (e.g., anal region).

With complicated sinus or fistulous tracts and multiple abscesses, it may be helpful to explore the limits of these cavities. The most appropriate catheter to use is a Meditech steerable catheter, and it may be helpful to seal the skin with stomadhesive as previously described. The catheter is positioned a short way under the skin, and the patient

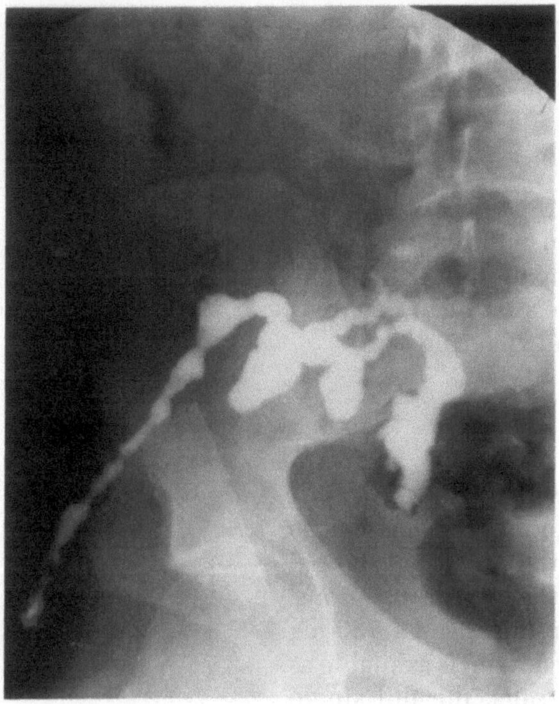
A

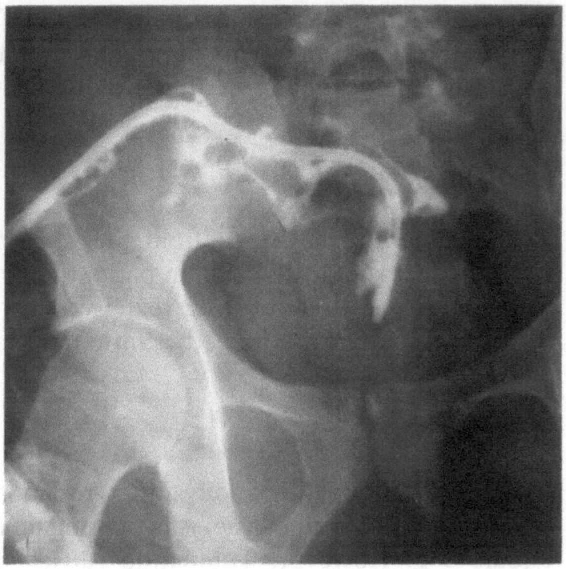
B

Fig. 6.3. A complex sinus tract is opacified with contrast (**A**). With Meditech steerable catheter, most distal recesses of cavity can be reached and drained (**B**).

holds the stomadhesive in position. A small amount of contrast is injected, and the catheter is steered and advanced to follow the tracts of contrast to explore the further recesses of the abscess cavities (Fig. 6.3). In discussion with the referring surgeon, drainage catheters may then be left in abscess cavities as required.

Oral Cholecystography: Operative and Postoperative Cholangiography

Oral Cholecystography

Indications

Oral cholecystography (OCG) was introduced in 1924 and since has been found to be an accurate method of detecting gallstones with reported accuracy rates of up to 98% [1,2,3], particularly if a double dose is used as a routine, with tomography for poor or nonvisualization.

Real-time ultrasonography has largely replaced oral cholecystography as the primary examination for detecting gallbladder disease, with accuracy rates also greater than 90% [4,5,6,7,8]. We have found OCG a useful supplementary examination in patients in whom sonography is found to be inadequate because of patient obesity or anatomy, or when the ultrasound results need to be confirmed. In children we find sonography sufficiently accurate and at the Hospital for Sick Children, we no longer perform OCG.

With the development of biliary lithotripsy a new interest has evolved in oral cholecystography. Oral cholecystography helps quantitate number of stones, size of stones, and presence or absence of calcification. Lithotripsy may be precluded if there are more than three stones, the stones are 30 mm or greater in diameter, in the presence of gallstone calcification or nonfunctioning OCG [9].

Contraindications and Precautions

Technical failure may result from poor absorption of the contrast material. The test is of little value in patients with impaired liver function. There is a small risk of drug toxicity after ingestion of the contrast material, usually experienced as mild nausea and vomiting.

Materials

Oral biliary contrast iopanoic acid, tyropanoate sodium.

Iopanoic acid (Telepaque) is in 500-mg tablet form; a full single dose equals 3 g. However, Telepaque causes diarrhea in a substantial minority of patients. There are two other satisfactory preparations. Tyropanoate sodium (Bilopaque sodium) is produced as a 750-mg capsule; a full single dose equals 3 g. Ipodate (Oragrafin) is available as sodium (regular) or calcium (rapid-absorption) salts; the full single dose is 3 g.

Patient Preparation

Two-day fat-free diet, double-dosing oral biliary contrast on 2 consecutive days, and clear fluids from midnight until 6 hours before the study, at which time the patient is kept in a fasting state.

□ *Procedure*

Step 1. The examination is started with the patient erect, arms above the head. Under fluoroscopic guidance, two films are taken in the erect position with varying degrees of obliquity (Fig. 6.4). The gallbladder should not be obscured by overlying ribs, feces, or gas. Compression is used over the lower part of the gallbladder.

Step 2. The patient is now put into the Trendelenburg position, supine with the arms above the head. A film is obtained centering over the neck of the gallbladder (Fig. 6.5).

Step 3. A fourth film is taken in the right lateral decubitus position, centering over the lateral border of the gallbladder.

Step 4. If there is apparent nonvisualization of the gallbladder, right posterior oblique (RPO) tomograms should be obtained (Fig. 6.6). This will frequently show that there is opacification, and may reveal calculi that were not visible on spot films.

Step 5. For assessment of gallbladder emptying, the patient is given one-half of a can of Ensure, and after 20 minutes two erect postfat films in different obliquities, or one erect and one supine film, are taken (Fig. 6.7). Administration of fat by mouth will cause the normal gall-

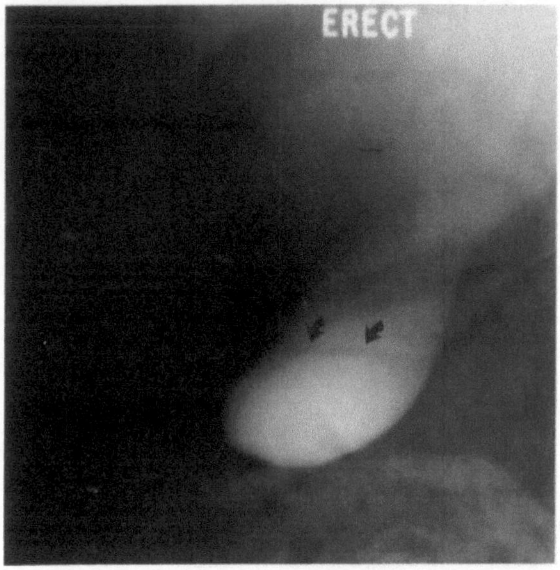

Fig. 6.4

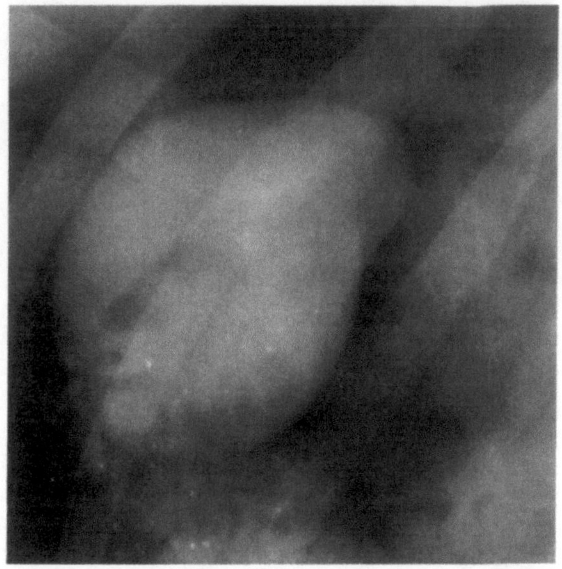

Fig. 6.5

Fig. 6.4. Oral cholecystogram. Erect film identifies series of floating gallstones (*arrow*).

Fig. 6.5. Oral cholecystogram. Trendelenburg position. Particles of contrast are seen within bowel. Optimum obliquity should be selected to minimize overlap of gallbladder and bowel.

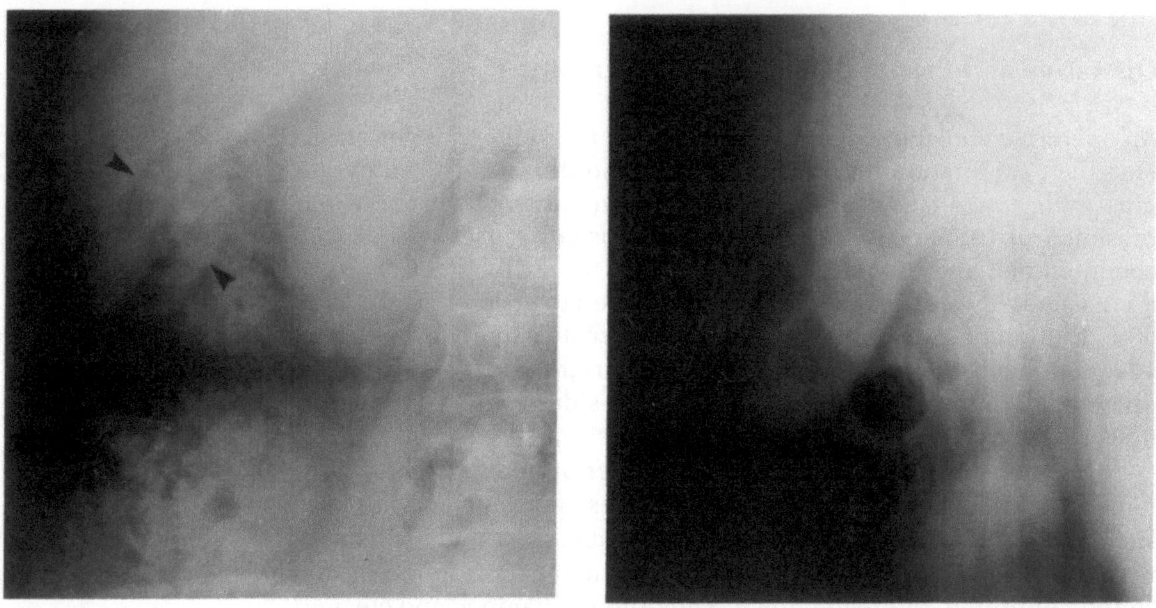

A B

Fig. 6.6. Oral cholecystogram. Extremely poor visualization of gallbladder on a conventional spot film (**A**). Gallbladder is demonstrated by *arrowheads*. Anteroposterior tomographic slice through gallbladder (**B**) clearly demonstrates presence of multiple stones.

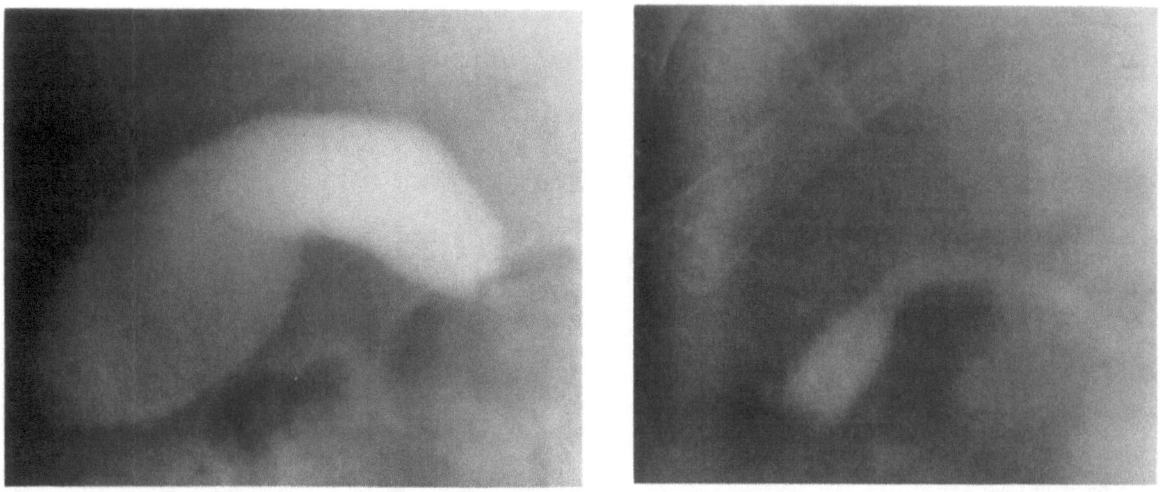

Fig. 6.7. Oral cholecystogram. Clearly visualized, well-distended gallbladder (A) is almost completely emptied following contraction provoked by fatty meal (B).

bladder to contract. This will sometimes improve visualization of a poorly opacified gallbladder, accentuate the features of adenomyomatosis, and often demonstrate the bile duct if a film is taken 15 to 20 minutes after the fat has been given.

De Lacey et al. [10] recently reported the usefulness of fluoroscopic OCG for the detection of acalculous adenomyomatosis and many polyps that would not be detected on ultrasound.

Operative and Postoperative Cholangiography

An operative cholangiogram is performed by the surgeon before common duct exploration for possible choledocholithiasis. The study begins with a scout film of the right upper quadrant to exclude the presence of calcified stones. A needle is usually inserted into the common duct and may also be inserted into the gallbladder or cystic duct. Enough water-soluble contrast is injected to opacify the ducts. A 50% dilution of sodium or meglumine diatrizoate usually provides an adequate density for the study. Films of the right upper quadrant are obtained with the patient in an oblique right-side-down position (Fig. 6.8) [11], or by tube angling if a C-arm unit is available.

Postoperative t-tube cholangiography is performed to exclude a retained common bile duct calculus or to assess for any complications such as a bile leak before removal of the t-tube. The study is usually performed 7 to 10 days after surgery. The patient is positioned supine slightly obliqued, right-side-down. The t-tube is clamped and cleaned with Savlon or Proviodine. A water-soluble contrast infusion is prepared (usually a 50% dilution). The infusion is connected to the t-tube either end to end with an appropriate-size connector or into the side of the t-tube through a butterfly needle. Care must be taken to exclude air bubbles from the connecting system as the air will make interpretation of the subsequent films very difficult. Filling is observed under

Fig. 6.8
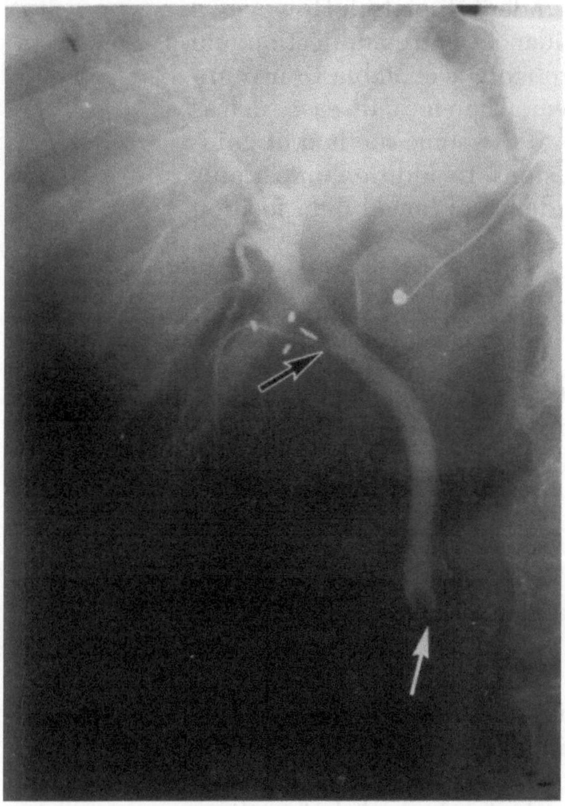

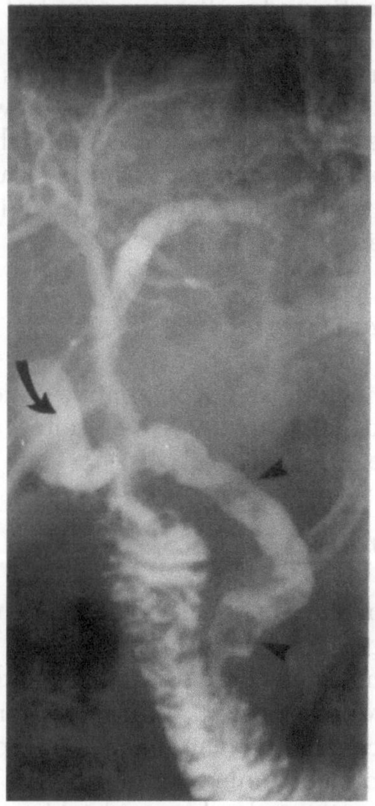
Fig. 6.9

Fig. 6.8. Operative cholangiogram. In operating suite, contrast medium was injected into biliary tree through needle (*straight arrow*) introduced into common bile duct. Retained calculus (*curved arrow*) is seen in distal common bile duct.

Fig. 6.9. T-tube cholangiogram. Contrast has been infused through t-tube (*curved arrow*) and is outlining dilated biliary tract and multiple common bile duct stones (*arrowheads*).

fluoroscopic control and spot films are taken (Fig. 6.9) in various obliquities and with elevation of the head of the table. Although contrast medium may also be injected with a syringe, there is evidence to suggest that allowing the contrast to drip under gravitational forces helps to prevent overfilling, pain, and ascending cholangitis [12].

An alternative approach in patients with clinically suspected common bile duct calculi is to perform a preoperative ERCP and sphincterotomy, making it unnecessary for surgical common bile duct exploration.

Liver Biopsy

Percutaneous

Indications

Liver biopsy may be undertaken for diffuse or focal disease. For diffuse disease, a random liver biopsy is usually performed from the right side. For focal disease, fine-needle aspiration cytology is often carried out directly under ultrasound control or under CT control. However, a core biopsy may also be taken under guidance. The complication rate of liver biopsy is very low, and it is probably acceptable to use unguided biopsy for diffuse disease; however, when focal disease such as metastasis is suspected, it is preferable to use some method of guidance to look for and then sample focal lesions. In addition, in patients with cirrhosis there is an increased incidence of bowel interposition between liver and chest wall.

Contraindications

These include an uncooperative patient who cannot suspend respiration, coagulopathy, massive ascites, empyema, and possibly hydatid disease.

Preparation

Liver biopsy is normally performed on an outpatient basis, but with 6 hours postprocedural supervision.

An informed consent is taken and the risks, which include bleeding (approximately 0.2%), biliary peritonitis (more likely in obstructive jaundice), and pneumothorax, are explained. Pain and fainting are the most common minor complications.

The patient should avoid taking aspirin for 1 week before liver biopsy. CBC, platelets, prothrombin time, and partial thromboplastin time should all be done and be normal before liver biopsy is carried out. If there is a coagulopathy, or platelets are very low, transjugular biopsy should be considered [13].

Local anesthetic is used; this is usually xylocaine although bupivacaine has a longer duration of action. Liver biopsy is often performed without sedation, but it is kinder to give a mild sedation such as fentanyl or diazepam immediately before the procedure.

□ *Procedure*

The skin is cleaned initially with Proviodine. Site: Tap out the upper limit of dullnes on expiration in the midaxillary line, and choose a spot one rib space below this upper limit (Fig. 6.10). The biopsy is performed on expiration. The examiner should have the patient practice breathing in, breathing right out, and then suspending respiration in expiration. Many patients will take an inspiration automatically at this point and need to be trained to stop at the end of expiration and then hold their breath for 2 to 3 seconds while the biopsy is taken. Local anesthetic is administered at this time.

The skin is stabbed with a scalpel blade to avoid the biopsy needle being gripped by the skin. The needle most frequently used is the Jamshidi, 16-gauge, a disposable needle of Menghini type. Disposable needles are sharper and more certainly sterile. The Jamshidi needle is advanced to the liver capsule, and as soon as any caudad movement of the needle occurs on inspiration (from the needle being just within the

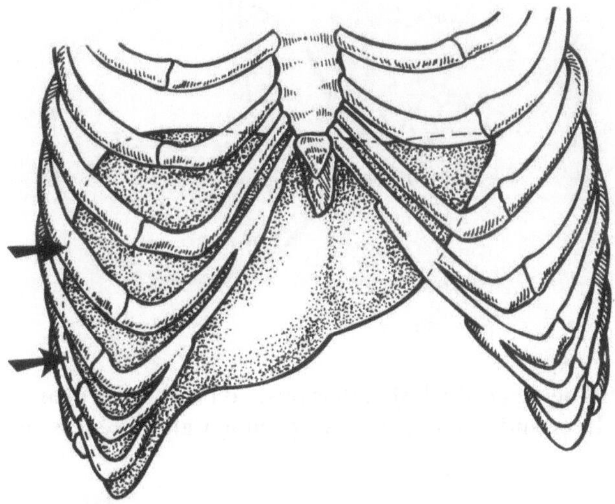

Fig. 6.10. The pleural space extends much lower (*arrows*) than one usually expects. This should be taken into consideration when choosing site for percutaneous biopsy to prevent puncture of pleura.

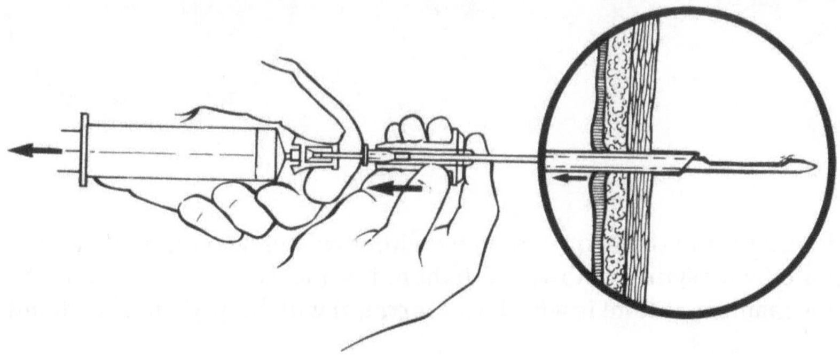

Fig. 6.11. Trucut needle is introduced into liver; when appropriate depth has been reached, sheath is withdrawn (*arrows*) with suction being applied with syringe at same time. This exposes recess on stilette where specimen becomes attached as result of suction.

liver), a small amount (1 ml) of saline is injected to clear the needle tip, suction is exerted on the syringe plunger, which is then locked, and the needle is then advanced 1 to 2 in. into the liver. The whole system is then withdrawn, still under suction, and the plunger is slowly released. Gentle syringe pressure is used while slowly withdrawing the needle over a piece of gauze to expel the core, which is then transferred to the sample pot. Up to three passes may be used to obtain a good specimen.

The Trucut needle is also acceptable (Fig. 6.11–6.13), and the Trucut in the "Biopty gun" provides a very rapid automatic firing system, which ensures a good core specimen every time. As the Trucut needle has a fairly large bore, if a patient has a bleeding disorder or an abnormal clotting mechanism, the tract is plugged with gelfoam particles as the needle is withdrawn (Fig. 6.14 and 6.15). The Roth biopsy gun (Cook Inc.) (Fig. 6.16) is a biopsy device similar to the Biopty gun; it uses a Trucut type of needle, and has the advantage of being able to

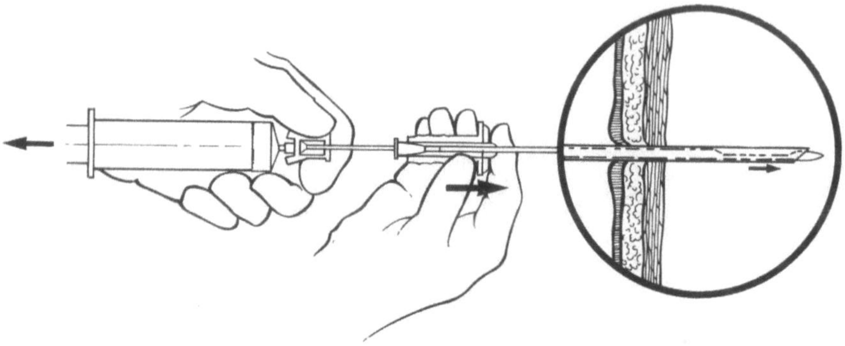

Fig. 6.12. With suction still being applied, sheath is pushed back (arrows) over stilette, cutting through liver and leaving biopsy specimen along recess on stilette.

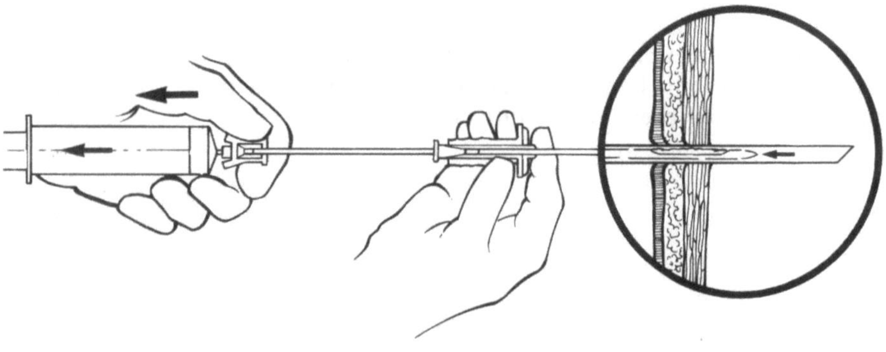

Fig. 6.13. Stilette and sheath may then be withdrawn with continuous suction being applied with syringe. However, if there is some concern about patient's clotting mechanism, stilette is withdrawn (*arrows*) with biopsy and sheath left in place.

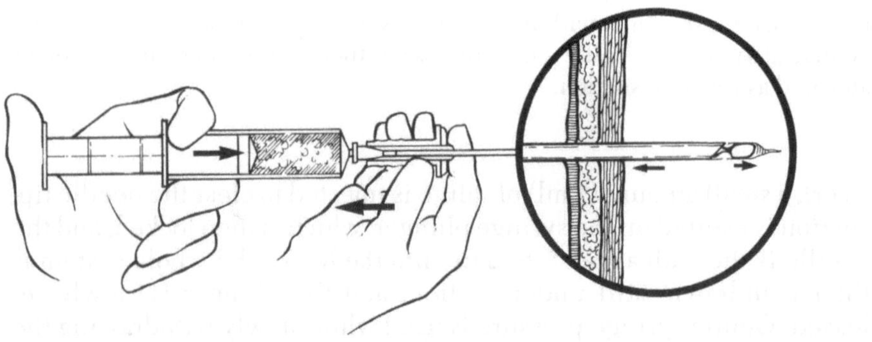

Fig. 6.14. In patient with abnormal clotting mechanism, gelfoam particles are introduced into biopsy tract.

sample tissue from the area surrounding the needle tip without advancing further when the mechanism is triggered. The Biopty gun, on the other hand, has a biopsy needle that moves further into the lesion when it is fired, limiting the amount of control you have on the position of the tip by the throw built into the model of biopty gun that is being used.

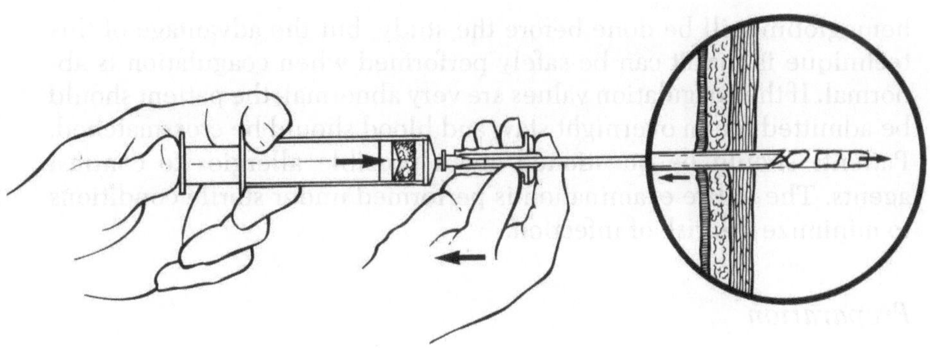

Fig. 6.15. Sheath is removed in stepwise manner leaving gelfoam particles along biopsy tract.

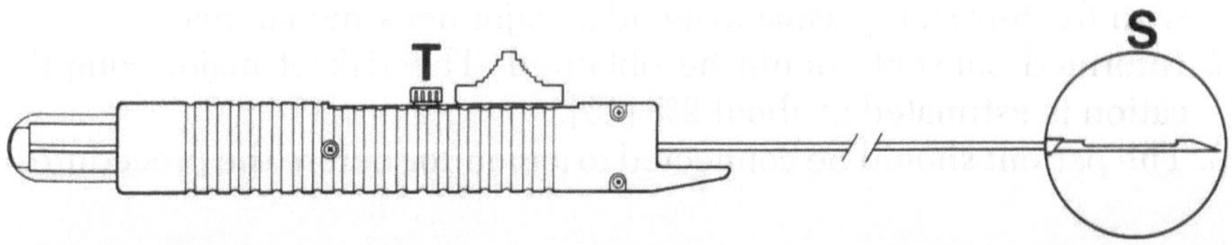

Fig. 6.16. Roth biopsy device. T, trigger button; S, tissue stilette. [Courtesy of Cook Canada (Inc).]

Postprocedure Care

1. Vital signs are recorded every 15 min for an hour, then every 30 min for hours, and hourly until the patient is discharged.
2. One dose of an analgesic is permitted. If the patient requires a second analgesic, the physician should consider why this is necessary and look for any evidence of any complications as well as considering admission overnight for observation.
3. If the patient is well 6 hours after the procedure, the patient may be allowed to go home to rest and instructed not to go out on the town that night. The following day, however, normal activity may be resumed.

Transjugular

Indications

A transjugular liver biopsy is performed whenever a liver biopsy is required but a percutaneous approach is contraindicated. This would include patients with abnormal liver function, elevated prothrombin time (PT) or partial thromboplastin time (PTT), and patients with abdominal ascites [14]. A transjugular biopsy may also be considered if tissue from a particular area deep to the surface is desired.

Precautions and Contraindications

Patients with liver or biliary duct abnormalities may have abnormal serum levels of clotting factors. Bleeding times, PT, PTT, Platelet, and hemoglobin will be done before the study, but the advantage of this technique is that it can be safely performed when coagulation is abnormal. If the coagulation values are very abnormal, the patient should be admitted for an overnight stay, and blood should be crossmatched. Patients should be questioned about possible allergies to contrast agents. The entire examination is performed under sterile conditions to minimize the risk of infection.

Preparation

1. The patient's PTT and PT should always be checked. In most cases these values will be abnormal. However, this should not be a deterrent unless there are difficulties in obtaining hemostasis after a venepuncture. In this case it may be prudent to cover the patient with fresh-frozen plasma to avoid a major neck hematoma.
2. Informed consent should be obtained. The risk of major complication is estimated at about 2% [15].
3. The patient should be connected to a monitor before the procedure.

Technique

The biopsy must be done on a tilting fluoroscopic table. The patient's shoulders are elevated with a linear pad so that they are about 10 cm above the table top. The shoulders should be high enough so that the head hangs lower than the anterior surface of the chest wall. This position stretches the vessels of the neck and assist in immobilizing them. It also straightens them so that there is a straight passage down the internal jugular vein to the superior vena cava.

The table is then tilted into a 30° Trendelenburg position. This position encourages the internal jugular vein to become engorged. While this is being achieved, an intravenous line is inserted into an arm vein and run at a level to keep the vessel open. You may administer sedation through this line if necessary.

After about 10 minutes the internal jugular vein is sufficiently engorged for it to be easily punctured.

The neck is prepared using Proviodine. The head is covered with a cap or towels and sterile drapes are placed around the puncture site. The patient's head is turned slightly to the left to make the right internal jugular puncture easier (Fig. 6.17).

The puncture site is chosen by locating the position of the common carotid artery and identifying a point about 2 cm below the angle of the jaw and just lateral to the carotid artery (Fig. 6.18). The internal jugular is situated lateral and deep to the carotid artery (Fig. 6.19). Once a suitable puncture site has been located, the area is infiltrated with 2% Xylocaine. The infiltration should be fairly deep. During the injection of the local anesthetic it is useful to try to locate the position of the internal jugular vein. The vein is then punctured using the Seldinger technique (Fig. 6.20). A guide wire is introduced down to the inferior vena cava and the dilator with its sheath is introduced over it. The dilator is then removed and the 9 French catheter that is part of the Cook transjugular biopsy set is introduced over the guide wire. It is

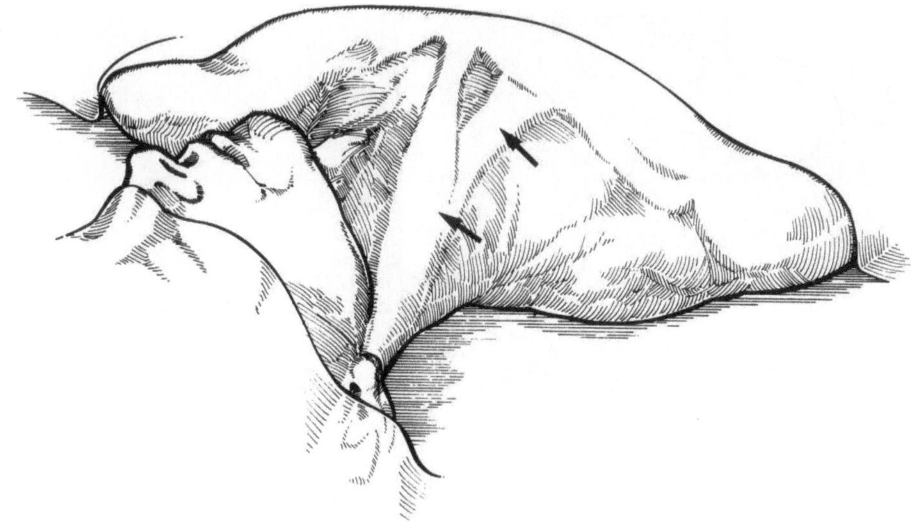

Fig. 6.17. Patient is positioned in slight Trendelenburg position; head is tilted slightly in direction away from radiologist. Sternocleidomastoid muscle (*arrows*) is easily identified.

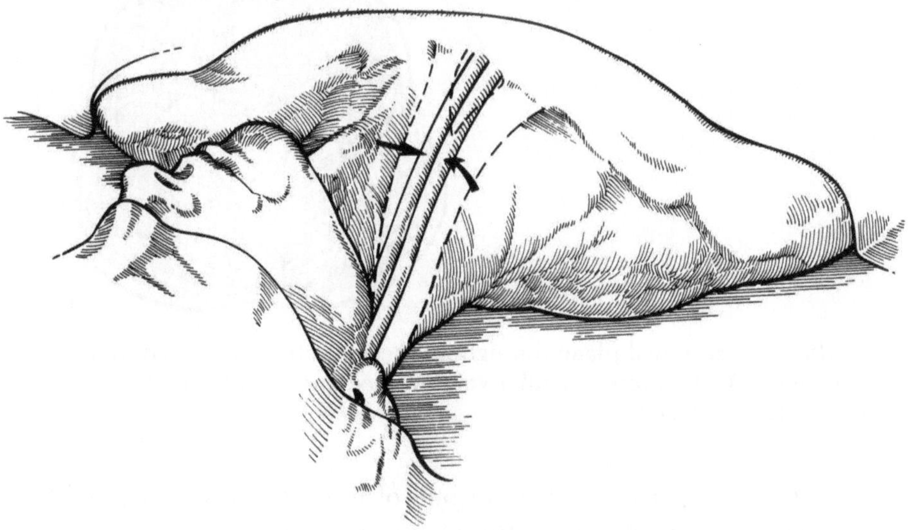

Fig. 6.18. Internal jugular vein (*curved arrow*) lies lateral to carotid artery (*straight arrow*). Position of artery is located by palpation.

useful to use this method because the curve at the end of the catheter occasionally becomes caught up in the right atrium, making entry into the inferior vena cava difficult.

When the catheter is in the inferior vena cava, the guide wire is removed and one of the hepatic veins catheterized (Fig. 6.21). It is usually safer to catheterize the right hepatic vein as there is more tissue on this side. However, there is no absolute contraindication to catheterizing the left lobe, if you are careful and do not puncture the liver capsule during the biopsy procedure. A preliminary CT scan or ultrasound examination will give information as to whether the patient has cirrhosis with a small atrophied right lobe and an enlarged left lobe.

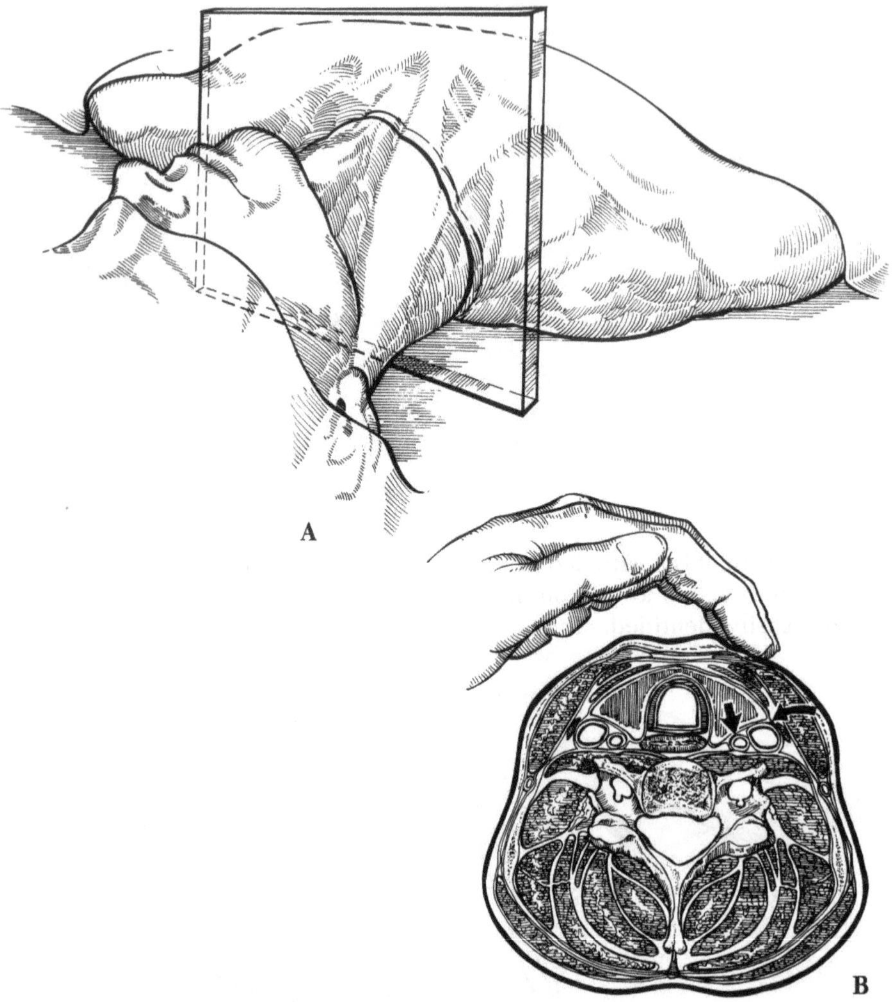

Fig. 6.19. Cross-sectional plane through midneck has been obtained to illustrate anatomy (**A**). Position of jugular vein (*curved arrow*) is lateral to carotid artery (*straight arrow*) (**B**).

When the catheter is in place in one of the branches of the right hepatic vein, and confirmed with an injection of contrast medium, wedged and free hepatic vein pressures are recorded. The biopsy needle is then introduced with a 30-ml syringe with 10 ml of saline attached. A biopsy is then taken by inserting the needle into the liver substance while the patient stops breathing, and applying suction with the syringe. The needle is then removed with the syringe attached. The specimen is removed from the needle by blowing it out with a syringe and clean saline. The specimen is sent to pathology in formaldehyde unless you want electron microscopy as well. In the latter case, a separate specimen is sent in glutaraldehyde. If culture and sensitivity is also required, a specimen is sent in a sterile container to microbiology. You can make several passes with the needle if the specimens are not adequate. The use of the sheath for introduction reduces trauma to the puncture site. After the biopsies have been obtained, it is wise to inject contrast medium into the hepatic vein where the biop-

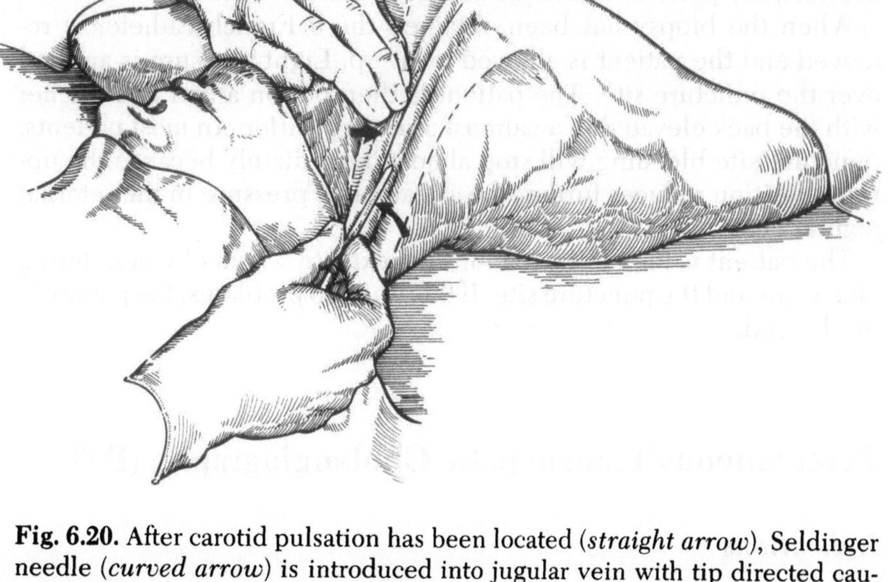

Fig. 6.20. After carotid pulsation has been located (*straight arrow*), Seldinger needle (*curved arrow*) is introduced into jugular vein with tip directed caudally and toward ipsilateral midclavicle.

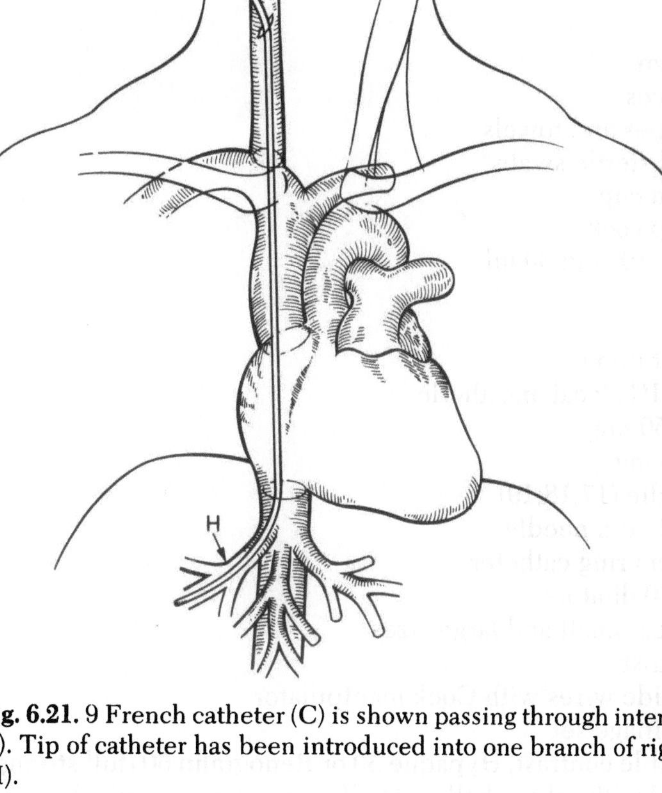

Fig. 6.21. 9 French catheter (C) is shown passing through internal jugular vein (J). Tip of catheter has been introduced into one branch of right hepatic vein (H).

sies have been taken to ensure that the liver capsule has not been penetrated. If it has been punctured and there is extravasation of contrast, the perforation can be plugged with gelfoam.

When the biopsy has been obtained the 9 French catheter is removed and the patient is allowed to sit up. Light pressure is applied over the puncture site. The patient is then put on a bed or stretcher with the back elevated in an almost upright position. In most patients, puncture site bleeding will stop almost immediately because the upright position reduces further the already low pressure in the internal jugular vein.

The patient is then followed for the next 2 to 4 hours by monitoring vital signs and the puncture site. If there are no problems, the patient is discharged.

Percutaneous Transhepatic Cholangiography (PTC)

Indications

The procedure is performed in patients with obstructive jaundice secondary to obstruction of the biliary tract, to determine the etiology and exact anatomical position of the obstruction, and as a preliminary step to insertion of a biliary drainage catheter.

Materials

1. Sterile gown
2. Sterile gloves
3. Sterile drapes and towels
4. Savlon and sterile swabs
5. Preparation cup
6. Saline, stop cock
7. Syringes 5, 10, and 30 ml
8. Scalpel
9. Forceps
10. Extension tubing
11. Xylocaine 1%, local anesthetic
12. Demerol, 50 mg
13. Valium, 10 mg
14. Chiba needle (17,18,19)
15. 9-in. portal vein needle
16. P8 3G 50-cm ring catheter
17. #9 and #10 dilators
18. Guide wires, small and large sizes
    Lundequist
    Short guide wires with Cook manipulator
19. Biliary drainage set
20. Water-soluble contrast, Hypaque 50 or Renografin 60 (full strength and diluted with saline, half and half), or nonionic equivalent if in hospital use.

Precautions and Contraindications

A patient with liver or biliary duct abnormalities may have abnormal serum levels of clotting factors. Bleeding times, PT, PTT, platelet, and hemoglobin should be taken before the study to ensure normal hemostasis. If the PT is slightly prolonged, it may be satisfactory to give vitamin K I.M. and postpone the procedure for 24 hours. With severe prolongation of PT, or with an urgent situation such as acute suppurative cholangitis, the procedure may be covered by the administration of fresh-frozen plasma. In these situations the advice and help of the hematology service should be obtained. The patient should be questioned about possible allergies to contrast agents. The entire examination is performed under sterile conditions to minimise the risk of infection.

Preparation

1. Check serum clotting factors, bleeding times, platelet, and hemoglobin
2. NPO after midnight
3. I.V. N/S to keep the vein open on the morning of examination
4. Demerol I.V. or other similar drug just before the procedure may be helpful. In children heavy sedation is generally necessary and younger children usually require general anaesthetic.
5. If an obstructed bile duct is suspected with jaundice, a prophylactic antibiotic should be given before the procedure, using either a combination such as ampicillin and gentamicin, or a broad-spectrum cephalosporin (cefoxitin).

□ *Procedure*

Step 1. In children it is useful to determine the site and depth of the porta hepatis before the procedure. We routinely mark the skin over the porta before the procedure. We also keep the ultrasound machine with sterile probe at the tableside for further localization as necessary.
Step 2. Preliminary fluroscopy is performed to choose a puncture site in the right midaxillary line. Although it may be difficult to avoid puncture of the pleura, to minimize the chance of puncturing the lung the costophrenic angles can first be plotted under ultrasound or fluoroscopic guidance. The puncture is then made below the costophrenic angle. This area is cleansed and draped.
Step 3. Local anesthetic is usually required for these examinations, although some children may need a general anesthetic. Local anesthetic is injected into the skin, subcutaneous tissue, and liver capsule. Xylocaine wears off within an hour or so, and many patients spend a very uncomfortable night after a percutaneous transhepatic procedure. Marcaine (bupivacaine) 0.5% with adrenaline provides local anesthesia for 8 to 12 hours and is a great improvement [13].
Step 4. A small incision with the scalpel is made in the skin at the selected needle entry site.
Step 5. The Chiba needle tip is introduced into the subcutaneous tissues. With suspended respiration the needle is advanced (under

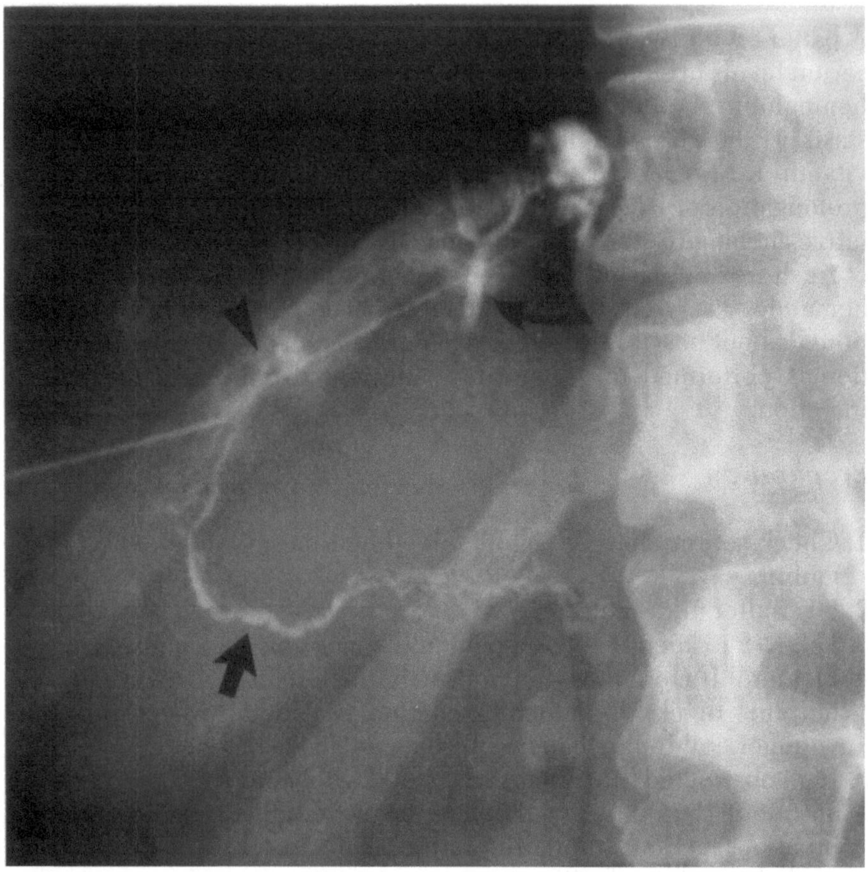

Fig. 6.22. Spot film shows contrast extravasation (*arrowhead*), contrast within lymphatics (*straight arrow*) and contrast within branch of portal vein (*curved arrow*).

fluoroscopic control) in the direction of the dome of the diaphragm.
Step 6. The stilette is removed leaving the sheath in position. The patient is allowed to resume shallow respiration.
Step 7. A 30-ml syringe containing the diluted contrast (25% Hypaque or 30% Renografin) is connected to a connecting tube with a one-way stopcock, and this is then attached to the sheath.
Step 8. The contrast is slowly injected under fluoroscopic control to see if the bile ducts are opacified (Fig. 6.22). (The normal anatomy of the liver is illustrated in Fig. 6.23.) If not, the needle is withdrawn in a step-by-step manner with injection of contrast after each withdrawal step until the tip of the needle comes to lie within a bile duct (Fig. 6.24). First pass is directed cephalad towards the upper margin of the body of T12 and stops about 3 cm short of the vertebral body. Four further passes may be made in the same horizontal plane, each a little more caudad and each inserted a shorter distance. If these are unsuccessful a further five passes may be made with more ventral angulation. Although there is no absolute maximum number of needle passes, most practitioners will stop at 10 to 15, as there is little increase in success beyond 10 passes.

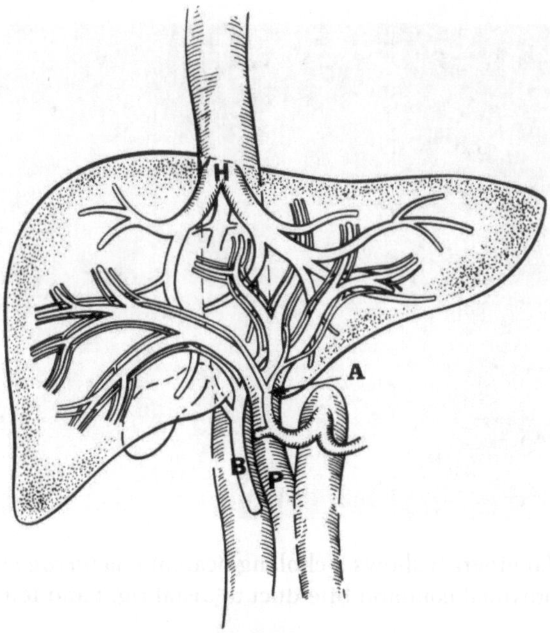

Fig. 6.23. Normal intrahepatic anatomy. Intrahepatic branches of hepatic vein (H), hepatic artery (A), portal vein (P), and biliary system (B) can be followed by tracing branches from these vessels through liver.

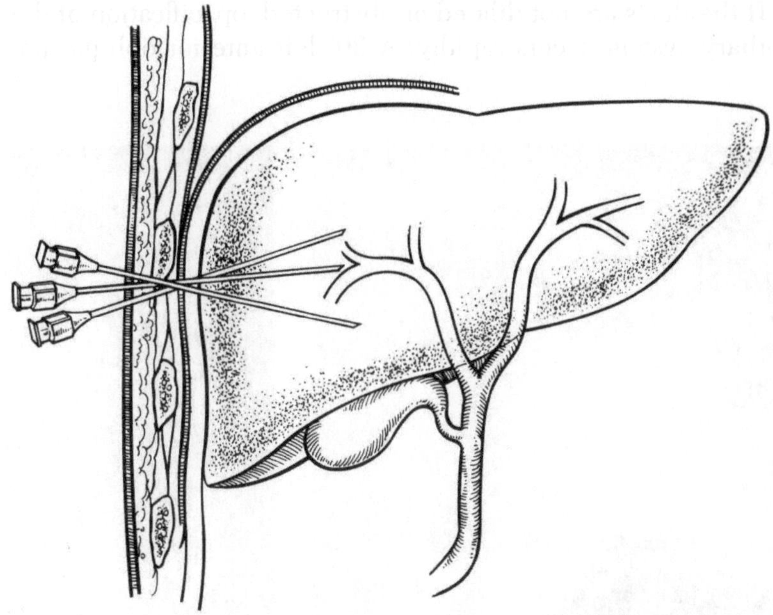

Fig. 6.24. Diagrammatic sketch of several punctures being made, with contrast medium being injected after each withdrawal, until needle tip comes to lie within biliary system.

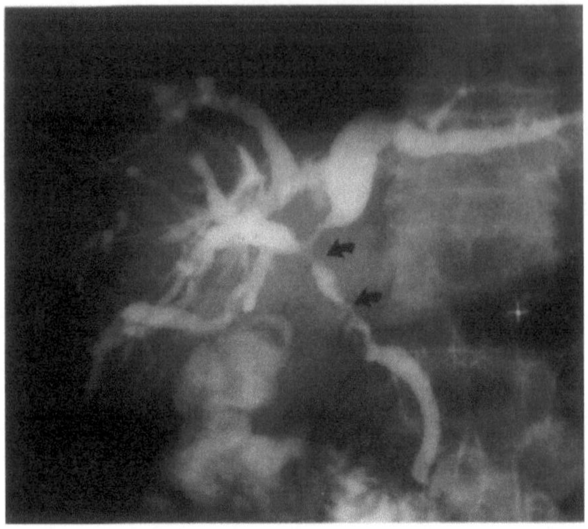

Fig. 6.25. Percutaneous cholangiogram shows a cholangiocarcinoma (*arrows*) extending proximally from proximal common bile duct to distal right and left hepatic ducts.

Step 9. When the bile duct is visualized, further contrast is injected under fluoroscopic control with spot films taken in multiple projection. Once a dilated duct starts to fill, 30% contrast is injected. Only the minimal amount of contrast needed to obtain opacification of the ducts is used. If the ducts are not dilated or obstructed, opacification of the whole biliary system occurs rapidly. A 30° left anterior oblique po-

A

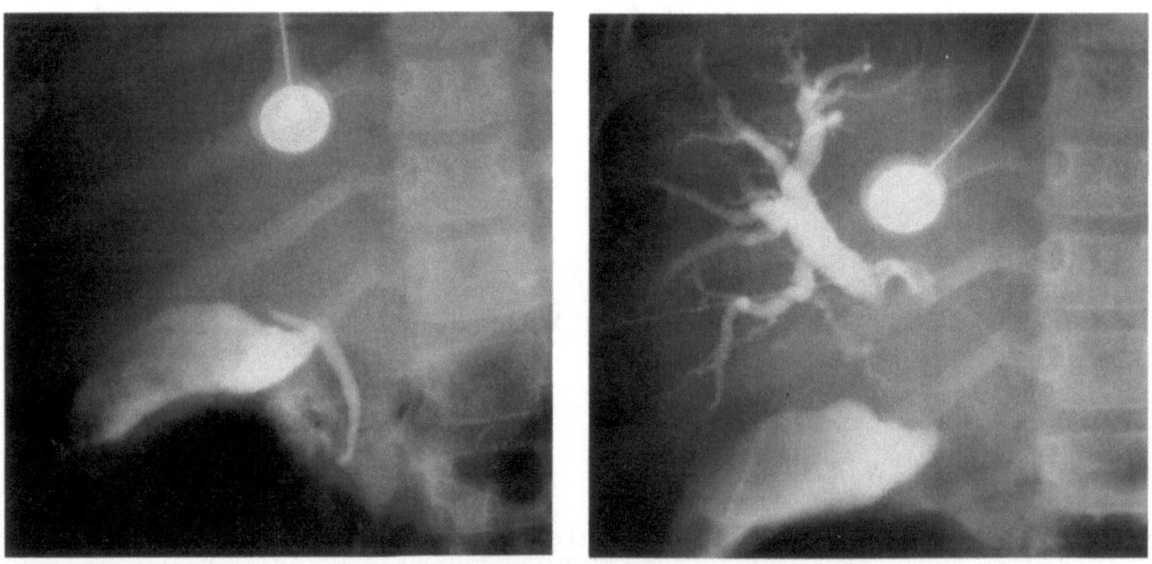

B

Fig. 6.26. Combined approach to visualization of obstructed biliary tract. ERCP examination (**A**) shows filling of gallbladder but abrupt termination of common bile duct just proximal to cystic duct. PTC (**B**) was performed with good filling of dilated right biliary system but no filling of left. PTC needle was withdrawn and repositioned within dilated left hepatic duct (**C**). Composite image (**D**) shows missing segment (*arrows*) caused by tumor of biliary tract.

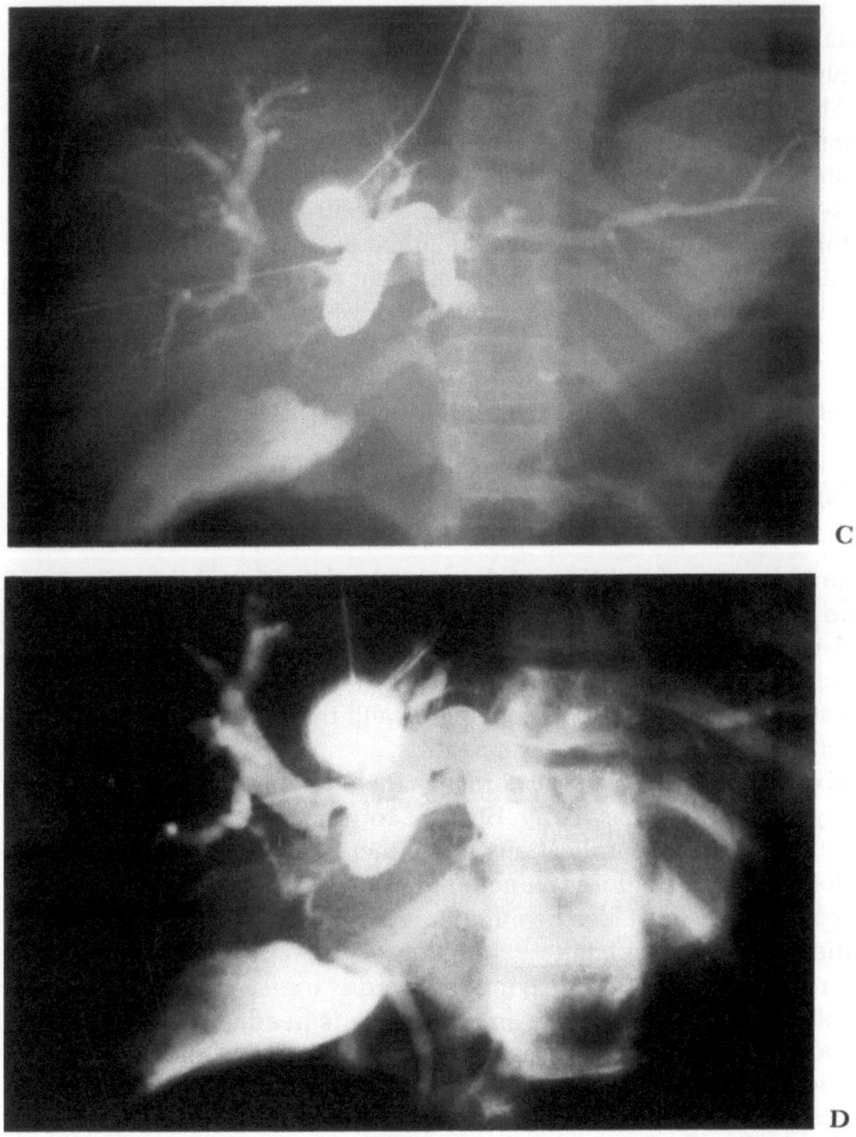

Fig. 6.26

sition will show the Common Bile Duct (CBD) clear of the spine, and 60° right anterior oblique positioning will visualize the right and left hepatic duct confluence (Fig. 6.25).

With the patient supine a falsely high point of obstruction may be diagnosed. The patient may have to be turned to the left, and the table head elevated to 45°, to run the contrast medium down to a point of obstruction. If the duct is dilated, it may be simpler to pass the guide wire followed by 3 or 5 French catheter before identifying the obstruction point. The catheter permits withdrawal of some bile before more contrast is injected, so as to avoid overinjection of an obstructed system, which often leads to bacteremia. If after puncture of the right biliary system the left biliary tree is not visualized despite changing the patient's position, a separate puncture of the left system may be necessary to exclude an obstructing lesion at the level of the confluence of the ducts (Fig. 6.26).

Postexamination Care

Vital signs are observed closely. The complications of this procedure include [18]:

Major: Sepsis, biliary peritonitis, bleeding, and pneumothorax. All are rare with simple PTC, but are more likely to occur if an obstructed system is found and not drained. The patient should therefore be observed for rising pulse or temperature, falling blood pressure, respiratory difficulty, or increasing abdominal or shoulder tip pain.

Minor: Local pain is the most common, and is almost abolished by the use of bupivacaine as previously discussed.

Endoscopic Retrograde Cholangiopancreatography

Diagnostic ERCP

The indications for this procedure are the detection and treatment of bile duct stones, the imaging of the bile duct in jaundice, the assessment of chronic pancreatitis, and, occasionally, the investigation of obscure upper abdominal pain. Emergency indications are the treatment of acute suppurative cholangitis and the relief of impacted bile duct stone in acute biliary pancreatitis.

Explanation and consent normally include consent for sphincterotomy if a duct stone is likely. Because torrential hemorrhage and perforation are rare complications of sphincterotomy, a surgical consultation is required before sphincterotomy is considered. The possibility of pancreatitis must also be mentioned as it occurs in at least 1 in 500 patients, and can be fatal.

Premedication before leaving the ward is unnecessary for most patients, but heavier sedation and analgesia is needed than for routine upper GI endoscopy. Diazepam (or Diazemuls) and Demerol are convenient mixture; use 10 mg and 50 mg, respectively, for a healthy adult, but as little as 3 mg and 20 mg, respectively, for an elderly or frail individual with poor respiratory reserve.

After intubation, the stomach is emptied of fluid to diminish the risk of aspiration, and a cursory examination of stomach and duodenum is made as the scope is advanced to the second part of the duodenum. (Of patients with obscure upper abdominal pain having ERCP, 4% in one series had a peptic ulcer.) Once the endoscope tip is in the second part of the duodenum, the scope is withdrawn with a clockwise rotation to reduce the length of instrument in the patient from about 80 or 90 cm to 65 cm. Very slow further withdrawal brings the papilla into view, usually with 58 to 62 cm of endoscope inserted. Intravenous glucagon, 0.5 mg, will produce sphincter relaxation and aid cannulation, with a right-angle direction of the cannula toward the two-o'clock position of the field of view favoring the pancreas and a retrograde direction towards the eleven-o'clock position favoring the bile duct.

When the pancreas is injected, the radiologist should observe filling carefully to be sure there is no pancreas divisum as 0.5 ml may then be enough to fill the duct system (Fig. 6.27). The patient should be turned

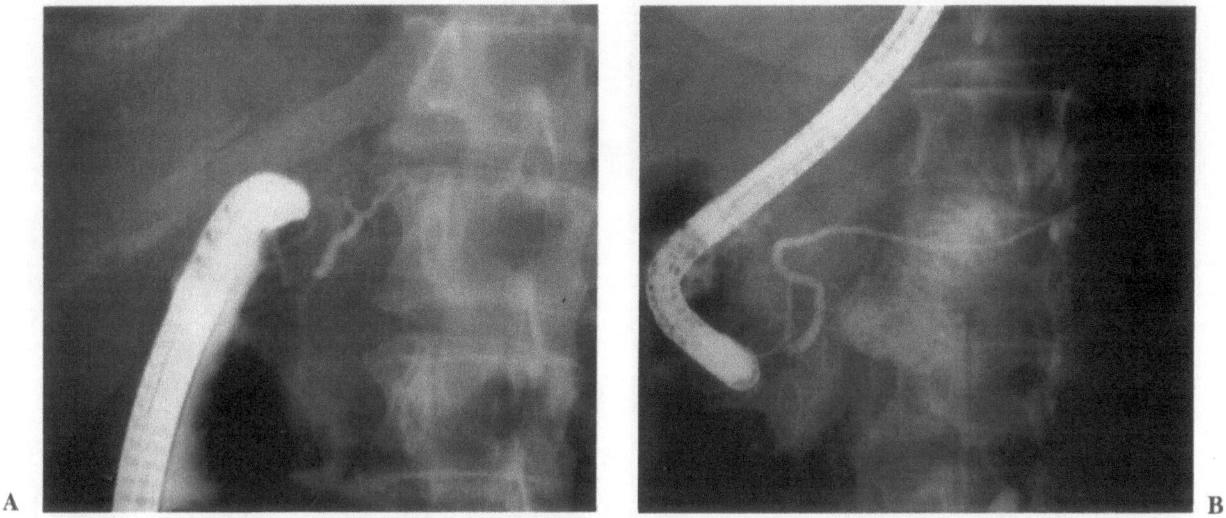

Fig. 6.27. ERCP. A. Contract opacification of separate small duct of pancreas divisum. B. Normal appearance of pancreatic duct (B).

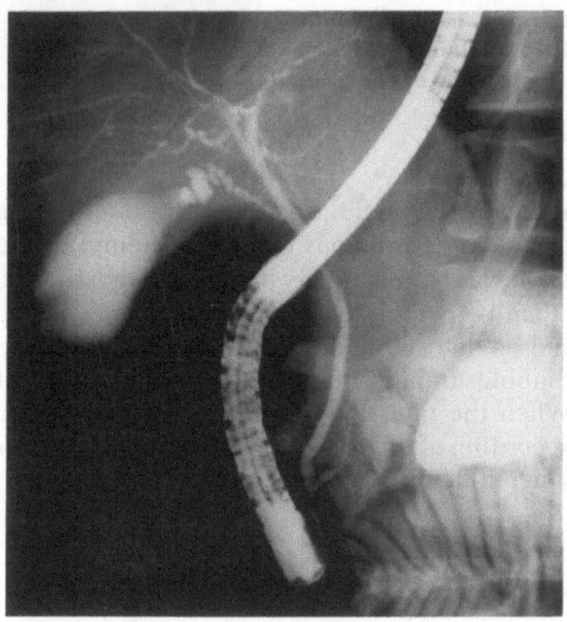

Fig. 6.28. ERCP. Opacification of normal nondilated biliary tree with contrast also filling cystic duct and gallbladder.

fully prone for the pancreatic films, and if a 10 × 12 in. film is used, it should be turned sideways so that the pancreatic tail is included.

When the bile duct is filled, careful observation is made for bubbles or small stones being washed up into the intrahepatic ducts. Contrast is heavier than bile, and in the prone position the mid common hepatic duct and left lobe will fill preferentially; when the patient is supine, the right lobe and common bile duct will outline best (Fig. 6.28). After

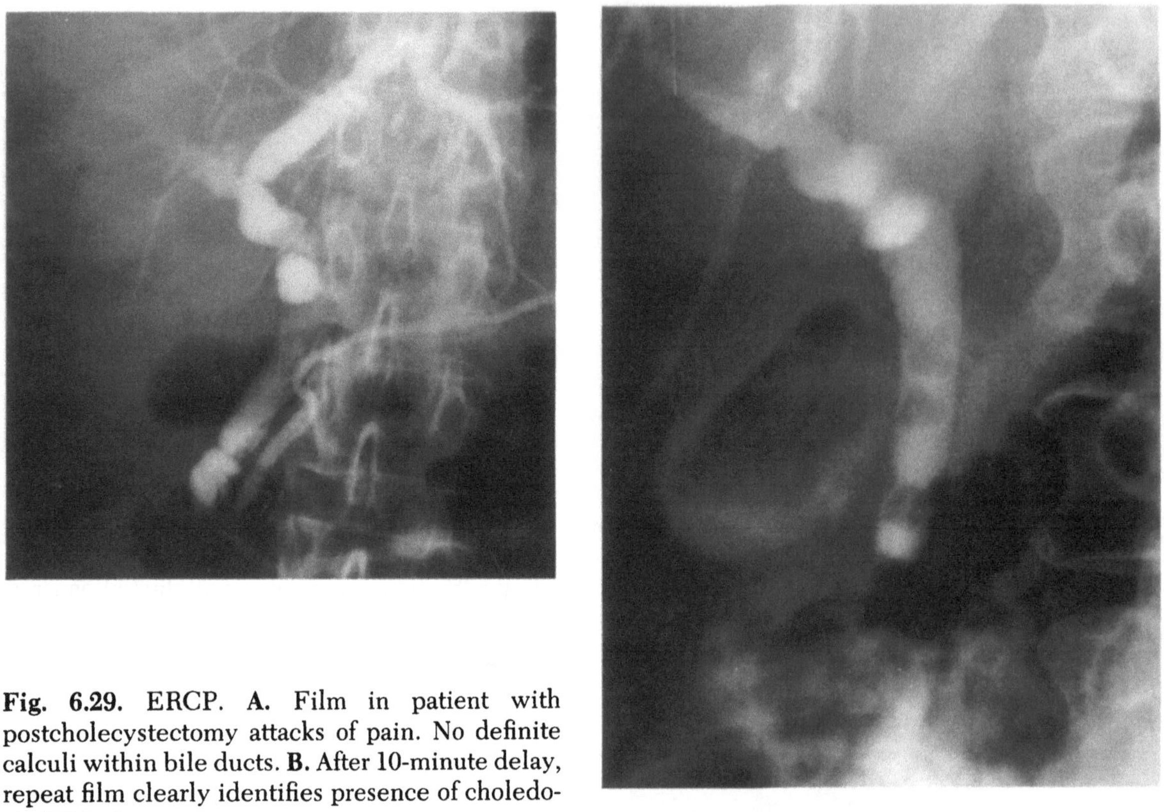

A

B

Fig. 6.29. ERCP. **A.** Film in patient with postcholecystectomy attacks of pain. No definite calculi within bile ducts. **B.** After 10-minute delay, repeat film clearly identifies presence of choledocholithiasis.

about 10 minutes, mixing occurs (Fig. 6.29), and the whole duct system will fill evenly if there has been a previous cholecystectomy; in the presence of a gallbladder, however, the duct system may empty into it, so that duct films must then be completed early. Small stones in the gallbladder may layer and be detectable only with a horizontal beam film. Distinguishing air bubbles from stones is sometimes difficult, but gravity usually helps. When the question of obstruction is raised, a short segment of video recording of the opening and closing sphincter is sometimes more convincing than still films.

Endoscopic Sphincterotomy (ES)

Indications for sphincterotomy include removal of bile duct stones, prophylactic incision in an elderly patient with recent passage of stones and further stones in the gall bladder, if there is a relative contraindication to surgery, acute cholangitis, acute biliary pancreatitis not settling or with further stones in the bile duct, and ampullary tumors.

There is no indication for sphincterotomy or precut to facilitate a purely diagnostic but difficult ERCP. The risks are greater than those of percutaneous transhepatic cholangiography. Clotting factors and platelet count are checked, and the risks of the procedure explained. These may either be spelt out in detail for those that want it (2% chance of bleeding, 1% chance of perforation, 0.5% chance of death) or put as a relative risk for those who want a less detailed accounting (five to six

A 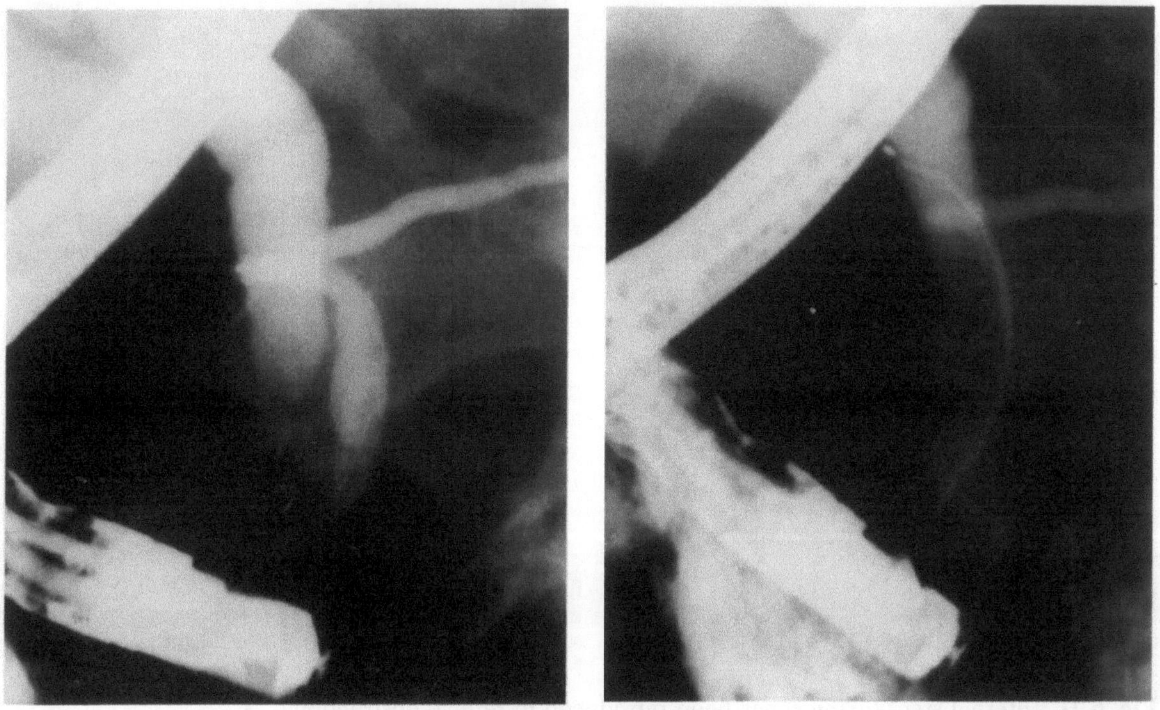 B

Fig. 6.30. ERCP, sphincterotomy. Papillotome has been inserted for sphincterotomy, but fluoroscopic check reveals that it is in pancreatic duct (**A**), a potentially lethal situation. Reinsertion achieves the desired position (**B**) and sphincterotomy can proceed safely.

times safer than open surgery to explore the bile duct and remove stones in an elderly patient).

The papillotome is introduced into the opacified bile duct and its position deeply within the bile duct (and not the pancreatic duct) is confirmed by fluoroscopy, or if necessary by film (Fig. 6.30). The wire is bowed, and with about one-quarter to one-third of the wire within the papilla, a cutting current at 60–70 watts is applied in short bursts. An attempt is made to cut in small controlled increments to a total length of 1 to 1.2 cm on average, but a little longer if the duct is considerably dilated and larger stones are present. Stones are then removed with dormier basket or balloon catheter. If stone removal is not possible, the duct may be protected against stone impaction by either placement of a transnasal biliary drainage catheter or by placing an internal stent (Fig. 6.31). The catheter is suitable for younger patients in whom one wishes to reattempt stone removal or try stone dissolution. The stent is better for older patients who may pull out a nasal catheter, and who may satisfactorily be left permanently with a straight stent protecting the duct.

Patients with a Billroth II anatomy present a special problem. The pediatric colonoscope is well suited to biliary cannulation for these patients. Sphincterotomy can usually be achieved with the standard papillotome, but instead of the wire being pulled for bowing, it is pushed, which makes it bow into the lumen of the duodenum and provides a leading edge that produces a sphincterotomy in the appropriate vertical direction.

Fig. 6.31

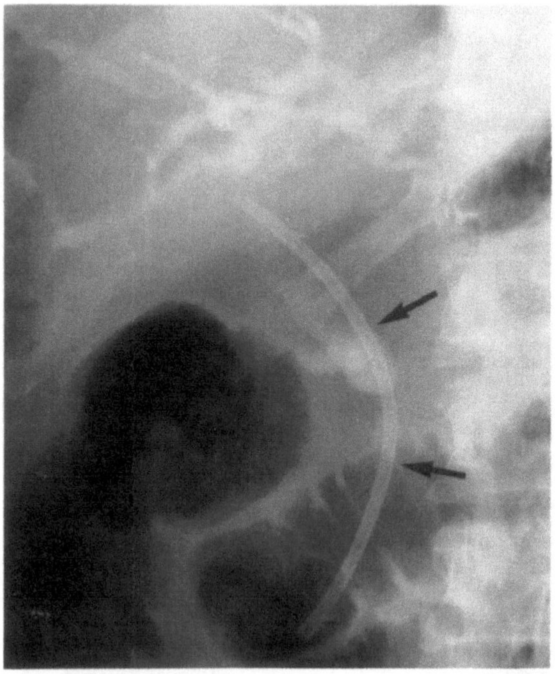

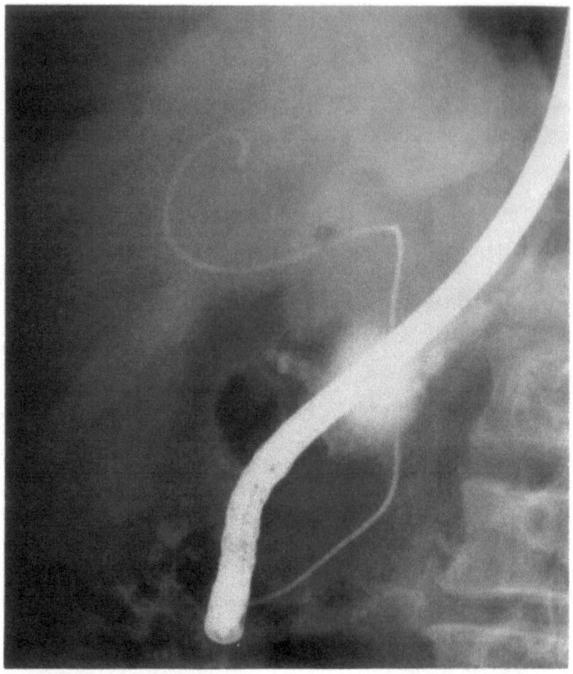

Fig. 6.

Fig. 6.31. Internal stent (*arrows*) has been introduced to relieve obstruction caused by malignant lesion. Proximal portion lies within biliary tree proximal to obstruction. Distal end lies within duodenum.

Fig. 6.32. 12 French stent is positioned within biliary tree endoscopically.

Stents

Stents are placed in the bile duct to palliate strictures or protect against stone impaction, and are placed over guide wires after sphincterotomy. Ten French straight stents are the current standard for stricture palliation, but newer instruments are permitting 12 French stents to be placed, which may provide longer palliation (Fig. 6.32). Stents usually occlude within 3 months and often sooner, and are not yet a very satisfactory form of long-term palliation.

Combined Techniques

ERCP, sphincterotomy, and stent placement all sometimes fail. The insertion of a transhepatic biliary catheter into the duodenum allows the endoscopic procedure to be successfully completed. Alternatively a guide wire inserted transhepatically can be pulled up the esophagus endoscopically, so that large stents up to 14 French can be passed down over a guide wire and placed across a biliary stricture with only a 3 or 5 French tract through the liver. This combined approach promises to be a great advance in biliary palliation.

Gastrostomy

Radiological

Indications

To provide a portal of nutrition into the alimentary tract in patients with normal stomach, small, and large bowel, but who are unable to take oral foods because they have:

a. neurological problems (central inability to swallow)
b. muscle disorders with abnormal swallowing mechanism
c. esophageal obstruction.

Precautions

As with all percutaneous procedures, a normal PT and PTT is mandatory. The risk of the procedure is decreased by using pre study ultrasound to mark the inferior border of the liver.

Materials

1. Fluoroscopy and ultrasound
2. Nasogastric tube with guide wire
3. 50-ml syringe, 5-ml syringe, and 20-gauge needle
4. 22-gauge skinny needle with 20-gauge sheath
5. Omnipaque
6. 0.046-cm guide wire with short flexible tip
7. Teflon dilators (up to 9 French)
8. 0.097-cm J-tip guide wire (145 cm long)
9. 9 French Kifa catheter with a curved tip and two or three sideholes
10. Savlon
11. 1% Xylocaine
12. Molnar disc

Patient Preparation
NPO overnight.

□ *Procedure*

1. With the patient sitting on the fluoroscopic table, a nasogastric tube is introduced and the tip positioned in the stomach. The patient then lies down prone and air is insufflated into the stomach (Fig. 6.33).
2. The lower edge of the liver can be marked using ultrasound.
3. Under fluoroscopic control a puncture site over the stomach body is selected.
4. The skin is now washed with Savlon and frozen with 1% Xylocaine.

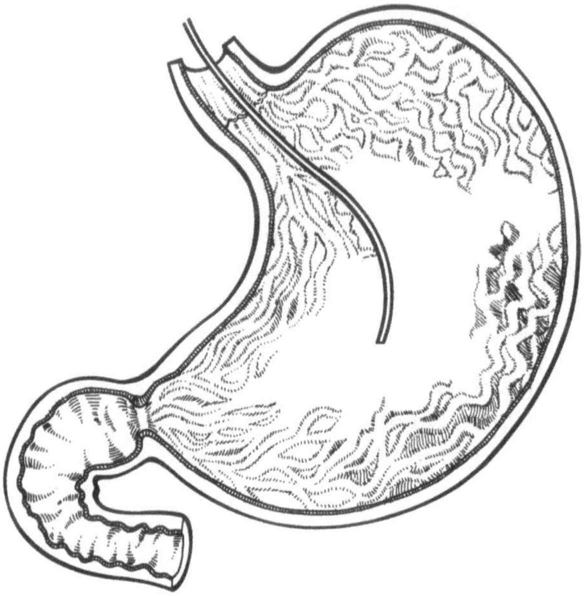

Fig. 6.33. Nasogastric tube has been introduced into stomach and stomach is distended with air.

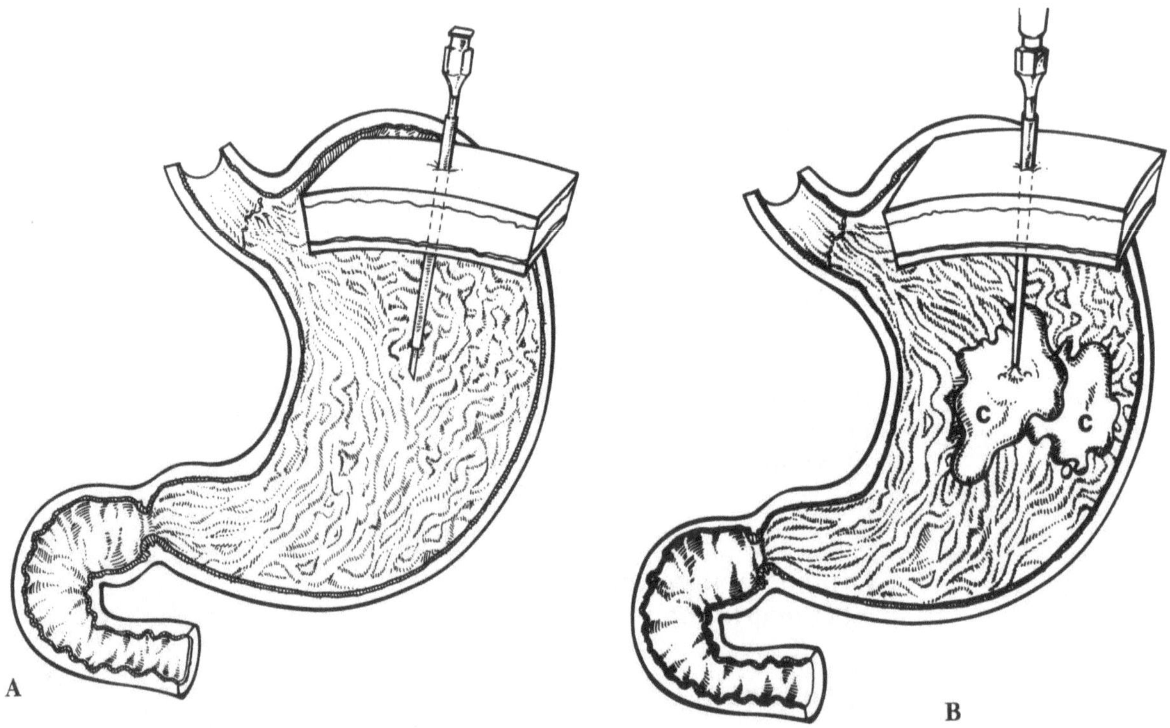

Fig. 6.34. Skinny needle with 20-gauge sheath is introduced percutaneously into distended stomach (**A**). Skinny needle is withdrawn and sheath left in place within gastric cavity (**B**). Contrast medium (C) is injected through sheath under fluoroscopic control to confirm position of its tip.

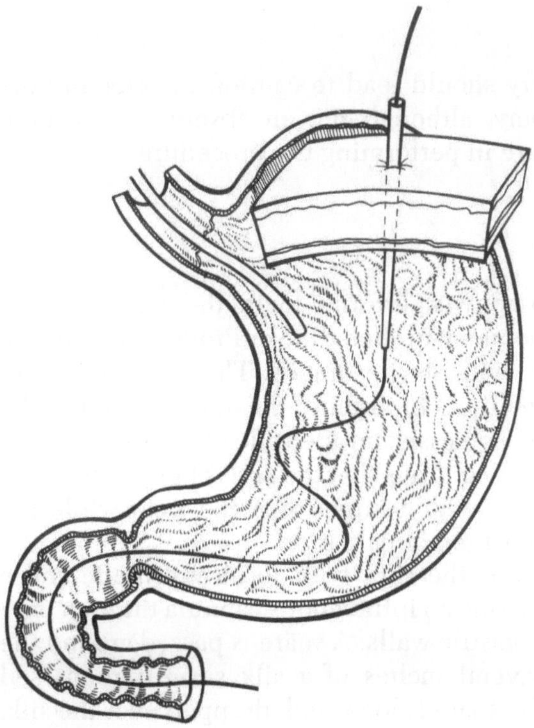

Fig. 6.35. Guide wire is now passed into stomach and then more distally into duodenum through sheath. Gastrostomy catheter may now be introduced.

5. A 22-gauge skinny needle with a 20-gauge sheath is now passed into the stomach (Fig. 6.34A).
6. The position of the sheath inside the stomach is confirmed by injecting Omnipaque through the sheath into the stomach (Fig. 6.34B).
7. The short, flexible-tip, 0.046-cm guide wire is introduced through the sheath into the duodenum (Fig. 6.35).
8. The sheath is withdrawn and the needle tract is expanded with the Teflon dilators up to 9 French.
9. The 0.046 guide is removed and 0.097-cm J-tip guide is introduced.
10. The 9 French dilator is withdrawn and the 9 French Kifa catheter is now advanced.
11. Both the 9 French Kifa catheter and the guide wire are advanced through the pylorus into the duodenum and subsequently passed by the ligament of Treitz. (See section on enteroclysis p. 47.)
12. The guide is now removed and the catheter is fixed to the skin using a Molnar disc.

Endoscopic

Indications

As for the radiological technique; inability to swallow from neuromuscular disease, oropharyngeal or esophageal tumors, or trauma. Difficulty in swallowing because of stroke is the most frequent indication.

Precautions

Previous abdominal surgery should lead to caution in selecting the site, and partial gastrectomy, although not an absolute indication, should lead to particular care in performing the procedure.

☐ *Procedure*

After initial sedation, endoscopy is performed with the patient supine after first preparing the abdomen with Betadine or Proviodine solution and covering the abdomen with sterile drapes. The room lights are dimmed, and the endoscope tip is brought to the anterior wall of the lower body of the stomach. The assistant identifies the position from the transilluminated light and confirms that the site is below the costal margin. The assistant presses with a finger over the light while the endoscopist identifies the position of palpation.

The assistant then prepares the skin with local anesthetic and a scalpel blade stab before passing an intravenous cannula through both the anterior abdominal and gastric walls. A snare is passed around the cannula and tightened. Several inches of a silk suture are passed through the cannula, and the snare is loosened, dropped over the silk, and retightened. The endoscope, snare, and silk are then withdrawn through the mouth. The silk is tied securely to the end of the gastrostomy tube, and the abdominal end of the silk is then pulled to drag the gastrostomy down the esophagus and out through the abdominal wall. A flange or mushroom presses the gastric wall to the abdominal wall, and the final positioning of this is usually done under endoscopic control by reintroducing the endoscope. A crossbar is positioned around the gastrostomy tube against the abdominal wall to secure it in position. A variety of commercial gastrostomy tubes are now available from companies such as Wilson-Cook and Microvasive. Some are designed particularly for patients with esophageal strictures too narrow for the normal mushroom end to pass. Others are designed for distal passage to the jejunum.

Complications

Complications occur in 5 to 15% of patients, and infection around the tube is the most common. Pneumoperitoneum is common and usually not of clinical significance. Separation of the stomach from the abdominal wall is rare, as are gastrocolic fistula and necrotizing fasciitis. The procedure is as safe as the traditional surgical approach, and cheaper and more convenient.

Computed Tomography

The newer generation of faster CT scanners (2 seconds) with better resolution now allows improved imaging of the GI tract and a more complete evaluation of its pathology. CT is the only technique that allows visualization of so many different aspects of GI disease, such as bowel wall thickening, local invasion, lymph node involvement, vascular invasion, and fistula formation as well as metastases to the liver. In children, these indications for the evaluation of gastrointestinal tract are less common. In addition, young children between the ages of 1 and 5 years often require sedation, which makes the procedure even more invasive.

For optimal visualization of different parts of the gastrointestinal tract, a variety of techniques have been developed. There is a standard technique for routine evaluation, but additional views with more contrast, occasionally with changes in patient position, may be performed to provide greater detail of specific anatomical areas.

The basic examination consists of opacification of the bowel lumen and abdominal vasculature. The bowel lumen may be opacified with either a water-soluble contrast or a barium-based suspension [20]. Iodinated water soluble solutions are used in a 2% to 3% concentration. The available water-soluble solutions (Gastrografin and Hypaque powder) need flavoring agents as they have an unpleasant taste. An iodinated water-soluble agent that will be released in North America in the future is virtually tasteless in a 2% to 3% solution. This contrast agent, Telebrix 38 (Mallinckrodt), is available only as a research drug [21]. The Montreal Children's Hospital is using it, and we also have had great success with it [20]. The barium-based products taste better and are readily available commercially in 1.2% to 2% suspensions. The commercial preparations contain suspending agents that avoid flocculation and ensure a homogeneous distribution in the lumen of the bowel. If there is flocculation, streak artifacts may occur in areas with a high concentration of barium. Our preferred barium-based oral contrast is currently Tomocat (Mallinckrodt) because patients prefer its taste over the other suspensions; it has a good transit time through the bowel, and coats as well as any of the others.

A routine scan of the abdomen requires 1000 to 1500 ml of oral contrast. About 800 to 1000 ml is given 45 to 60 minutes before the examination. A further 250 ml is given 15 minutes before the examination and a further 250 ml just before scanning. Appropriate lower doses of contrast are selected for the pediatric patients.

The use of intravenous contrast should be an integral part of any CT examination of the abdomen. It not only helps to identify the normal vasculature but also abnormal vascularity and any invasion of the vessels. The contrast may be delivered as a rapid bolus or as a rapid infusion. A total of 40 to 45 g of iodide should be given. The ideal delivery system is an infusion pump set at 2 to 3 ml per second [22,23]. With pump injections, the site of injection during the first half of the injection should be observed to ensure that there is no interstitial leakage, especially if a smaller or peripheral vessel is being used. The scanning begins after 40 ml has been injected and continues during the rest of the procedure.

Esophagus

The esophagus is opacified with a barium-based paste. This adheres to the wall permitting easy identification of tumors (Fig. 6.36) and the

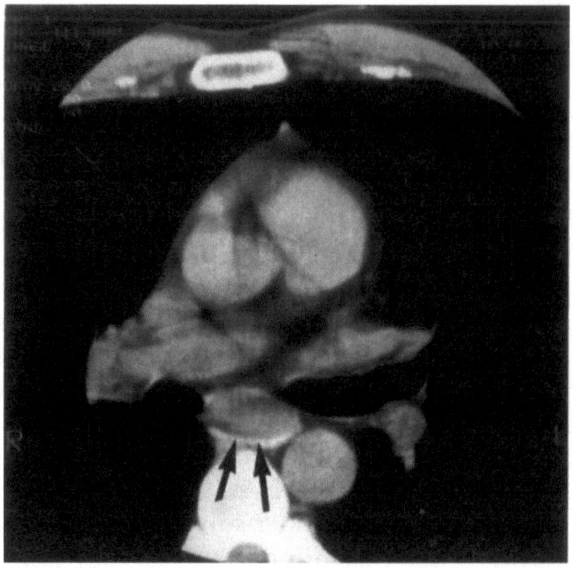

Fig. 6.36. CT of esophagus. Esophageal lesion (leiomyoma) is seen within esophagus. Compressed lumen of esophagus is outlined with contrast medium (*arrows*).

assessment of any extravasation from ulcerating tumors. If the esophagus is being examined with the rest of the GI tract, the oral contrast to opacify the bowel is given first, followed by esophageal barium paste just before scanning begins through the chest. The gastroesophageal area if not well distended can be liable to misinterpretation. There may be focal thickening of the wall of the cardia or a pseudotumor appearance as a result of poor distension (Fig. 6.37). These situations can be elucidated by reexamination with additional contrast and placing the patient in the left posterior oblique or prone position [24].

Stomach and Duodenum

The stomach is optimally examined with air as a contrast agent. The air is given to the patient in the form of gas granules (Baros, E-Z-gas), the same type of gas agent that is used for double-contrast studies of the upper GI tract. The gas agent is given to the patient just before scanning, and may be given with the last cup of barium. If the scan time is longer than 2 seconds, the gas agent should be given about 15 minutes after the last cup of barium because the positive contrast produces streak artifacts on the longer scan times.

The patient's position is changed according to the area of the stomach that is to be visualized. Usually the body, antrum, and pyloric area are adequately distended in the supine position. The fundus is optimally visualized in the right lateral decubitus position. The cardia, esophagogastric junction, and lesser curve can be seen in the left lateral decubitis position, but they are imaged better in the right lateral decubitus. The antrum and duodenum are shown best in the left lateral

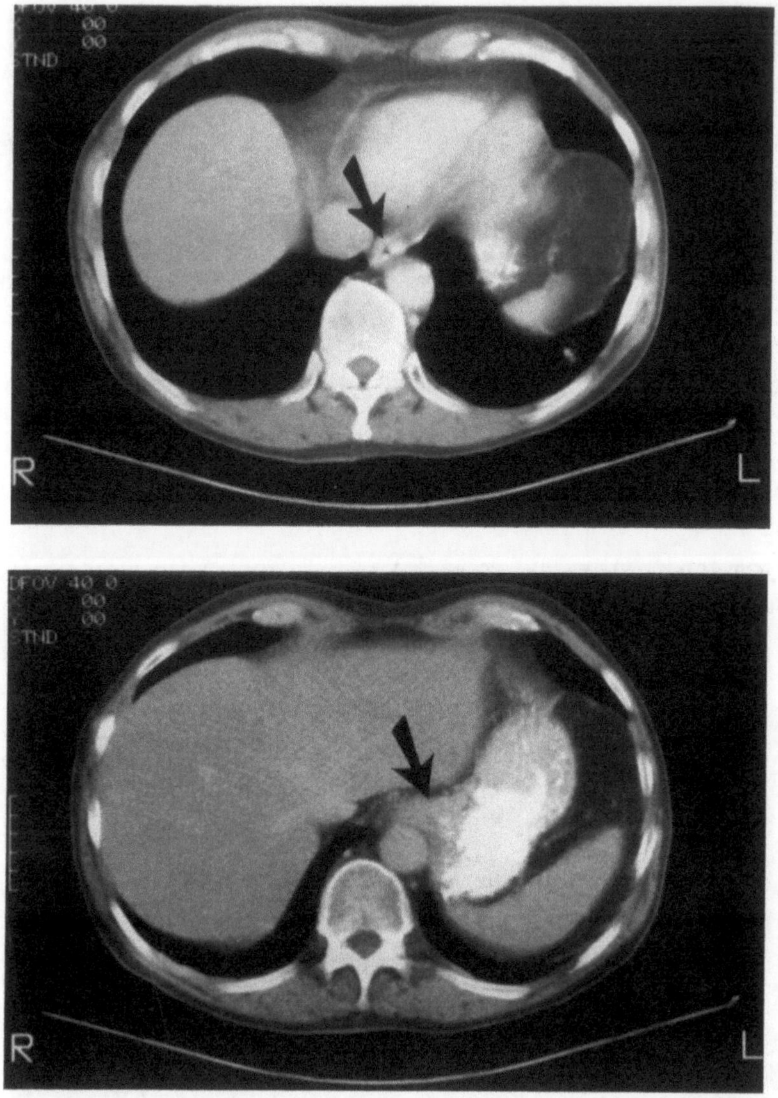

A

B

Fig. 6.37. Malignancies of esophagus can be extremely difficult to identify. **A.** They may be seen in proximal esophagus as thickened wall (*arrow*). If malignancy extends lower down to cardia, it could easily be mistaken for hiatal hernia. **B.** Lower esophageal carcinoma (*arrow*) is seen extending into cardiac region of stomach.

decubitus position. Good distension and relaxation of the duodenum, as well as the stomach, are obtained if glucagon (0.1 mg) or Buscopan (20 mg) is given intravenously just before scanning begins.

For the best results, the stomach should not contain food; therefore, the patient must be kept NPO for 6 hours before the scan until the oral contrast is given. This allows accurate assessment of not only the bowel wall thickness but also mucosal lesions, provided the stomach is well distended (Fig. 6.38). Occasionally, contrast in the stomach is the same density as the stomach tumor, preventing asssessment of wall thickness. Giving the patient 500 ml of water and rescanning allows the thickened stomach wall to be differentiated from gastric contents.

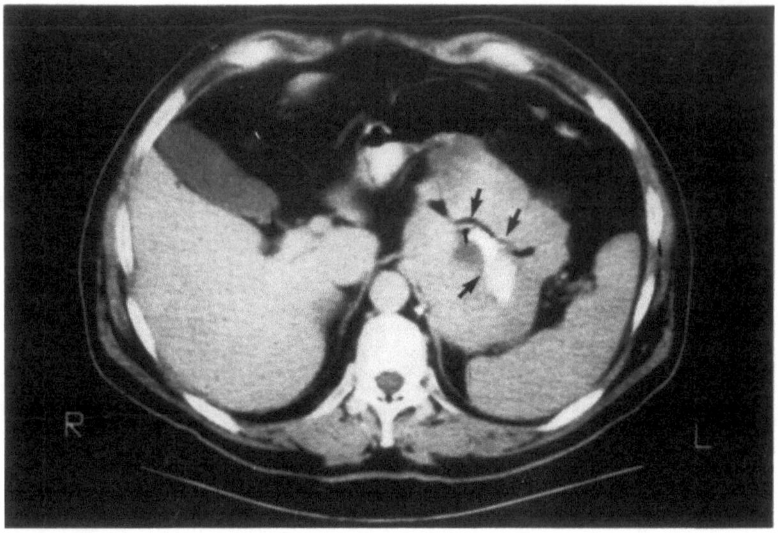

Fig. 6.38. CT of stomach. Lumen of stomach is seen outlined with barium and gas (*arrows*) in patient with leiomyoma of stomach.

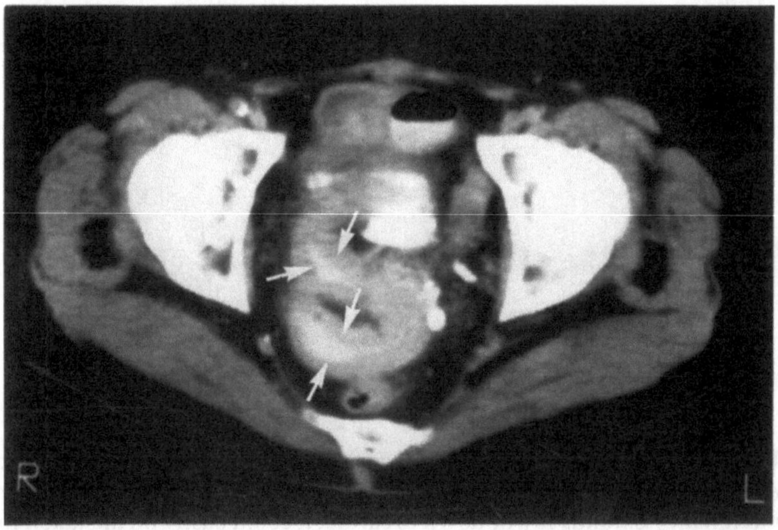

Fig. 6.39. CT of small bowel. Barium within small bowel helps to identify marked mucosal thickening and irregularity (*arrows*) in patient with Crohn's disease.

Small Bowel

In the examination of the small bowel itself (Fig. 6.39), CT has limited value. The jejunum and ileum if well opacified are seen, but mucosal lesions are difficult to identify unless there is a marked wall thickening. To achieve good visualization, at least 1 liter of oral contrast has to be given about 40 minutes to 1 hour before the study to opacify the distal bowel. The proximal small bowel is opacified with a cup of

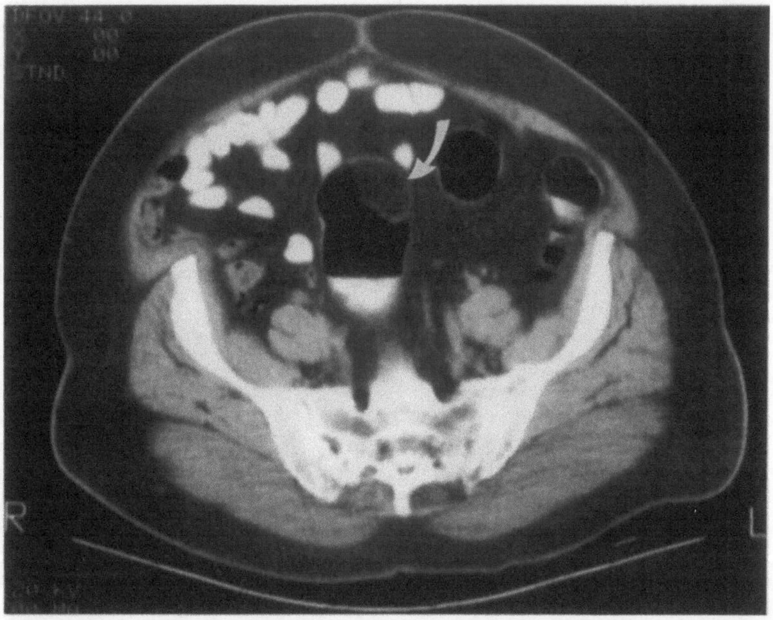

Fig. 6.40. Rectum has been opacified both with barium and air insufflation. In this patient, air insufflation clearly demonstrates lipoma (*curved arrow*) in anterolateral wall of rectum. (Courtesy of Dr. J. Kwok-Liu, St. Joseph's Hospital, Hamilton.)

barium about 5 minutes before the examination begins. If the small bowel is well opacified, mesenteric lesions are easily seen, and in Crohn's disease fistulae and abscesses are particularly well demonstrated.

Colon and Rectum

Good opacification of the colon and rectum is reliably achieved only if about 1000 ml of oral contrast is given 12 to 24 hours before the study [22]. This is not always possible, and rectal introduction of contrast is usually acceptable. Rectal insufflation of air also aids in identifying pathology related to the colon and rectum [25] (Fig. 6.40). The colon usually contains a lot of stool, which may slow the transit of the oral contrast medium with segments of large bowel remaining unopacified. If this occurs it may occasionally be difficult to differentiate an abscess or a partially necrotic mass from a colon full of stool. Therefore, it is a good idea to either ensure complete opacification of the colon or have the large bowel cleansed before the study so that there is minimal or no residual stool. If the bowel is clean, then air insufflation per rectum is also more useful in assessment of the colon. The large bowel can be cleansed with a propylene glycol preparation such as Golytely, Lyteprep, or Kleenprep [26]; Citromag works equally well. The decision on the preparation to use depends on cost and patient preference.

Patients who are having a CT examination for the investigation of colon carcinoma, follow-up of previous colonic surgery, diverticulitis,

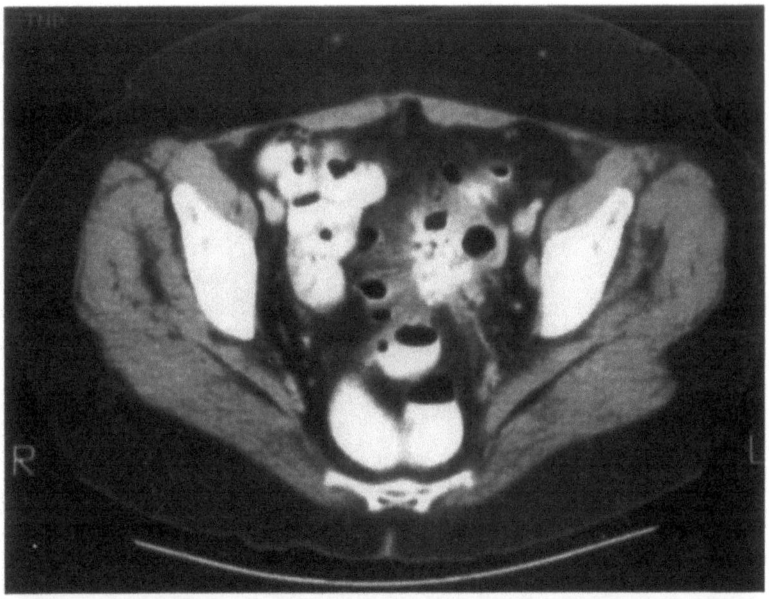

A

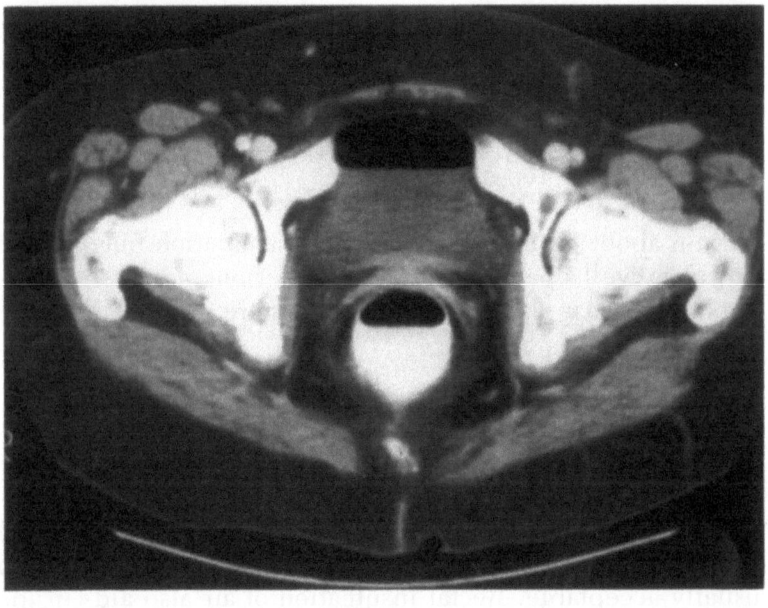

B

Fig. 6.41. CT of pelvis. Patient was examined after oral and rectal contrast. Rectal air was also insufflated. **A.** Extensive diverticular disease is seen within sigmoid colon. **B.** Air–fluid level was identified within bladder as consistent with colovesical fistula that was not suspected clinically.

pelvic mass, and genitourinary neoplasm will have air insufflation of the colon as part of a CT study [27]. The air is administered with a 14 French catheter. The volume introduced is determined by the level of patient tolerance. As this air is introduced without fluoroscopy, it is useful to use a pressure gauge in series with the insufflator so that the intracolonic pressure does not exceed 30 cm of water [28]. Carbon dioxide may be preferable as it is absorbed more quickly and causes less cramping.

Pelvis

For assessment of pelvic masses, scanning may be performed in the supine or prone position if air insufflation is used, (Fig. 6.41). The prone position allows the air to rise to the superiorly located rectosigmoid where maximal distension assists in outlining the colon better in relationship to the mass. In female patients a vaginal tampon is useful in the further delineation of pelvic pathology.

Liver

Dynamic incremental scanning is the procedure of choice for liver CT. Rapid sequential scanning produces images during the phase of maximal contrast difference between normally enhancing tissue and pathological lesion, which may enhance either less or more [20]. We do not routinely use an initial unenhanced scan unless hyperdense or isodense lesions such as metastases from islet cell tumors or carcinoid, are suspected [30].

If a patient is referred with a clinically suspected hemangioma an unenhanced scan is performed initially for localisation of the lesion. The scanner is then set up for nonincremental scanning at a representative level through the mass, and 100 ml of contrast is injected as a bolus. The injection is completed within 1 minute. Scans are made at 15 and 30 seconds and at 1, 2, 3 and 5 minutes. The lesion will be seen to opacify from the periphery inward (Fig. 6.42). If the lesion is still increasing in density or has not completely filled centrally, further delayed scans through the area are performed up to 20 minutes. For routine liver scanning, contiguous 15-mm-thick scans are acceptable. However, when trying to exclude specific pathology with confidence, such as excluding colon metastases before colon cancer resection, slice thickness may also be reduced to 10 mm with increased sensitivity. If CT is being performed to assess a specific previously localized lesion, 10-mm-thick scans will usually suffice, but to avoid partial volume effect, for example with small cysts, 5-mm scans may be worthwhile.

Pancreas

In delineating tumors of the pancreas, especially small lesions, thin slices are essential. However, the study is started with 15-mm contiguous unenhanced scans through the upper abdomen to localize the pancreas, and 5-mm contiguous scans [31] are now obtained after 150 ml of intravenous contrast medium injection. Smaller lesions are also more easily seen with dynamic scanning after rapid infusion of intravenous contrast. The contrast may be introduced by hand or with a power injector at 2 ml per second. A total of 150 ml is used in a pancreatic protocol. The scanning is begun after 50 to 75 ml has been introduced, which ensures total opacification of all the vascular structures in the pancreatic area as well as the pancreas itself (Fig. 6.43).

Lesions in the head of the pancreas may be difficult to see if the duodenum is not well opacified. The stomach and duodenum may be distended with oral gas granules and the patient placed in the left

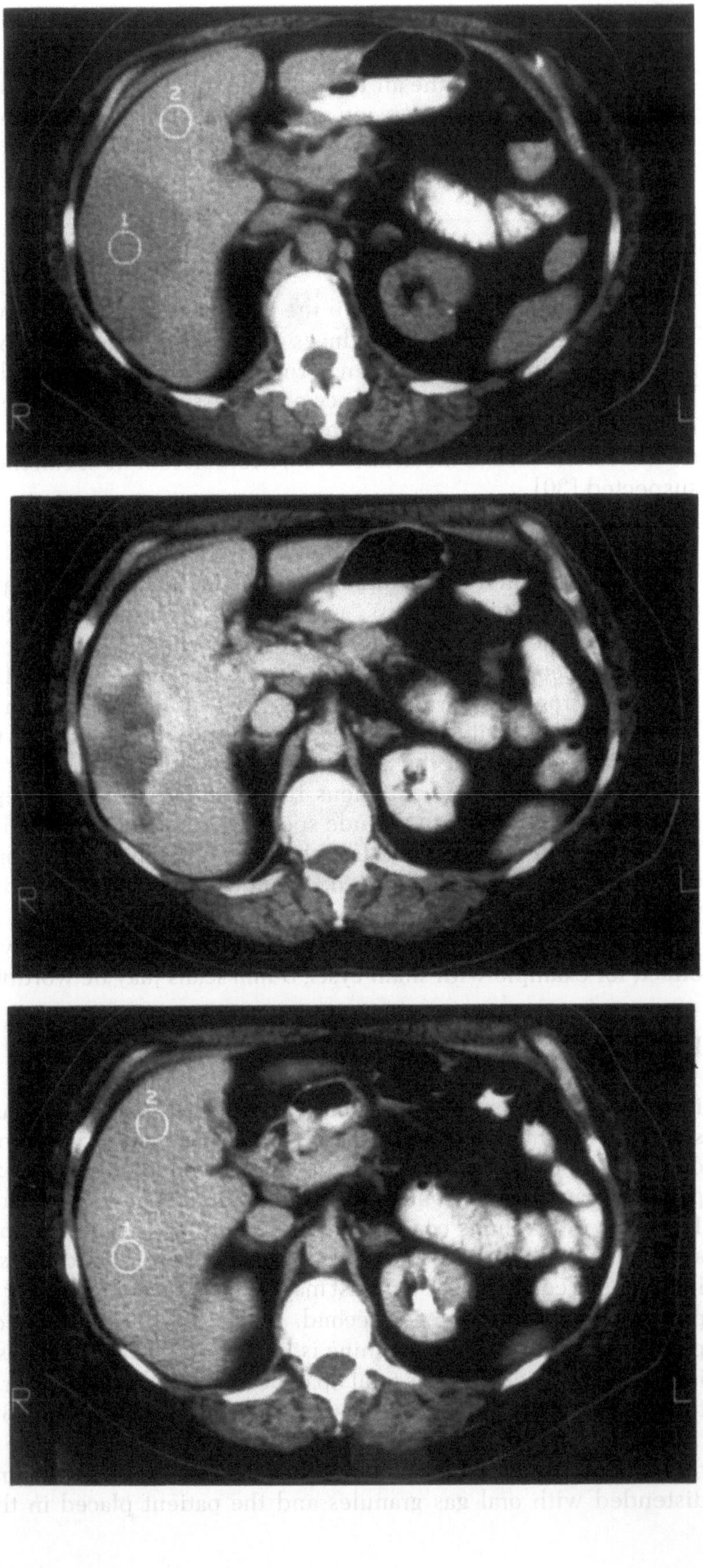

A

B

C

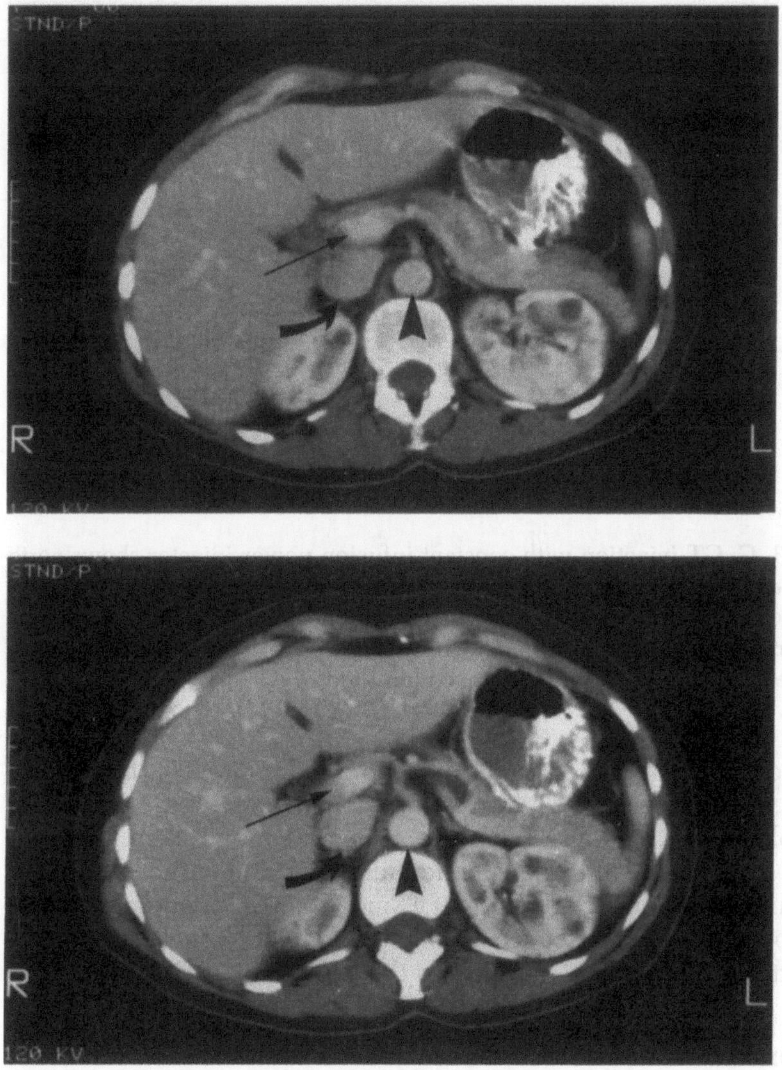

A

B

Fig. 6.43. A. CT performed through pancreatic area with constant infusion of contrast clearly demonstrates vascular anatomy; superior mesenteric vein with splenic vein joining it (*long arrow*), aorta and superior mesenteric artery arising from it (*arrowhead*), and inferior vena cava (*curved arrow*). **B.** CT with constant infusion with pump shows aorta, celiac trunk, and its hepatic and splenic branches (*arrowhead*), portal vein (*long arrow*) and inferior vena cava (*curved arrow*) (*continued.*)

Fig. 6.42. A. Unenhanced scan of liver shows low attenuation lesion within posterior segment of right lobe. When contrast is injected, lesion is seen to enhance from periphery inward (**B**). **C.** 20-minute delayed scan shows complete homogeneous enhancement of lesion consistent with diagnosis of hemangioma.

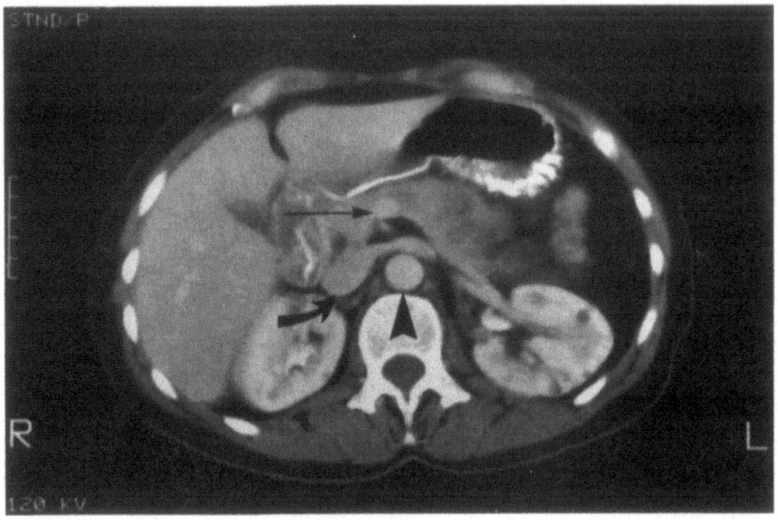

C

Fig. 6.43. C. CT injection with constant-infusion power injector shows aorta (*arrowhead*), inferior vena cava with left renal vein joining it (*curved arrow*), and superior mesenteric vein (*long arrow*). Identification of these vessels is important for assessing the pancreas. In all three slices through same patient, multiple cysts in both kidneys are also identified.

lateral decubitus position to distend the duodenum. The last cup of barium, together with gas granules, must be given with the patient on the table and just before scanning. Scans are now taken with the patient lying on the left side. Duodenum distension will be improved and maintained during the study if a smooth muscle relaxant such as glucagon (0.1 mg) or Buscopan (20 mg) is given intravenously immediately after the last cup of barium and the gas agent [32,33].

References

1. Baker HL, Hodgson JR (1960). Further studies on the accuracy of oral cholecystography. Radiology 74:239–245.
2. Ochsner SF (1970). Performance and reliability of cholecystography South Med J 63:1268–1272.
3. Vas W, Salem S (1980). Cholecystosonography in diagnosis of cholelithiasis: pathologic and radiographic correlation. J Can Assoc Radiol 31:116–119.
4. Bartrum RJ, Harte CC, Foote SR (1977). Ultrasonic and radiographic cholecystography. N Engl J Med 296:538–541.
5. Daly R, Arnaud JP, Turbelin JM, Adloff M (1981). Comparative study of sonography and oral cholecystography in gallbladder lithiasis detection. J Radiol 62:235–237.
6. Hessler PC, Hill DS, Detorie FM, Rocco AF (1981). High accuracy sonographic recognition of gallstones. AJR 136:517–520.
7. Lau SWL (1981). Diagnosis of cholelithiasis: comparison between oral cholyecystography and ultrasonography. Australas Radiol 25:48–51.
8. Gelfand DW, Wolfman NT, Ott DJ, Watson NE, Chen YM, Dale WJ (1988). Oral cholecystography vs gallbladder sonography: a prospective, blinded reappraisal. AJR 151:69–72.
9. Sackmann M, Delius M, Sauerbruch T, Holl J, Weber W, Ippisch E, Hage-

lauer U, Wess O, Hepp W, Brendel W, Paumgartner G (1988). Shock-wave lithotripsy of gallbladder stones: the first 175 patients. N Engl J Med 318:393–397.
10. DeLacey G, Twomey B, Gajjar B, Levi J, Cox AG (1984). Should cholecystography or ultrasound be the primary investigation for gallbladder disease? Lancet i:205–207.
11. Goldberg HI (1976). Operative and postoperative cholecystocholangiography. Semin Roentgenol 11:203–211.
12. Messmer JM, Bradley JJ, Cho SR, Turner MA (1986) Bacteraemia following T-tube cholangiography: hand injection vs. gravity infusion technique. Gastrointest Radiol 11:298 (Abstr).
13. Lieberman RP, Sledor PR (1986). Pain control after percutaneous biliary drainage: local infiltration with bupivacaine and adrenaline. AJR 146:595–596.
14. Roesch J, Lakin PC, Antonovic R (1973). Transjugular approach to liver biopsy and transhepatic cholangiography. N Engl J Med 289:227–231.
15. Gamble P, Colapinto RF, Stronell RD, Colman JC, Blendis L (1985). Transjugular liver biopsy: a review of 461 biopsies. Radiology 157:589–593.
16. Ferrucci JT, Mueller PR, Harbin WP (1980). Percutaneous transhepatic biliary drainage: technique, results, and applications. Radiology 135:1–13.
17. Fraser GM, Cruikshank JG, Sumerling MD, Buist TA (1978) Percutaneous transhepatic cholangiography with the Chiba needle. Clin Radiol 29:101–112.
18. Harbin WP, Mueller PR, Ferrucci JT (1980). Transhepatic cholangiography: complications and use patterns of the fine-needle technique. Radiology 135:15–22.
19. Jain S, Long RG, Scott J, Dick R, Sherlock S (1977). percutaneous transhepatic cholangiography using the 'Chiba' needle—80 cases. Br J Radiol 50:175–180.
20. Azouz EM, Hassell P, Nogrady MB, DiPaolo M (1982). Bowel opacification using 'Telebrix 38' for CT scanning. J Can Assoc Radiol 33:233–235.
21. Mitchell DG, Bjorgvinsson E, ter Meulen D, Lane P, Greberman M, Friedman AC (1985). Gastrografin versus dilute barium for colonic CT examination: a blind, randomised study. J Comput Assist Tomogr 9:451–453.
22. McCarthy S, Moss AA (1984). The use of a flow rate injector for contrast-enhanced computer tomography. Radiology 151:800.
23. Shepard JO, Dedrick CG, Spizarny DL, McLoud TC (1986). Dynamic incremental computed tomography of the pulmonary hila using a flow-rate injector. J Comput Assist Tomogr 10:369–371.
24. Meyers MA (1986). Computed Tomography of the Gastrointestinal Tract, Including the Peritoneal Cavity and Mesentery. New York: Springer-Verlag, p. 7.
25. Sanders RC, McNeil BJ, Finberg HJ, Hessel SJ, Siegelman SS, Adams DF, Alderson PO, Abrams HL (1983). A preoperative study of computed tomography and ultrasound in the detection and staging of pelvic masses. Radiology 146:439–442.
26. Fitzsimons P, Shorvon P, Frost RA, Stevenson GW (1987). A comparison of Golytely and standard preparation for barium enema. J Can Assoc Radiol 38:109–112.
27. Megibow AJ, Zerhouni EA, Hulnick DH, Beranbaum ER, Balthazar EJ (1984). Air insufflation of the colon as an adjunct to computed tomography of the pelvis. J Comput Assist Tomogr 8:797–800.
28. Megibow AJ, Balthazar EJ (1986). Computed Tomography of the Gastrointestinal Tract. St. Louis: Mosby, p. 23.
29. Foley WD, Berland CC, Lawson TC, Smith DR, Thorsen MK (1983). Contrast enhancement technique for dynamic hepatic computed tomographic scanning. Radiology 147:797–803.

30. Megibow AJ, Balthazar EJ (1986). Computed Tomography of the Gastrointestinal Tract. St. Louis: Mosby, p. 14.
31. Hosoki T (1983). Dynamic CT of pancreatic tumors. AJR 140:959–965.
32. Feczko PJ, Simms SM, Iorio J, Halpert R (1983). Gastroduodenal response to low dose glucagon. AJR 140:935–940.
33. Miller RE, Chernish SM, Greenman GF, Maglinte DDT, Rosenak BD, Brunelle RL (1982). Gastroduodenal response to minute doses of glucagon. Radiology 143:317–320.

CHAPTER 7

Technical Aspects of Imaging of the Gastrointestinal Tract

The Technologists's Role

Radiological technology is a rapidly growing and changing profession, and dedicated technologists should continually strive to improve their knowledge, understanding, and skills. As health care professionals, they have an important role to play on the radiological team.

An essential factor in producing the best GI examination possible is a strong working relationship between the radiologist and the technologist. A morning of barium exams may be seen as a tedious, busy, and repetitive session unless there is a sense of involvement and commitment in being an active member of the GI team. The team spirit is engendered by participating in educational seminars, GI rounds, reporting sessions, and general discussion on procedures.

A GI technologist should be able to anticipate the radiologist's needs during fluoroscopy and be totally familiar with all procedures. Any changes from the routine as a result of variations in anatomy and pathology should be understood and allowances made for differences in the technique. Not only will the patient benefit from this harmonious and cooperative working arrangement, but both room and fluoroscopy time will be dramatically reduced.

Organization

A permanent staff member designated as being in charge of the GI area is essential in achieving this dedicated approach. Departments vary greatly in size, layout, and the number of patients so staffing structure must be tailored to the individual institution. One senior or charge person, with junior technologists rotating through the area for a minimum of 2 weeks at a time, is ideal. This may be impractical in smaller hospitals; in that case, a designated charge person responsible for updating procedures and technique charts and for training staff is advisable.

Radiation Protection

Adequate radiation protection methods must be employed if assistance is required in the room during fluoroscopy. The design of radiographic rooms ranges from the conventional room with undertable tube to the newer remote control units. All require staff to spend time in the room during fluoroscopy. It is essential that adequate methods of radiation protection are available. A full lead apron with a 0.5-mm thickness of lead equivalent in the front is a must. Aprons with a 0.5-mm front and 0.25-mm lead equivalent at the back afford adequate protection and are more comfortable to wear. They should have both Velcro and buckle fasteners to allow the technologist good mobility without fear of the jacket coming open. A belt around the waist allows some of the weight to be taken off the shoulders. Thyroid collars and lead glasses should also be worn, especially if using a unit with an overtable tube. Routine testing and measurement of doses should be performed on the equipment and the technologists made aware of the results. A map of the room showing the safest place to stand, away from the direct beam, is a good reminder to have posted on the control panel.

Patient Preparation

The technologist should always question patients on the adequacy of preparation before taking them into the x-ray room. The questions should be open ended, and never leading. Ask how much they managed to drink of the polyethylene glycol preparation for barium enemas, and for a description of the final bowel movement. Leading questions such as "Did you drink at least half," and "Were the bowel movements clear," are likely to elicit a favorable response but not necessarily the correct one. An accurate assessment of bowel preparation at this stage can save valuable room time and save the patient from beginning what would probably prove to be an inadequate examination. The technologist, knowing the radiologist's criteria, should be able to order colon washouts or reschedule the examination as necessary. An assessment of the patient's physical condition at this stage may indicate that a single-contrast enema may be more appropriate and the necessary preparations should then be made.

Communication

If a patient leaves the department feeling confused, neglected, or misunderstood, he may choose not to continue with any more diagnostic tests. Clear, concise, and effective communication is essential between the health care worker and the patient to ensure cooperation and to preserve the patient's dignity. On entering the x-ray room, the procedure should always be explained carefully allowing time for questions. Frequently patients will feel far more comfortable expressing fears and concerns before the radiologist enters the room.

Communication with the ward staff is equally important. How many times do inpatients arrive in the department inadequately prepared for their exam? Unless the nursing staff has some understanding of the radiological procedures and the need for what are often rigorous preparations, their cooperation will not be assured. Both in-service education and tours of the department for the ward nurses help increase their awareness of the complexity of procedures today. Accurate detailed instructions sent to the ward for each patient appointment are far more personal and effective than a standard preparation book. Any time the department changes its methods of patient preparation, it is essential to spend time in effective communication with ward staff. Again, the advisability of having one senior technologist or charge nurse handle these levels of communication has proven to be essential.

Technical Factors and Equipment

Grid

A 10:1 grid with 103 lines per inch provides adequate cleanup of scatter and allows moderate latitude for centering and measurement of the focal film distance. A grid with a higher ratio would prove to be more difficult to work with because of the decreased latitude in accuracy, and would give a higher tube loading and radiation dose with very little benefit in quality of the film. It will act effectively in the kilovolt (kV) range of all GI studies.

Film/Screen Combination

The choice of film screen combination is critical to GI radiography.

High Speed	• To eliminate the effects of both voluntary and involuntary movement on the sharpness of the image. • To allow the use of a small focal spot to help increase image sharpness.
Wide Exposure Latitude	• To demonstrate satisfactorily areas of markedly different x-ray absorption as in barium and air.
Moderate Contrast	• Good contrast decreases as latitude increases. The film should exhibit a moderate degree of contrast between the blacks and whites.
Good Resolution	• Identification of small mucosal lesions requires good resolution.

A 400 speed system utilizing rare earth screens and a latitude film meets these criteria.

High-kV Techniques (Kilovolts)

The kV chosen should be appropriate to meet the following criteria.

Long-Scale Contrast	• To exhibit detail over a wide variety of density ranges from barium to air and over differing ranges of body part thickness.

Good Penetration	• A hard beam allows penetration of the dense barium.
Low Patient Dose	• Low milliamp (mA) values will decrease the entrance radiation dose to the patient.
Low Tube Loading	• The heat units to the anode are also reduced.

When the unit allows it, 105 to 110 kV for double contrast and 120 kV for single contrast will meet these criteria. For other GI studies, 85 to 95 kV is usually adequate.

The Barium Kitchen

As in any home, the kitchen is a focal part of the unit. The recipes for each barium suspension should be well documented, easy to follow, and readily displayed for the technologists. Preparation of the barium suspension may follow the manufacturer's instructions or be adapted slightly by the radiologist. Unlike the home kitchen, individual interpretation or experimentation with a proven recipe by the staff is detrimental to the consistency of the product. Junior or inexperienced staff members should never be allowed to prepare the barium without complete instructions and supervision.

Measuring and mixing are the two most critical factors affecting the barium suspension. Barium supplied in large containers must be weighed on a scale, never measured by volume. Measuring by cups can be highly inaccurate and lead to widely divergent results. One cup of one brand of barium will never weigh the same as 1 cup of an alternate brand. Even when using the same barium, it is very easy to obtain varying amounts in a "cup" depending on the leveling of the cup, the amount of compacting of the barium both in the cup and in the original container, and the consistency of the barium, either dry and loose or heavy and dense.

An accurate standard method for obtaining reproducible results is essential. The two systems most commonly used are the weight/weight and weight/volume percentage methods. Most literature and papers on GI studies will always refer to the w/w or w/v of the supension. The higher the w/w or w/v, the greater the density of the barium suspension and the more "contrasty" the radiograph. The thickness and viscosity of the suspension also will increase as the percentage increases. For example:

$$\%\text{w/w} = \frac{\text{Weight of the barium sulfate in suspension} \times 100}{\text{Weight of barium sulfate} + \text{weight of water}}$$

$$\%\text{w/v} = \frac{\text{Weight of barium sulfate in suspension} \times 100}{\text{Volume of total suspension}}$$

It is important to remember that barium sulfate is insoluble in water and does not form a solution with water but a suspension; one gram (1 g) of barium sulfate displaces approximately 0.25 ml of water.

Expertise in the mixing of barium is required. Most bariums are now easily dispersible in water and do not require the use of an electric mixer. Rigorous mixing either by hand or mixer is likely to cause the formation of foam. If foam is present, the barium suspension will not coat the mucosal walls evenly. Firm but gentle shaking or mixing of the water and barium allows an even suspension without flocculation or foam. If barium is mixed ahead of time it should be gently remixed just before use. Some bariums tend to form sediment fairly rapidly.

Specific Tips for Technologists During a Barium Enema

During the Examination

Note should be taken of the patient's body type, the structure of the bowel, especially the sigmoid colon, and the positon of the flexures and transverse colon. Familiarity with the procedure allows the technologist to anticipate when to clamp the barium, when an antispasmodic drug is indicated, and when the table position will be changed.

Overheads

There are three essential factors for ensuring good overhead films.

Speed	• Especially if using carbon dioxide, which is absorbed far more rapidly than air. Two technologists working together are a great asset although a luxury most departments cannot provide. • Familiarity with the routine and experience will also greatly decrease the time needed for overheads.
Accuracy	• Correct measurement of the focal film distance. • Correct centering to the grid and to the patient. • Positioning: often it is far easier for a patient with a distended abdomen to naturally try and adjust themselves to a slightly oblique position.
Observation	• Assessment of the patient during fluoroscopy will help the technologist when it comes to positioning for the overheads.

Specific Radiographs

Anteroposterior (AP)

To include the flexures, center at approximately the iliac crest; this will vary with the body habitus. Larger patients may need the cassette placed crosswise to ensure all the flexures are covered. The centering point may need to be adjusted if the flexures are higher or lower than average. Whenever possible the entire bowel from the anorectal area to the tip of the flexures should be included.

Posteroanterior (PA)

To include the rectum, center approximately at the iliac crest but check the level of the anus against the bottom of the cassette to ensure that all the rectum is included. The density setting on the automatic exposure device may need to be decreased if the barium-filled transverse colon is thought to be lying directly beneath the photocell.

Prone Angled

This is frequently the most difficult projection for the technologist. The extreme obliquity of the central ray causes several problems, one of which is the exposure difference between the top and bottom of the film. Another is the large amount of abdomen the beam must traverse, resulting in increased scatter to the distal part of the cassette.

The focal film distance must be measured. It is totally impossible to estimate with the central ray angled 40° to the feet. For an accurate measurement, the bucky tray should be pulled out toward the technologist and the angled tube brought over above the cassette. The central ray should pass through the (anterior superior iliac spine (A.S.I.S.) The easiest way to do this is for the techologist to place a hand at the same angle as the central ray and rest it against the A.S.I.S., adjusting the centering until the light beam passes along the line of the hand.

Accurate collimation is critical to decrease the effects of scatter. Again, observation during fluoroscopy helps assess the length of the unfolded sigmoid colon. The collimated area on the patient's back will be quite small because of the large distance between it and the film.

Lateral Rectum

The patient should lie in the left lateral position with the arms and legs bent for stability. Center to the middle of the rectum, checking the level of the anus against the lower edge of the cassette. Collimation is again critical to reduce the effects of scatter from the size of the hips. A contoured piece of lead may be placed on the table around the rectum to absorb any scattered radiation. This will increase the visibility of detail on the image.

Decubitus Films

Previous studies have shown that, in some hospitals, more than 50% of decubitus films were either over- or underexposed, contributing to a significant percentage of missed lesions. An independent ceiling-suspended bucky grid with an automatic exposure device and a self-centering tube is the ideal setup for these radiographs, but probably not readily available in most hospitals. A stationary grid with an independent ceiling-suspended tube is the type of equipment usually available.

A filter can compensate for the increased absorption of the beam by the dependent soft tissue. Various types are available. The most effective device, requiring the least increase in tube loading or dose to the patient, is a half-Plexiglass filter. When correctly attached to the tube, it allows the exposure to be adequate to penetrate the dependent side of the abdomen but filters enough of the beam that the nondependent side is not overpenetrated. The filter can be attached to a Plexiglass insert that is inserted into the tube head before making an exposure. Alternatively, strips of Velcro on the insert and strips of Velcro on the bottom of the tube head can be used. The Velcro method allows more flexibility in positioning the filter, depending on the size of the patient, but provides more wear and tear on the filter if it is not removed and put away immediately after use. The filter is positioned with the bottom edge just slightly below the midline of the patient.

Another method of obtaining optimum density on both sides is to always have the abdomen tightly compressed against the grid for each decubitus film. The patient should be positioned in the true lateral position with the knees slightly bent for stability. A foam block should be placed underneath the side to ensure the entire abdomen is included on the film. Between exposures the tube must be moved to the opposite side of the table to enable the patient's abdomen to once more be positioned against the grid. This method is more time consuming but advisable and rewarding, particularly on larger patients.

A detailed technique chart with abdominal measurements and body type listed (for example, solid, flabby) should be available for each GI room. Taking the patient's abdominal measurement with calipers before the bowel becomes distended with air will give a more accurate measurement.

Accurate centering to the grid and the midline of the patient, plus tight collimation, all contribute to an optimal radiograph.

Equipment

Cassette holder. Should have a good solid construction; there is an L-shaped model in which the base slides directly underneath the patient and the perpendicular part holds the cassette. The patient's weight ensures the cassette is totally stable. The grid should be positioned to allow the grid lines to run parallel to the short axis of the cassette, allowing ease of centering of the central ray.

Table top. Should be flat to allow correct placement of the cassette holder and foam block. Positioning is very difficult with the curved type.

CHAPTER 8

Pharmacology

Drugs that may be used in the Gastrointestinal Radiology department include:

1. metoclopramide HCl
2. glucagon
3. Buscopan
4. edrophonium chloride
5. fentanyl
6. meperidine
7. diazepam
8. lidocaine
9. phentolamine

Please refer to product monographs before administration.

1. *Metoclopramide HCL* (Maxeran) is a benzamide derivative that modifies gastrointestinal tract activity and that has a central antiemetic effect. The antiemetic effect is through an action on the chemoreceptor trigger zone. The effect on the gastrointestinal tract is probably through antidopaminergic activity.

Metoclopramide affects the motility of the entire GI tract [1]. It increases resting pressure in the lower esophageal sphincter with increased strength of the peristaltic contractions in the esophagus, stomach, and small intestine. This results in faster gastric emptying and shorter small bowel transit times.

Peak plasma levels occur between 45 to 90 minutes after oral ingestion and within minutes of intravenous injection. The half-life is approximately 3 to 5 hours.

Metoclopramide, with its accelerating effects on the GI tract, has been found most useful in expediting small bowel meal and small bowel examinations (page 53). It is administered intravenously at a dose of 5 to 10 mg. In enteroclysis, it is particularly useful if overdistension has caused temporary paralysis of the small bowel. If a patient presents for a barium meal having had a coffee or other drink in the morning, 10 mg of metoclopramide either intravenously or orally as a syrup and a 1-hour delay will usually produce an empty stomach.

Adverse efects include drowsiness and fatigue; therefore, patients should be cautioned about driving if these effects occur. In children, metoclopramide can produce extrapyramidal effects with Parkinsonian-like rigidity, usually on prolonged or high dosage, and should be used with caution, especially in small children.

2. *Glucagon* is a naturally occurring polypeptide hormone produced by the alpha cells of the islands of Langerhans in the pancreas. Glucagon exerts an action on liver glycogen, converting it to glucose and therefore increasing blood glucose levels. When administered intravenously, glucagon causes relaxation of smooth muscle in the GI tract [2].

Glucagon decreases the pressure of the lower esophageal sphincter and sphincter of Oddi, and causes hypotonia of the stomach, duodenum, small bowel, and colon.There is also some evidence suggesting gulcagon transiently impairs peristalsis of the body of the esophagus.

Glucagon is administered intravenously at a dose of 0.1 to 1 mg. Lyophilized glucagon must be dissolved in a solvent before injection. The time of onset of action is usually within 1 minute, with the effect lasting up to 20 minutes after a 1-mg dose. Glucagon can also be injected intramuscularly, but the onset of action can be delayed up to 10 minutes. The half-life in plasma is 3 to 6 minutes.

In a low dose of 0.1 to 0.2 mg intravenously, glucagon produces a short-lived atony of the stomach and duodenum, and is helpful in barium meal examinations, especially for hypotonic duodenograms. At a dose of 0.5 mg, it appears to produce considerable relaxation of the sphincter of Oddi and is useful in facilitating selective cannulation of the common bile duct during ERCP. At a dose of 0.5 to 1 mg intravenously, it produces atony of the colon and reduces symptoms of spasm, allowing for improved double-contrast barium enema studies.

Symptoms of abdominal pain, nausea, and vomiting may be produced; these are rarely seen with doses less than 0.75 mg intravenously, but are common with doses greater than 1 mg. Glucagon is contraindicated in patients with insulinomas and by releasing catecholamines may cause a hypertensive crisis in patients with pheochromocytomas. Phentolamine and glucose should be readily available in departments in which glucagon is used routinely.

3. *Hyoscine butylbromide* (Buscopan) is a spasmolytic drug that exerts its central and peripheral action through inhibition of cholinergic receptors. The anticholinergic effect in the GI tract causes paralysis of the esophagus, stomach, duodenum, small bowel, and colon.

Buscopan is the agent of choice for hypotonic duodenal studies. It is administered intravenously at a dose of 10 to 20 mg. The drug works almost immediately with the duration of effect of 10 to 20 minutes. Smaller doses are also effective, but have a shorter duration of action and should be reserved for patients who are most cooperative and can move quickly. A 20-mg dose can be administered for prevention of colonic spasm during double-contrast barium enemas. Many endoscopists use Buscopan routinely for ERCP and during upper GI endoscopy, as it is useful to produce gastric paralysis to aid guided biopsy in patients whose stomach is rather active.

The adverse effects of Buscopan include tachycardia and blurred vision. The blurred vision has been reported in 10%–37% of patients after a 20-mg I.V. injection. The visual blurring lasts about 20 to 30 minutes, rarely persisting several hours [3–6]. Patients should be warned of this effect and should not drive until the effect has worn off.

Buscopan is contraindicated in patients with acute angle glaucoma. Pro-Banthine is well known to cause urinary retention, and in theory the shorter acting Buscopan might also do so. However, in 20 years of using Buscopan routinely we have never encountered a urinary problem with this drug, presumably because it has a shorter duration of action.

4. *Edrophonium chloride* (Tensilon) is a short and rapid-acting cholinergic drug. By inhibiting cholinesterase activity it attenutates the effect of acetylcholine and restores normal muscle activity in patients with myasthenia gravis. In susceptible patients it appears to trigger nonperistaltic esophageal activity and is used for this purpose in manometry laboratories. It may also have a role in precipitating this same type of motor activity in the esophagus during a barium swallow in patients with chest pain in whom an esophageal cause for the pain is being sought.

Edrophonium is administered intravenously; its effect is seen within 30 seconds and lasting about 10 minutes.

Tensilon is contraindicated in patients with mechanical intestinal and urinary tract obstruction and with hypersensitivity to anticholinesterase agents. Adverse effects include bradycardia and hypotension, increased salivation and GI secretion, nausea, vomiting, and diarrhea.

5. *Fentanyl citrate* (Sublimaze) is a narcotic analgesic agent with action similar to morphine and meperidine. At a dose of 100 μg intravenously (2 ml), it produces a brief sense of relaxation and analgesia. For this reason it is an ideal drug to make slightly unpleasant short procedures easier and better tolerated by the patients. It is ideal for routine upper GI endoscopy and for facilitating intubation during enteroclysis.

When given at 50 to 100μg I.V., it works almost immediately with duration of action lasting 30 to 60 minutes. Two hours after injection there is still considerable impairment of driving ability [7], although patients feel normal. It is therefore not suitable for patients who have to drive following a procedure.

Fentanyl is contraindicated in patients with shock and septicemia. It may produce muscle rigidity, euphoria, pupil dilatation, bradycardia, and bronchoconstriction. As with other narcotics, it can cause respiratory depression that is dose related. Larger doses can lead to apnea, and a narcotic antagonist such as naloxone, as well as resuscitation equipment, should be readily available.

6. *Meperidine HCl* (Demerol) is a narcotic analgesic with limited use in barium examinations, but it is used routinely for endoscopy and interventional procedures. The drug is administered I.V. or I.M. at a dose of 25 to 50 mg. Contraindications and adverse effects similar to fentanyl are seen. Meperidine should be administered with caution.

7. *Diazepam* is used as an anxiolytic sedative agent. It can be used instead of fentanyl to facilitate endoscopy, intubation for enteroclysis, or interventional procedures. Diazepam can be administered I.M., I.V., or per os before the examination.

Diazepam should not be given to patients in shock or to elderly and very ill patients. Administration should also be avoided in patients with psychiatric disorders. It can cause drowsiness and ataxia, and patients should be advised against driving after a Valium injection. [7]. Doses as low as 2.5 mg I.V. can cause respiratory arrest in patients with chronic lung disease, or the elderly. An agent to reverse its respiratory depressant effect is not currently available, but is shortly to be released (Flumazenil).

Valium can cause phlebitis after injection, and a newer fat-soluble derivative is now available that avoids this painful complication and is therefore preferred (Diazemuls).

8. *Lidocaine HCl* (Xylocaine) is a local anesthetic. Its effect is almost immediate and lasts 90 to 120 minutes. Hypersensitivity to lidocaine can occur. It is contraindicated in shock or heart block, and can cause drowsiness and lassitude. Lidocaine injectible is available in 0.5%, 1%, and 2% solutions with or without epinphrine. We have found that 1% works best; the 2% solution stings, and 0.5% has a very poor effect.

Other local anesthetics are also useful. Mepivacaine HCl (Carbocaine) has been found useful because its action is more prolonged than that of lidocaine. Bupivacaine HCl (Marcaine) with adrenaline 1:200,000 has been found to be effective for pain control after transhepatic procedures [8], and is therefore now the agent of choice.

9. *Phentolamine* (Rogitine) is an alpha-adrenergic blocking agent. Its use in radiology is limited to treatment of hypertensive episodes induced by glucagon injection. Phentolamine is injected at a dose of 5 mg I.V. All alpha-blocking agents are contraindicated in patients with myocardial infarction or coronary insufficiency because tachycardia, cardiac, arrhythmias, and hypotension can occur.

References

1. James WB, Melrose AG (1969). Metoclopramide in gastro-intestinal radiology. Clin Radiol 20:57–60.
2. Kreel L (1975). Pharmacoradiology in barium examinations with special reference to glucagon. Br J Radiol 48:691–703.
3. Mehlfeld G, Bleichert A (1986). The problem of the impairment of the action of parasympatholytic substances. Opthalmologic criteria and methods. Arzneimittelforschung 36:271–273.
4. Mehlfeld G, Bleichert A (1986). The effect of anticholinergic drugs on the inner eye muscles. Graefes Arch Clin Exp Ophthalmol 224:92–95.
5. Ayre-Smith G (1976). Hyoscine-*n*-butylbromide (Buscopan) as a duodenal relaxant in tubeless duodenography. Acta Radiol [Diagn] (Stockh) 17:701–714.
6. Hupscher DN, Dommerholt O (1984). Action and side effects of small doses of Buscopan in gastroduodenal radiology: a prospective study in 300 patients. Diagn Imag Clin Med 53:77–86.
7. Stevenson GW, Pathria MN, Lamping DL, Buck L, Rosenbloom D (1986). Driving ability after intravenous Fentanyl or Diazepam: a controlled double-blind study. Invest Radiol 21:717–719.
8. Lieberman RP, Sledor PR (1986). Pain control after percutaneous biliary drainage: local infiltration with bupivacaine and adrenaline. AJR 146:595–596.

APPENDIX I

Products and Manufacturers

1. Barium products

A. Upper GI tract

a. E-Z-HD (E-Z-Em). Contains 98% barium sulfate (340 g), simethicone, and other additives; addition of 65 ml of water produces 135 ml of suspension of 85% w/w or 250% w/v

b. Liquid Sol-O-Pake (E-Z-Em), 45% w/w or 72% w/v barium sulfate suspension

c. HD 200 Plus (E-Z-Em)-225% w/v.

d. Novopaque, 40% w/w or 60% w/v barium sulfate suspension with sodium saccharine flavouring. This is a pre-mixed liquid barium in 355 ml cans or 3.71 litre containers.

e. Micropaque 92% w/v. No longer available in Canada.

f. Polibar powder. (E-Z-Em) Supplied in a 100-g jug; suspension from 27% w/w to 50% w/w can be obtained with appropriate quantity of water

g. Baricon (E-Z-Em). Contains 95% barium sulfate (340 g). Addition of 70 ml of water produces 83 w/w suspension

B. Small bowel

a. Ultra-R (E-Z-Em), 95% barium sulfate powder with simethicone and additives. Can be diluted to 45%, 50%, 55%, or 60% w/w (72%–110% w/v)

b. Enterobar (E-Z-Em), 50% w/v barium suspension

C. Double-contrast colon

a. HD85 (E-Z-Em), 85% w/v suspension (2000 ml)

b. Polibar Liquid (E-Z-Em), 55% w/w or 100% w/v barium sulfate suspension (1900 ml)

c. Liquid Polibar Plus (E-Z-Em), 57% w/w or 105% w/v suspension

d. Colobar (E-Z-Em), 56% w/w or 100% w/v barium sulfate suspension (2000 ml)

D. Single-contrast colon

a. Polibar Liquid (E-Z-Em). Dilute 1 volume Polibar Liquid with 5 volumes of water to obtain 15.4% w/w or 17.5% w/v suspension

b. Baroperse Enema Kit (E-Z-Em). Contains 340 g Barosperse

c. Unibar 100 (E-Z-Em), 56% w/w or 100% w/v barium sulfate suspension (2000 ml)

d. Unibar 110 (E-Z-Em), 60% w/w or 110% w/v suspension (2000 ml)

E. Barium suspension for CT

a. Baro-cat (E-Z-Em), 1.5% w/w barium suspension

b. E-Z-Cat (E-Z-Em), 4.5% w/w concentration; dilutes to 1.1% w/w suspension (225 ml)

c. Readi-Cat (E-Z-Em), 1.2% w/w barium sulfate suspension (450 ml, 2000 ml)

d. Esopho-Cat (E-Z-Em), 3% w/w barium sulfate paste for coating of esophagus

2. Water-soluble contrast for upper GI tract in adults only (very dangerous in children)

a. Gastrografin (adults only)

b. Hypaque (Winthrop)

c. Renografin (Squibb)

d. Omnipaque (Winthrop)

e. Isovue (Squibb)

f. Ioxyglate, Hexabrix (Mallinckrodt)

g. Hypaque powder for oral CT contrast (Winthrop)

3. Effervescent Tablets

a. E-Z-Gas2, effervescent granules (E-Z-Em). Contain sodium bicarbonate 2.21 g, citric acid 1.53 g, simethicone 0.02 g; produce no less than 400 ml CO_2

b. Unik-Zoru, tablets or granules (E-Z-Em). Produce 280 μg of gas per dose

c. Baros, granules (E-Z-Em)

4. Methylcellulose

a. Enterocel (E-Z-Em), 500-ml concentration of methylcellulose

b. MC (E-Z-Em), 1% w/v hydroxypropylmethylcellulose solution

5. Enteroclysis catheters

a. Maglinte enteroclysis catheter (Cook Inc, E-Z-Em), 155 cm × 13 French catheter with balloon and torque cable

b. Gianturco catheter (Cook Inc.). Has flexible guide for stiffening and torque control

c. Bilbao Dotter catheter (Cook Inc.). Has a curved tip for directional control. 12 and 14 Fr available in various lengths

d. Muller catheter. (Cook Inc.) Has variable curve tip control

6. Enema tubes and tips

Various enema bags with various sizes, tips with and without cuff are supplied by E-Z-Em. Cuffs should not be used in children

7. Film.

a. T-Mat L Film (Eastman Kodak)

b. Cronex 7 Film (Dupont)

c. High-Ortho Film (Konica)

d. Fuji Xray Film (Fuji)

Various products are available that are suitable for examination of the gastrointestinal tract. This appendix lists only the products with which the authors have clinical experience.

APPENDIX II

Further Reading

1. Margulis AR, Burhenne HJ, eds (1988). Alimentary Tract Radiology, 4th Ed. St. Louis: C.V. Mosby.
2. Meyers MA (1986). Computed Tomography of the Gastrointestinal Tract including the Peritoneal Cavity and Mesentery. New York: Springer-Verlag.
3. Gelfand DW (1984). Gastrointestinal Radiology: Performing and Interpreting Fluoroscopic Examinations. New York: Churchill Livingstone.
4. Kelvin FM, Gardiner R (1987). Clinical Imaging of the Colon and Rectum. New York: Raven Press.
5. Laufer I, ed (1979). Double Contrast Gastrointestinal Radiology, with Endoscopic Correlation. Philadelphia: W.B. Saunders.
6. Nolan JD (1980). The Double Contrast Barium Meal: a Radiological Atlas. Aylesbury: HM & M.
7. Hunt RH, Waye JD (1981). Colonoscopy: Technique, Clinical Practice and Colour Atlas. London: Chapman and Hall.
8. Blackstone MO (1984). Endoscopic Interpretation: Normal and Pathologic Appearances of the Gastrointestinal Tract. New York: Raven Press.
9. Cotton PB, Williams CB (1984). Practical Gastrointestinal Endoscopy. Oxford: Blackwell Scientific.
10. Nahum H, Fekete F, margulis AR (1976). Radiology of the Postoperative Digestive Tract, Trans AE Oestreich. New York: Masson.
11. Binelson J. Castell DO (1988). Disease-A-Month. Esophageal Motility Disorders, Vol. 34(6). Chicago: YearBook Medical Publications.
12. Oudkerk M (1981). Infusion rate in enteroclysis examination. Thesis. Leiden, The Netherlands: Leiden University.
13. Megibow AJ, Balthazar JE, eds (1986). Computed Tomography of the Gastrointestinal Tract. St. Louis: C.V. Mosby
14. Felson B (1976). Roentgenology of the Gallbladder and Biliary Tract. Orlando: Grune and Stratton.
15. Shirakabe H (1971). Double Contrast Studies of the Stomach. Tokyo: Bunrodo Co. Ltd.
16. Op Den Orth JO (1979). The Standard Biphasic Contrast Examination of the Stomach and Duodenum (Series in Radiology: Radiological examination of the GI tract). The Hague: M. Nijhoff.
17. Simpkins KC, ed (1988). The alimentary tract: the hollow organs and salivary glands. In: A Textbook of Radiological Diagnosis, 5th Ed, Vol. 4. London: HK Lewis.
18. Sherlock S (1981). Diseases of the Liver and Biliary System, 6th Ed. Oxford: Blackwell Scientific.

19. Fishman EK, Jones B (1988). Computed Tomography of the Gastrointestinal Tract. New York: Churchill Livingstone.
20. Ponsky JL, Gauderer MWL, Stellato TA, Aszodi A (1985). Percutaneous approaches to enteral alimentation. Am J Surg 149:102–115.
21. Farrar CW (1979). Patterns of sigmoid colon and their implications for barium enema radiography. Med Radiogr Photogr 55:1–28.

Index

MIX
Papier aus verantwortungsvollen Quellen
Paper from responsible sources
FSC® C105338

If you have any concerns about our products,
you can contact us on
ProductSafety@springernature.com

In case Publisher is established outside the EU,
the EU authorized representative is:
Springer Nature Customer Service Center GmbH
Europaplatz 3, 69115 Heidelberg, Germany

Printed by Libri Plureos GmbH
in Hamburg, Germany